Nutritional Anthropology

Nutritional Anthropology

Editor

Francis E. Johnston

Department of Anthropology
University of Pennsylvania
Philadelphia, Pennsylvania

Alan R. Liss, Inc., New York

Address all Inquiries to the Publisher
Alan R. Liss, Inc., 41 East 11th Street, New York, NY 10003

Library of Congress Cataloging-in-Publication Data

Nutritional anthropology.

    Bibliography: p.
    Includes index.
      1. Nutrition.   2. Nutrition—Social aspects.
3. Food habits. I. Johnston, Francis E., 1931–
QP141.N85 1987   613.2   87–4037
ISBN 0–8451–4216–X

Contents

SECTION IV: ANTHROPOLOGY, NUTRITION, AND ECOLOGY

Contributors

Linda S. Adair, Department of Anthropology, Rice University, Houston, TX 77251 **[119]**

Manuel Amador, Instituto Superior de Ciencias Médicas de La Habana, Havana 16, Cuba **[255]**

Jorge Bacallao, Instituto Superior de Ciencias Médicas de La Habana, Havana 16, Cuba **[255]**

Cynthia M. Beall, Department of Anthropology, Case Western Reserve University, Cleveland, OH 44106 **[197]**

Claude Bouchard, Physical Activity Sciences Laboratory and Center for Research on Nutrition, Laval University, Quebec, Canada G1K 7P4 **[101]**

Kathleen D. Gordon, Department of Anthropology, National Museum of Natural History, Smithsonian Institution, Washington, DC 20560 **[3]**

Judith Gussler, Ross Laboratories, Columbus, OH 43216 **[155]**

John H. Himes, Department of Health and Nutrition Sciences, Brooklyn College, City University of New York, Brooklyn, NY 11210 **[85]**

Francis E. Johnston, Department of Anthropology, University of Pennsylvania, Philadelphia, PA 19104 **[ix]**

Solomon H. Katz, Krogman Growth Center, University of Pennsylvania, Philadelphia, PA 19103 **[41]**

Robert M. Malina, Department of Anthropology, University of Texas, Austin, TX 78712 **[173]**

Manuel Peña, Instituto Superior de Ciencias Médicas de La Habana, Havana 16, Cuba **[255]**

Ernesto Pollitt, School of Public Health, The University of Texas Health Science Center, Houston, TX 77225; present address: Department of Applied Behavioral Sciences, University of California, Davis, CA 95616 **[225]**

Sara A. Quandt, Departments of Anthropology and Nutrition and Food Science, University of Kentucky, Lexington, KY 40506-0024 **[67]**

John W. Townsend, The Population Council, 11560 Mexico D.F., Mexico **[277]**

Angelo Tremblay, Physical Activity Sciences Laboratory and Center for Research on Nutrition, Laval University, Quebec, Canada G1K 7P4 **[101]**

The number in brackets is the opening page number of the contributor's article.

Preface

It is no wonder that nutritonal anthropology has emerged as an important focus in anthropological research. The centrality of food in anthropological thinking has been obvious for decades and the result has been an increasing emphasis upon nutritional concerns in explaining variability in human biology, behavior, and culture. It is now obvious that perhaps no force has been more powerful in shaping the human species than that generated by the need to assimilate physiologically those substances which have evolved as essential nutrients in hominids of the past and present.

Kreuter [1980] describes nutrition as a *process* and as a *science*. It is the process by which humans utilize food to meet the requirements of biological and behavioral functioning, and it is that science which studies the body's "chemical processing and biological use of food." That being the case, nutritional anthropology is that branch of anthropology which deals with nutrition as a process and as a science, but from the perspective of our own discipline. The anthropological perspective is one which seeks to understand human biological and cultural variability by analyzing the differences within and among human groups, past and present. With respect to nutrition, it is advisable to separate nutritional anthropology from the study of the anthropology of food. The former brings anthropological concerns to the study of nutrition and hence has a clear, and usually predominant, biological focus, since nutrition is defined in biological terms. The latter brings anthropological concerns to the study of food and, since food is defined culturally (rather than biologically), has a predominant social and cultural focus. Even such a separation breaks down when put to the test, for a number of anthropologists seek consciously to locate their research as near the union of these two areas of study as possible.

The original articles in this book, when taken together, indicate the biological predominance of nutritional anthropology as an area of study. Yet they themselves encompass a broad approach to the subject matter, ranging from evolutionary concerns to a consideration of ways to help alleviate the nutritional problems of the Third World. A number of chapters deal with the scientific methodology practiced by researchers while others cover the human life cycle.

Collectively, they provide a picture of nutritional anthropology as seen by a sample of those working actively in this area of science. Though the majority of contributors are anthropologists by training, others have developed their perspective through their research, a perspective which is no less valid nor valuable than that of those with degrees in anthropology. The picture of nutritional anthropology presented is one of science, of research, of analysis, and of concern with human problems. The field is a vital one, important not only to anthropology but to researchers, clinicians, and planners in other disciplines as well. It has only begun to develop.

Francis E. Johnston

REFERENCES

Kreuter PA (1980): "Nutrition in Perspective." Englewood Cliffs, NJ: Prentice-Hall.

SECTION I:
EVOLUTION, ADAPTATION, AND VARIATION

Nutritional Anthropology, pages 3-39
© 1987 Alan R. Liss, Inc.

Evolutionary Perspectives on Human Diet

Kathleen D. Gordon, PhD

Department of Anthropology, Smithsonian Institution, Washington, D.C. 20560

INTRODUCTION

Why should we be concerned about evolutionary changes in human diet? Why is this such an active field of inquiry? The most obvious reason is that modern human subsistence behavior is so dramatically different from that of all other primates, including our closest relatives the apes, that changes in diet and food procurement must have been important factors in the evolutionary changes leading to modern man. How an animal makes a living in large part determines other aspects of its behavior, reproduction, and social organization. Furthermore, it has recently been proposed by Martin [1983] that the unique developmental and evolutionary features of the large human brain could only have come about as a result of some important changes in type and quality of the diets of early hominids, in order for the high energetic cost of expanding brain tissue to have been affordable. Thus, attempts to reconstruct the diet of our antecedents are not only intended to determine their nutritional "niche," but are also essential to understanding the other aspects of anatomy, social behavior, ecology, and demography that distinguish *Homo sapiens* from other animals.

Three general phases can be recognized in the evolution of hominid subsistence behavior. The first involves a shift from an unprocessed primarily vegetarian diet to one that relied on nonoral food preparation techniques and included significant proportions of meat, changes that must have occurred between the late Miocene and early Pleistocene. During the second phase, specialized hunting and gathering strategies, which may have begun with *Homo erectus*, were perfected and continued through the end of the Pleistocene, persisting in some regions up to historic times. The third phase spans the transition made by various human populations from hunting and gathering to more intensive control over plant and animal resources through domestication. This change occurred in different regions of the world at different times, but generally at or after the end of the last glacial period.

In this chapter I will survey briefly the current evidence we now have of the subsistence activities characteristic of each of these periods. The various methods used by prehistorians and paleoanthropologists to reconstruct past diets and the limitations of those methods have been discussed by numerous authors [Dennell, 1979; Freeman, 1981; Gilbert and Mielke, 1985; Isaac and Crader, 1981; Wing and Brown, 1979]. Direct evidence about human diet is exceedingly rare in the prehistoric record and is found only in such indisputable food remains as the stomach contents of corpses preserved under unique circumstances [Glob, 1969], or human coprolites [de Lumley, 1969; Boaz and Gauld, 1979]. More abundant indirect or circumstantial evidence comes from several different sources. Some derives from techniques based on aspects of morphology or biochemistry of fossil hominid remains themselves (such as dental morphology and wear, both gross and microscopic; jaw mechanics; ratios of trace elements and stable isotopes in bone). Other information comes from the analysis of cultural and food debris and other material associated with human activities (functional analyses of stone tools; lithic use-wear; faunal analysis; study of bone breakage, cutmarks and other sorts of damage to faunal material; stratigraphic and paleoecological studies of archeological sites). Comparative behavioral studies provide a third line of evidence (comparative primate behavior; ethnographic studies of living and historic hunting and gathering peoples). Because of the limitations and difficulties associated with each type of data, no single method or study should be considered definitive. However, when the full suite of available information is analyzed, some consensus about the prehistory of human diet may be achieved.

THE EARLY HOMINIDS: CARNIVORES OR VEGETARIANS?

Almost everyone who studies early hominids has at some point speculated about what they ate. The striking anatomy of the australopithecines' absolutely and relatively huge flat cheek teeth with thick enamel, coupled with small or even diminutive anterior teeth and very reduced canines, has intrigued workers since the discovery of the Taung cranium. Furthermore, the knowledge that *Homo sapiens* is the only primate who hunts regularly for a living has been projected back onto the early fossil record, far beyond unequivocal archeological evidence, in an effort to determine when meat-eating and hunting first became a part of the human or protohuman subsistence repertoire. Although diet in the earliest phases of hominid evolution is a topic of intense interest, regrettably it is also the period about which we have the least abundant and most ambiguous evidence. While the variety and sophistication of techniques upon which we base dietary reconstructions today have improved over the years [e.g., Brain, 1969; 1970; 1978; 1981; Grine, 1981; Isaac 1978a,b; 1981; Isaac and Crader, 1981; Potts and Shipman, 1981; Schoeninger 1979, 1982; Shipman, 1984, 1986; Walker, 1980, 1981; Walker et al., 1978], many areas of uncertainty remain. These uncertainties derive not only from biases in the preserved evidence itself but also to some extent from the category of evidence used. For instance, based on anatomical analogies with other mammals, emphasis on the comparative morphology of australopithecine teeth and jaws biases the inquiry toward identification of those plant foods that would require so robust a masticatory system. Emphasis on the behavioral consequences of hunting and its presumed importance in determining human social organization has led other researchers to comb the faunal and archaeological evidence for indications of when and how hominid involvement with animal foods began. Consequently, depending on whether one's starting point is morphology or behavior, different dietary elements may be emphasized and different data sets used in the reconstruction of hominid dietary behavior.

The earliest characterization of the diet and behavior of *Australopithecus* was that of Dart [1940, 1949, 1953, 1957, 1962] who found evidence in the South African cave breccias that convinced him that *Australopithecus africanus* was a hunter who killed his food and occasionally his conspecifics. Although subsequent investigation of his "osteodontokeratic culture" did not support these claims [Brain, 1969, 1970, 1972, 1978, 1981; Klein, 1975; Sutcliffe, 1972; but see also Brain, 1984, 1985; Lewin, 1984], the image of early hominids as predatory carnivores has persisted, and much popular speculation about the evolution of human social behavior and organization draws breath from this early portrayal [Ardrey, 1961, 1976]. The presumption of hominid carnivory has also had far-reaching effects on the way in which questions about human cultural and biological evolution have been framed and investigated by the scientific community, and reconstructions of early hominid behavior have drawn heavily on analogy with modern social carnivores [Cachel, 1975; Schaller and Lowther, 1969; Thompson, 1975, 1976]. The assumption that procurement of meat necessarily requires or involves hunting has in turn led to speculations about the development of communication, group cooperation, and pair-bonding in early hominids, as outgrowths of the hunting way of life [Washburn and Lancaster, 1968; Campbell, 1966].

Thus, discussions about the diet and subsistence behavior of early hominids are typically complex and multipronged. In essence however, leaving aside other adaptive questions about hominid behavior and their relation to diet, the discussion has focused on four major questions: 1) What was the basic diet of early hominids—primarily carnivorous, primarily vegetarian, or generally omnivorous? 2) If there was a significant animal protein component to early hominid diets, how was it obtained—by deliberate hunting, by "collecting" small slow-moving prey, or by scavenging? 3) If the dental specializations of early hominids were related to vegetarian adaptations, what kind of plant material necessitated the relatively large flat teeth and robust jaws which characterize (with variations of degree) all the early species known so far? and 4) Is there any evidence to support the hypothesis of dietary differentiation among the various species of Hominidae known in Plio-Pleistocene times?

One difficulty in answering the first question lies to some extent in definitions. The terms "vegetarian," "carnivore," and "omnivore" are not usually used rigorously, and in fact two or more of these may describe the same species, depending on the perspective of the observer and the population examined. Generally, for instance, modern apes rely most heavily on plant foods, some exclusively so. However, though chimpanzees are generally classified as frugivores, they take a significant amount of animal protein either in the form of insects or hunted prey (approximately 17% of their annual feeding time budget, from data in Teleki [1981]). Relative to gorillas or gibbons, they may be better described as omnivores [Teleki, 1973, 1981]. In comparison, some modern humans and Upper Paleolithic populations with well-organized hunting adaptations might be labeled "carnivores." But even a casual glance at the spectrum of modern human diets shows a remarkable range of feeding strategies, from the high meat diets of the Eskimo to the strict vegetarian diets of some groups on the Indian subcontinent, with every possible combination in between [Arnott, 1975; Brothwell and Brothwell, 1969; Farb and Armelagos, 1980; Lee, 1968]. The more closely primate diets are examined, the better the case becomes for viewing primates as "an order of omnivores" [Harding, 1981]. The narrow dietary niches typical of equids, bovids, or carnivores simply do not exist in primates generally, and scanning the fossil record for signs of such specializations in past hominids is likely to be unrewarding. In view of the unique and unprecedented dietary diversity and opportunism that characterize modern *Homo sapiens*, it seems reasonable to assume that early hominids had relatively unspecialized feeding habits as well. Omnivory in the very broadest sense probably characterized all of these early species, with diets which varied in time and space, as opportunities permitted.

Evidence about carnivory in early hominids comes from studies of archeological material and faunal remains, and from signs of human modification or damage to animal bones. The occurrence of hominid remains alone with bones of other animals, in the absence of tools, is in itself equivocal. It is difficult to determine whether other animals in the deposits were hominid food debris, or if, as was probably the case with some of the South African cave deposits, the hominids themselves were victims of predation [Brain, 1981]. Most of the evidence for early meat consumption comes from the Pliocene and Lower Pleistocene of East and South Africa. Although other regions have been reported to show signs of hominid occupation during the lower Pleistocene, these occurrences have often been in the form of hominid remains without any associated archaeological material, as in Java [Isaac and Crader, 1981]. Other sites may have faunal and cultural debris that is too sparse, or not well dated, or too incompletely analyzed to determine what activities are represented, such as the North African localities of Ain Hanech, Ternifine, Casablanca, and Melka Kunture' [Isaac and Crader, 1981].

In South Africa, hominid-bearing cave deposits generally have few deposits with numerous stone artifacts (except for Sterkfontein Member 5), although sporadic occurrences of stone and possible bone tools are reported from Swartkrans as well [Brain, 1984, 1985]. Bone accumulations at Makapan and in the older deposits at Swartkrans (Member 1) and Sterkfontein (Member 4) are very likely due to carnivore rather than hominid activity [Brain, 1969, 1970]. Tools, faunal remains, and hominid fossils have been recovered from younger deposits at both Swartkrans and Sterkfontein. Vrba [1975] has studied bovid remains at both sites and concluded that accumulations at Swartkans were due to hominid small-game hunting, while those at Sterkfontein were possibly more consistent with hominid scavenging activities. However, Isaac and Crader [1981] characterize this analysis as provocative but too untested as yet to be used in reconstructing early hominid diets.

A summary and evaluation of much of the evidence for hominid carnivory from East African sites at Olduvai and Koobi Fora is provided by Isaac and Crader [1981]. The strongest evidence comes from two types of sites, those with both relatively high densities of artifacts and faunal remains of several species (often termed "living floors" or "occupation" sites, the type "C" sites of Isaac and Crader [1981], and those with artifacts associated with the remains of a single animal or species ("butchery" sites, or Isaac and Crader's type "B" sites). Some of the best examples of the former, sites where hominids left tools and where abundant remains of many animals suggest that site use, if not actual occupation, may have occurred repeatedly or over some period of time, are the FLK Zinj floor at Olduvai [Leakey, 1971] and the KBS site (FxJjl) at Koobi Fora [Isaac, 1978b]. The size range of mammals represented is wide. Tool types are various and cores, debitage and unmodified raw materials ("manuports") are present as well. Some of the raw materials come from sources as far away as 2-3 kilometers [Potts, 1982, 1986]. However, there are some differences between these sites and known human occupation sites of Upper Pleistocene/Holocene times, and Potts has concluded that they were not in fact living sites or home bases, but processing sites used recurrently. Examples of possible butchery sites are the HAS hippo site at Koobi Fora (FXJj3) and FLK N, level and layer II. At each of these sites remains of one very large mammal (hippo, elephant, and deinothere, respectively) are found with artifacts, sometimes inside the skeleton itself. Although the activities of other carnivores as well are involved in site formation, at least at Olduvai [Potts, 1982, 1984; and see below], on the whole the evidence is convincing that by 1.6-1.8 million years (mys) BP (before present) hominids in East Africa were involved in procuring, transporting, and processing some animal remains for food.

What precise hominid activities contributed to such faunal accumulations is not so clear however, and this question has recently become the focus of paleoanthropological controversy. Since the earliest fossil hominid discoveries, the tendency has been to view all associated remains as the direct result of hominid predation, and some studies have taken hominid predation as a given upon which to base speculations about other aspects of early hominid behavior (Speth and Davis, 1976). However, as the science of paleoanthropology has become more sophisticated, other alternatives have been advanced to explain these assemblages as, for example, carnivore prey accumulating in natural catchments [Brain, 1981] or as the results of hydraulic conglomeration of hominid artifacts with other animal bones [Binford, 1977]. Even when hominid intervention is likely, as demonstrated by the appearance of cutmarks on animal bones [Bunn, 1981, 1983], it is not at all certain that the event being sampled was hominid hunting behavior. As Potts and Shipman [1981] have shown, cutmarks on animal bones from Olduvai frequently occurred in positions where meat was not likely to be found in much abundance, such as distal limb bones and podials. They theorized that other tissues such as hide or sinew might have been the goal, rather than meat. In the same study, they also demonstrated that hominids were not the sole utilizers of some animal carcasses. Carnivore tooth marks and stone tool cutmarks often occurred on the same bones. Occasionally, these marks overlapped, and when they did, it was possible to say which had been made first. In at least a few instances, hominids were not the first possessors of the carcass, since the cutmarks were often superimposed on previous carnivore gnaw marks. However the presence of hominid tool cutmarks in these assemblages cannot be accepted uncritically. Recent research has demonstrated that trampling on bone can produce scratches that exactly mimic the diagnostic characteristics of cutmarks [Behrensmeyer et al., 1986], suggesting that additional contextual information may be needed before the existence of "cutmarks" on bone associated with hominid sites can be taken as conclusive evidence of hominid processing activities.

The idea that hominids might have obtained meat by scavenging rather than hunting is not a new one. Many workers have at least considered the possibility [King, 1975; Peters and Mech, 1975; Read-Martin and Read, 1975; Szalay, 1975], often as a transitional phase between foraging and hunting. Potts [1983] has shown that if hominids at Olduvai were indeed scavenging rather than hunting, they were occasionally able to obtain early or at least intermediate access to carcasses, as shown by the relative frequencies of forelimb, hindlimb, and axial skeleton elements present. It would seem that lower Pleistocene hominids at Olduvai had already developed techniques for obtaining animal parts, by whatever means, and therefore the beginnings of this behavior must be sought in earlier time periods.

Shipman [1983, 1986] has undertaken a theoretical consideration of scavenging as a deliberate hominid strategy. Analysis of studies of modern scavengers led her to identify several characteristics which make scavenging a feasible feeding strategy. These include a low-cost mode of locomotion to cover large areas in search of carcasses, adaptations to improve vantage points for locating carcasses, a strategy for dealing with competition for carcasses from either the primary predator or other scavengers, and an alternative feeding strategy to fall back on between carcasses (required for an estimated minimum of 67% of the diet for a mammalian scavenger). She proposes that bipedalism provides a suitable means of locomotion and conveys an automatic improvement in vantage point for a scavenging hominid. Body size plays an important role in the type of competition strategy chosen, as well as the fall-back diet adopted. Small-bodied animals are at a disadvantage in overt competition to possess a carcass and so tend to specialize in stealth and avoidance, while larger animals that scavenge, such as lions, can successfully wrest kills from any predator. Larger scavengers will hunt to round out their diet; smaller ones tend to eat fruit and/or insects for the major part of their diet. Shipman assumes that average hominid body size in the Lower Pleistocene would have been around 35 kg, placing a hypothetical hominid scavenger in the "sneak" and "frugivore/insectivore" categories. The scavenging model she has proposed is both feasible and has some explanatory power in terms of other hominid adaptations. However, some refinements in its application may be necessary. At least some early hominids would have been a good deal larger in body size than 35 kg [Brown et al., 1985; Leakey and

Walker, 1985]. Further, the dental microwear evidence that she cites characterizing early hominids as frugivores [Walker, 1980, 1981] is very preliminary and has never been quantified. Lastly, it is hard to imagine even larger-bodied hominids, armed at best with sticks and rocks, deliberately engaging the formidable Pleistocene carnivores in competition over carcasses, or even exposing themselves to close contact with them. Scavenging can be risky business, and scavengers themselves often become prey. Hunting might have been less dangerous.

However difficult its execution, a hominid scavenging strategy has been shown by Blumenschine [Blumenschine, 1986; Bower, 1985] to be feasible even today in East African savannas. Blumenschine has surveyed predation and carcass distribution on the Serengeti to determine what conditions present the most favorable scavenging opportunities. While frequently only the brain and marrow remain of most prey after feeding by the primary predator, these are not inconsiderable sources of protein and fat for hominids able to break bone. The larger the prey animal, the greater the amount of flesh that may persist even after several days. Small-bodied animals, however, are almost completely devoured by primary predators. Predator species may also be an important variable. Lions are relatively inefficient consumers, and lion kills present more useful material to subsequent scavengers than do those of hyenas. Blumenschine discovered that carcass availability varies with season, and that a savanna like the Serengeti with large numbers of migratory species has periods of high nonpredation mortality which also generate resources for scavengers. Two interesting points emerge from this work. When small-bodied bovids are found in hominid sites, they are unlikely to have been brought in as scavenged remains, since these are usually totally consumed before the carcass is relinquished to scavengers. The second is that scavenging may not always require intense competition with large carnivores and primary predators, especially in seasons of high natural mortality in herbivore populations.

Some of the so-called "butchery" sites in East Africa may document either actual hominid kills or scavenged carrion. The BK and FLK N *Deinotherium* sites from Olduvai suggest that animals trapped due to natural causes were butchered by hominids, though whether the animals were killed first or died naturally is unclear. The BK site, which contains the remains of some 24 *Pelorovis* individuals, has been cited by Mary Leakey [1971] as evidence of an early Pleistocene game drive. While this conclusion is plausible, it is not the only possible explanation, and distinguishing causation from opportunistic exploitation by hominids of a naturally occurring event is beyond the resolution of the fossil record at this time.

Another question that cannot yet be answered is the determination of which hominid or hominids were responsible for the tool and animal bone accumulations. Tool manufacture and use have been generally attributed to the most advanced hominid present in tool-bearing deposits, and so at Olduvai it has been assumed that early artifact and bone assemblages document the cultural attainments of *Homo habilis*, rather than *Australopithecus boisei*. However, recent finds of *Homo erectus* from the west side of Lake Turkana, Kenya, dated at 1.6 mys [Brown et al., 1985; Leakey and Walker, 1985], indicate that *H. habilis* and *H. erectus* are contemporaneous in East Africa, and in the East Turkana region it has been suggested that possibly three [Walker and Leakey, 1978] or even four hominid species (Wood, 1985) may overlap in time. In South Africa, both *Homo erectus* and *H. habilis* are known from deposits containing tools and australopithecines as well, but their temporal relationships to one another are still uncertain [Brain, 1985; Clarke, 1985]. Clearly, any attempt to assign tool use to one of a range of possible hominid candidates is necessarily arbitrary and reflects only our preconceptions about cultural development and early hominids. Furthermore since rudimentary tool use and manufacture have been observed in other primate species [McGrew et al., 1979; Boesch and Boesch, 1981] there is little basis for assuming that tool-making was a rubicon attained only by the most cerebrally advanced hominids.

Stone tool use and manufacture has usually been assumed to reflect butchery of animal carcasses. However, the association of tools with preparation of meat or animal by-products is not a proven correlation. In southern Africa, stone tools appear in most levels of the deposits at Swartkrans (along with bone "digging tools"), but according to Brain cutmarks do not appear on any of the abundant faunal remains until the Early Stone Age member [Brain, 1985]. This would seem to imply that either the faunal material below this level was not collected or processed by hominids as food (assuming that such processing could always be detected), or that meat-eating, tool-using hominids simply did not use tools in processing animal parts until later time periods. In either case, the presence of tools is uncoupled from the evidence for butchery and meat consumption, which suggests that stone and bone tool use and manufacture probably predate human carnivory and were first developed to aid in acquiring or processing plant materials. In East Africa some tool occurrences that lack accompanying bone accumulations (type "A" sites, [Isaac, 1978a; Isaac and Crader, 1981]) have also been suggested as evidence of vegetable food procurement and processing.

New methods of analyzing stone tool function have provided some corroboration for this. While the analysis of tool types has yet to clarify the relationship between form and function [Toth, 1985; Lewin, 1986], microscopic wear on stone tool edges can provide information about what materials were actually processed with a tool. A study of use-wear on tools of the Karari Industry from Koobi Fora, dated at approximately 1.5 mys BP, was carried out by Keeley and Toth [1981] according to methods previously developed [Hayden, 1979; Keeley, 1980]. While some tool edges were found to show polishes similar to those produced experimentally by cutting meat and other animal soft tissues, other tools exhibited edge wear characteristic of use on wood and on soft plant materials. Kraybill [1977] points out the presence in deposits at Olduvai, Sterkfontein, and Makapan of tool types (spheroids, subspheroids, cuboids, and polyhedrons) that resemble tools used in the ethnographic present for pounding various plant food items. Lower Pleistocene stone tools seem to have been used to process a wide variety of materials, but the presence of tools in a deposit reveals little about who made them or used them, and only more intensive analyses of the tools themselves can clarify how they were used.

Despite the persistence of the dramatic and probably inaccurate "Man the Hunter" image, it has always been considered that some early hominids may have had specialized vegetarian diets. However, due to their poor preservation and underrepresentation in the fossil record, possible plant food components of early hominid diets are even more difficult to identify than faunal elements. Several types of actualistic studies provide the bulk of the admittedly circumstantial evidence for plant use by early hominids. For instance, the diets and subsistence strategies of modern hunter-gatherer peoples living at similar latitudes in similar environments to those occupied by early hominids have been studied intensively [Hayden, 1981; Lee, 1968; Lee and Devore, 1968]. Work among the !Kung San people of Botswana [Lee, 1968, 1979] revealed an unexpectedly high reliance on vegetable foods, which contribute approximately 67% of the total diet (by calories). Similar findings have been made for the Hadza [Woodburne, 1968], and Australian aborigines [Lee, 1968; Meggitt, 1962; Yengoyan, 1968]. Hunting is an unpredictable subsistence strategy even for modern hunters and would have been even less dependable for early hominids with less sophisticated technology and skills. In tropical and mid-latitude populations, the most common and reliable feeding strategy seems to be one based on high daily consumption of vegetable foods [Hayden, 1981; Woodburne, 1968], gathered primarily though not exclusively by women and children. These are supplemented by animal protein from both small slow-moving animals, which may be "collected" by anyone, and from larger animals actually hunted, usually by men only. Although meat is especially prized by most hunter-gatherers, it actually forms the smaller part of the diet in most living peoples with the exception of specialized hunters in Arctic and subarctic latitudes whose dependence on meat is unique. Hayden [1981] points out that fats are also highly prized by hunter-gatherers, and that ethnographers' preoccupations with hunting and meat consumption may have caused this to be overlooked. A subsistence base that provides a secure and dependable vegetable diet for all, while freeing some individuals from daily foraging activities in order to invest their time and effort in riskier and less reliable hunting activities, is what characterizes successful traditional hunter-gatherers of today.

Peters et al. [Peters and Maguire, 1981; Peters and O'Brien, 1981a,b; Peters et al., 1984] have focused on defining potential hominid plant foods by comparing modern primate diets. Surveying the currently available wild plant resources in Southern Africa and limited parts of East Africa, they have documented which are edible and are actually consumed by humans, chimpanzees and/or baboons [Peters and O'Brien, 1981a,b; 1982]. Although the authors' conclusions about potential competition for plant foods among the three species are problematic and not generally accepted, and the relevance of the contemporary flora to that of Plio-Pleistocene times may be questioned, their compilation has detailed some interesting species differences in patterns of plant food utilization. For instance, chimpanzees eat more seeds and pods than do sympatric humans, and in general the two hominoids utilize very few of the same species. Humans consume more kinds of leaves and shoots than do chimpanzees and also exploit underground storage organs, which chimpanzees do not utilize at all. Baboons are more similar to humans in most of these preferences.

More recent work by Sept [1986] has attempted to obtain detailed information about plant food availability in various ecologic zones in East Africa. She has collected data on seasonality of edible foods, on their distribution, and on normal annual variations in these resources. This information can be coupled with data about nutritional value and processing demands to arrive at estimates of the overall productivity of the various zones thought to have been inhabited by hominids in the past. Used in conjunction with paleoecological information about the habitats of early hominids [Behrensmeyer, 1978; Behrensmeyer and Cooke, 1985; Vrba, 1985] such approaches to past environments and food resources through the analysis of the present will yield more information in the future about the possible role of plant foods in the diet of early hominids.

Reconstructions of hominid feeding behavior based on analysis of hominid anatomy tend to reinforce the presumption of a largely vegetarian diet. Study of posterior dental morphology in *Australopithecus* leads to an impression of heavy mastication of some very resistant form of vegetal material. Low cusps are usually associated with molars adapted for crushing rather than shearing or slicing and would resist breakage better than higher cusps. Thickened enamel may also be a mechanism for withstanding forces which would tend to crack less heavily protected tooth crowns, or it might simply be a way of coping with highly abrasive foods. Tooth morphology and the type of tooth wear found in carnivores differs qualitatively from the patterns found in early hominids. Consequently, given the factors of phylogenetic heritage (i.e., apes are vegetarians) and the anatomical indications, the posterior dentition of early hominids seems to indicate a demanding vegetarian diet. "Demanding" can of course mean different things to different researchers. While Kay (1981) sees some of these characteristics, which are found also in earlier Miocene "ramapithecine" apes, as indications of resistance to intense but sporadic masticatory loads, Walker's analysis of australopithecine jaw mechanics leads him to conclude that early hominid dentitions were designed more to withstand longer durations of oral food-processing at not necessarily higher loads [Walker, 1981]. Only one worker has proposed that morphology of the *Australopithecus* dentition provides direct evidence of adaptations for carnivory [Szalay, 1975]. This is not widely accepted, however, and furthermore, microwear on teeth of *Australopithecus boisei* [Walker, 1980, 1981] shows no resemblance to that found on teeth of any modern carnivore yet studied (including cheetah, lion, and hyenas).

The chemical composition of fossil bone itself may soon provide evidence about the diet of early hominids. Strontium levels in bone can differentiate herbivores from carnivores [Schoeninger, 1979, 1982; Sillen, 1981; Sillen and Kavanaugh, 1982], and although post-depositional conditions may affect these values in some circumstances, it is possible that work now in progress may help to shed light on the diet or diets of early hominids. Similarly, stable isotopes which can be isolated from bone samples [DeNiro and Epstein, 1978; Van Der Merwe and Vogel, 1978] can distinguish between different types of herbivorous diets as well as between herbivore and carnivore [Schoeninger et al., 1983; Schoeninger and DeNiro, 1984; Ambrose and DeNiro 1986]. It has also been suggested that stable isotope ratios may enable workers to make quantitative estimates about the contribution of various foodstuffs to the diet, something which has been difficult to arrive at by more conventional means [Chisholm et al., 1983; Ambrose and DeNiro, 1986]. These methods should prove important in the future and have already yielded useful information about diet in later time periods [Schoeninger, 1979, 1981, 1982; Ambrose and DeNiro 1986], but attempts to apply them to the Plio-Pleistocene have not been conclusive as yet [Boaz and Hample 1978], due to the problems posed by diagenetic alteration of bone collagen [DeNiro, 1985; Sillen, 1985].

In an important synthesis of behavioral and anatomical evidence, Jolly (1970) argued that many differences between early hominids and living apes parallel those found between the gelada baboon, an animal adapted to semi-arid open-country environments and other baboons found in woodland savanna and forests. These characters included some aspects of habitat and social organization as well as anatomical traits of limbs, head, jaws, and teeth. He concluded that most of these traits were correlated with feeding behavior involving long bouts of sitting while manually gathering small, tough food items requiring little incisal preparation. He proposed that exploitation of seed crops of grasses and herbs (granivory) may have been the basal hominid adapatation, which predated bipedalism, tool use, and brain expansion and which could be seen to have influenced these later developments. This view of early hominids saw the australopithecines as specialized vegetarians feeding on savanna grass stands. Though many aspects of this scenario have been disputed or rejected in the ensuing years, the seed-eating hypothesis remains one of the most important syntheses about hominid feeding behavior. Various workers [Dunbar, 1976; Wallace 1975; Wolpoff, 1973] have since concluded that seeds were too seasonal to have formed the major component of the diet but found that small tough-object herbivory was still a reasonable possibility for early hominid diets.

Other resources found in semi-arid open country that might have been exploited by early hominids were discussed by Wolpoff [1973], and this scenario has recently been reinforced by possible evidence from Southern Africa [Brain, 1984, 1985; Lewin, 1984]. Underground roots and tubers are plentiful in both East and South African savanna grasslands, and, in fact, underground plant foods are abundant even in such apparently harsh environments as the Kalahari desert [Lee, 1968]. Warthogs also dig and consume underground plant parts, but they are only capable of reaching those within 6 to 8 inches of the soil surface. Brain has proposed that early hominids may have used bone digging sticks to obtain roots and tubers more easily and at greater soil depths than their warthog competitors. He has noted the presence in South African deposits of some possible utilized bone tools that exhibit microscopic abrasion patterns consistent with this hypothesis. The existence of other types of utilized bone tools recently confirmed in beds I and II at Olduvai [Shipman, 1984; Lewin, 1984] means that various hominid species may have possessed the technology necessary to exploit underground plant resources effectively.

The question of dietary divergence among early hominids has attracted much attention in the last 30 years. Broom and Robinson [Broom, 1950; Robinson, 1954b, 1956] had proposed generic distinctions between the gracile and robust australopithecines, based on differences in cranial and dental size and shape. Robinson [1954a, 1961, 1963] was the first to attribute these anatomical differences to fundamental differences in feeding behavior. He believed *Paranthropus* to be an herbivore, while *Australopithecus* would have been more omnivorous. He based this schema not only on the cranial and dental differences but also on purported differences in the amount of ante-mortem enamel chipping [Robinson, 1963]. Wallace [1973] and Tobias [1967] both discounted the evidence for differences in tooth damage, but Tobias at least seemed to concede that, questions of dubious taxonomy and enamel damage aside, dietary differences between the gracile and robust australopithecines (including *A. boisei*) may have existed.

The hypothesized taxonomic and ecological differences among the australopithecines have remained controversial. While some maintained that the morphology of the two taxa was not so different and that in fact the differences might be only due to sexual dimorphism [Brace, 1967, 1969, 1973; Wolpoff, 1971, 1974, 1976, 1978], others attributed the size and shape differences to allometric scaling (Pilbeam and Gould, 1974). Still others [Corruccini and Henderson, 1978; Creighton, 1980; Goldstein et al., 1978; Kay, 1975a,b; Wood and Stack, 1980] countered that comparisons with living mammals showed that gracile and robust australopithecines did not follow the usual pattern for allometric variants. Furthermore, the allometric argument is hope-lessly circular, since the way in which cheek teeth scale varies according to dietary habit. Consequently, it is not substantiated that the robust australopithecines had larger teeth solely because they were bigger animals. A dietary cause for the morphological differences remains a viable possibility. Dental microwear studies of deciduous teeth attributed to the two South African australopithecines have indicated some possible diet or processing differences between juveniles of the two species [Grine, 1981]. These differences also are present in adult australopithecines, according to more recent work by Grine [1986]. However, since newer dating of the difficult South African cave sites indicates that the robust and gracile forms may not have been contempora-neous after all [Grine, 1981; Brain, 1985; Vrba, 1985], some of the fervor of previous arguments has diminished, and it now appears that questions of diet in *Australopithecus* may involve change through time and space, rather than competition or character displacement in sympatric species. Furthermore, Grine has aptly pointed out that behavioral differences between gracile and robust forms need not have been as wide as those proposed by Robinson's original formulation of the dietary hypothesis. Vegetarian diets clearly can vary greatly, and while the skeletal and microwear evidence is suggestive of signifi-cant differences between the two, such differences could mean that robust australopithecines exploited vegetable foods which were simply different or more fibrous or smaller than those the gracile forms ate.

An even more fascinating question concerns the diets of the various hominids now known to be contemporaneous in East Africa. Some microwear studies have been carried out on teeth from Hadar, Laetoli, and Olduvai [Puech, 1984; Puech et al., 1983], from which the authors conclude that early hominids consumed highly acidic fruits and fibrous materials in sufficient quantities to erode enamel surfaces. But since these studies are unquantified and uncontrolled for taphonomic and other complicating factors, it is unwise to draw any conclusions from them. Preliminary microwear studies of the East African hominids have indicated that *A. boisei* shows frugivorelike abrasion patterns, while *H. erectus* teeth show signs of coarser grit in the diet [Walker, 1980, 1981]. However, this cannot be confirmed nor can the implications of these differences be assessed until these data are also expanded and quantified.

In summary, it seems most likely that all early hominids in Plio-Pleistocene times relied on significant amounts of vegetable foods and that at least some of these were resistant enough to require extraordinary amounts of oral processing. Animal protein from occasional fortuitous kills and "collected" animals and insects is likely to have been part of the diet as well, as they are in other living primates such as chimpanzees and baboons. Some food items, both vegetal and animal, may have required extractive technologies and implements not used by other primates in the same regions. There may have been some important differences among both australopithecines and early *Homo* species in the quality, type, amounts or possibly in processing techniques of these various foods, but vegetable foods are likely to have provided the bulk of the diet for all early hominids.

There is evidence that by 1.7 million years BP, at least one hominid species was involved in processing animal carcasses, either to scavenge meat and/or other useful tissues or as a result of actual hunting, but the identification of which species was or were involved is not possible at this time. Given the technological limitations of the available tool kit and the competition provided by other predators in the same environments, it is doubtful that any hominid of Pliocene/Lower Pleistocene times acquired or consumed significant amounts of meat from medium or large animals on a regular basis, although the possibility remains that even relatively small amounts of additional animal protein may have played an important nutritional role in early hominid diets. Since scavenging has now been reported for a variety of primates [Hasegawa et al., 1983; Strum, 1981; Sugardjito and Nurhuda, 1981], it is not possible to claim that this would have been a unique human adaptation. As with virtually all other behavioral characters that are used to differentiate modern man from apes, occasional scavenging appears to fall within the repertoires of several species. Two conditions, the ability to use tools to extract material from animal carcasses and the occupation of environments within which seasonal highs in natural mortality of herbivore populations would have provided some scavenging opportunities free of competition from primary predators, may have allowed hominids to exploit this strategy more intensively than other primates. A speculative scenario of the development of hominid scavenging skills can be envisioned, from occasional "late" scavenging of older carcasses to intermediate or early possession of carcasses or portions thereof, to the eventual decrease in scavenging as hunting of medium to large-size animals becomes more frequent and successful. However, at any given point in the Plio-Pleistocene, a combination of these differing levels of carcass control and processing would likely have been evident. Controversies now brewing that cast the question of hominid meat acquisition in terms of scavenging *versus* hunting miss the point for at least two reasons. Both behaviors, however incipient, were probably within the range of most or all early hominids. Secondly, as it is impossible to state with any certainty that only one hominid consumed meat, it is also impossible at this point to determine how two or more species living sympatrically might have varied in their patterns of animal protein acquisition and consumption. Answers to these questions must await further work and a denser fossil and archeological record.

THE MIDDLE AND UPPER PLEISTOCENE: REFINEMENT AND SPECIALIZATION

From the beginning of the Middle Pleistocene at about 700,000 years BP [Butzer, 1975], the emergence of hunting as a significant component of the hominid subsistence pattern seems indisputable. Sites preserving high densities of both stone artifacts and bone refuse become more numerous in Africa and for the first time are found extending into Europe and Asia as well [Isaac, 1971]. This increase in faunal remains is usually seen as related to more dependable hunting success, although it may also reflect increases in hominid population density or longer, more sedentary site occupations. During this period, several trends in hominid diet can be discerned.

One of the more evident changes in hunting patterns concerns the choice of prey species taken. Although many different mammal species are typically found in association with hominid remains or artifacts in both Early and Middle Pleistocene sites which are supposed to sample hominid hunting or scavenging [Horowitz et al., 1973; Isaac and Crader 1981; Klein, 1973, 1977, 1979; Kretzoi and Vert'es, 1965; Leakey, 1971; Wu and Lin, 1983], several authors have signaled a change apparent in the Middle and Upper Pleistocene toward hunting larger animals and also toward more dangerous and challenging prey

[Binford, 1968; Klein, 1977, 1979]. In East Africa, an Acheulian site complex at Olorgesailie, dated at somewhere between 700,000-400,000 years BP, preserves remains of approximately 90 individuals of an extinct species of giant gelada baboon (*Theropithecus oswaldi*). Although some have questioned the conclusion that the *Theropithecus* remains represent hominid food debris [Binford, 1977; Thackeray, 1981; Van Couvering and Stucky, 1981], original reports [Isaac, 1977] speculated that many of these presumably formidable baboons may have been killed at one time by hominids using group hunting techniques. Later studies of the faunal remains [Shipman et al., 1981] suggest instead that the mortality profile is more likely an attritional one, wherein relatively young individuals were selectively killed over some period of time. Even so, choosing as prey a baboon the size of a female gorilla has struck most observers as representing a considerable challenge to hominid hunting skill.

In southern Africa, Middle Pleistocene sites with good bone preservation are rare [Klein, 1977]. The few with faunal remains such as Pomongwe, The Cave of Hearths, and Elandsfontein, all show that a wide variety of herbivores were hunted or scavenged. Resolution is better in the Upper Pleistocene. In his studies of faunal remains from Middle (MSA) and Late Stone Age (LSA) sites (approximately 130,000 to 2,000 years BP), Klein [1979] has found shifts in type of prey species that led him to conclude that LSA hunters were more likely to hunt dangerous animals such as wild pigs, while MSA hunters more frequently hunted relatively docile bovids such as eland. Brooks [1984] also notes a similar faunal pattern in other southern African LSA sites. Later Pleistocene sites in Europe, particularly in Central European caves, give fairly compelling evidence that Mousterian peoples may have been able to kill large numbers of the extinct Pleistocene cave bear, although it is not impossible that hominids simply accumulated and stored the bones and skulls of animals already dead. If they were in fact hunted, it is unclear whether they were consumed as food or hunted primarily for ritual purposes [Howell, 1970].

During this period there is a tendency for carnivores, particularly large ones, to become increasingly rare in faunal remains from archeological sites. (The so-called Cave Bear Cult cited above is an exception to this pattern.) Carnivores are usually uncommon in faunal assemblages, at least in part due to their relative scarcity in living faunas. But Klein [1979] cites absence of carnivore remains in South African Middle Pleistocene sites as evidence of their avoidance by hominids. In contrast, his Upper Pleistocene Ukrainian sites showed relatively abundant remains of arctic fox and wolf, but the skeletons were found nearly intact, minus only their paws, which suggests that they were hunted for fur rather than food [Klein, 1973]. A shift in carnivore frequencies could mean simply a shift in ecology or behavior that made interaction with carnivores more unlikely, or it could signal a shift in predation patterns and/or diet. Avoidance of hunting carnivores as food is a characteristic generally shared by modern hunters [Hayden, 1981]. A possible functional explanation for this pattern and a hint at its beginnings is provided by the diseased *Homo erectus* skeleton KNM-ER 1808, from East Turkana, Kenya (dated at 1.8-1.5 myrs). The almost complete skeleton of this individual shows signs of extensive abnormal bone deposition on the limbs consistent with a diagnosis of chronic vitamin A poisoning [Walker et al., 1982]. Walker et al., hypothesize that hypervitaminosis A may have been a result of eating carnivore livers, which concentrate very high levels of the vitamin (unlike the livers of herbivores and man), during a period when hominids were only just beginning to include meat in their diet in any significant quantity and before they had learned what to avoid.

In addition to changes in prey species choice, there is also evidence for the development of selective hunting strategies in the Middle and Upper Pleistocene faunal accumulations. Many human occupation sites throughout the Old World record increases in the number of individuals of particular prey species taken, which presumably relates to changes either in technology and/or organization and strategy (Binford, 1968). It can be reasoned that the use of specialized techniques for gaining proximity to prey may have been part of hominid hunting behavior for some time. Such improvements in technique were probably necessary in order to increase hunting success. Even today, evidence from !Kung San hunters shows that some techniques are much more successful than others in providing meat, even with a relatively sophisticated weapons arsenal including poisoned arrows. Ethnographic data reveal that stalking prey yields on average only 2.6 kg of meat per man-day spent, while ambush strategies, including the use of stone hunting blinds, yield 15 kg of meat per man-day (Brooks, 1984; personal communication). Pit traps and game drives also increase the yield per unit of effort and minimize risks. The earliest hunting strategy to be adopted was probably the deliberate targeting of young or weakened animals. This pattern has been discerned by Vrba [1975] in the later deposits of South African caves, is apparent at Terra Amata [de Lumley, 1969] and continued, with modifications, up until the Late Stone Age of South Africa. Klein [1979, 1982] found that while eland and hartebeest were taken at almost any age, other bovids such as giant and Cape buffalo and roan and blue antelope were preferentially hunted while very young, and few prime-age adults are found in the faunal remains. He interprets this to indicate two different hunting strategies based on the differing size, temperament, and ecology of the two species-groups. In general, it seems that the presence of young individuals in an archeological deposit argues for hominid hunting rather than scavenging, because kills of juvenile animals are rapidly and completely consumed by primary predators, leaving virtually nothing available for later scavengers [Blumenschine, 1986; Klein, 1982].

Similar indications of growing sophistication in hunting strategy emerge from other localities in Europe. The sites of Torralba and Ambrona in Spain [Howell, 1966; Freeman and Howell, 1981, 1982; Howell and Freeman, 1982] have for many years been seen as examples of specialized elephant hunting. Remains of numerous elephants were found in situations suggesting game drives which trapped the victims in marshy valley bottoms where they were killed and butchered. Although the predominance of elephants has been overstated and the faunal accumulations may in part be due to natural death or nonhominid predation [Binford, 1981; Freeman, 1981; Shipman and Rose, 1983], the evidence is nonetheless convincing that Middle Pleistocene hominids, presumably *Homo erectus*, were able to use both fire and a complex understanding of geography and animal behavior to kill animals much larger than themselves and eventually in quantities unknown for other predators. At upper Pleistocene sites in the Ukraine, Klein [1973] has noted that although the numbers of different species utilized did not significantly decrease toward the end of the last glacial, upper Pleistocene populations seemed increasingly able to kill larger numbers of particular species, which implies the development of hunting strategies tailored to individual species. Such a change also means that relatively greater percentages of meat per capita would have come from fewer different animal species.

Indeed, the late Upper Paleolithic provides ample evidence that humans used specialized techniques to kill enormous numbers of animals. At Solutré in France at least 100,000 horse skeletons have been found at the base of the cliff, while Předmost, Czechoslovakia, preserves remains of more than 1,000 mammoths [Howell, 1970]. These and numerous other similar sites in both the Old and New Worlds have led some workers to explain the extinction of many large herbivorous species during or at the end of the Pleistocene as the result of human overkill [Klein, 1983; Martin, 1967; Martin and Wright, 1967]. While the evidence for this hypothesis has been critically reevaluated by Webster [1981] and the case for mass extinction as a direct result of human predation has been somewhat weakened, it is nonetheless apparent that hominids developed into formidable big-game hunters during the course of the Pleistocene and very likely played a significant role in species turn-over and extinction on all continents.

Studies that trace regional developments in subsistence throughout the middle and upper Pleistocene are rare, but one, the record of human diet on the Iberian Peninsula, has been summarized by Freeman [1981]. The changes he discerns between early and later sites there seem to apply generally, although in most other regions faunal remains have not been collected or studied as thoroughly in this time range. The Iberian Acheulian phase was one of opportunism rather than specialization in hunting. The range of species taken by hominids was much greater than that of any other predator, and prey size diversity was generally high. This was a relatively unselective approach to food procurement in which large-scale game drives may have been a factor. Mousterian times signal a change toward the use of more varied resources compared with Acheulian predecessors. Early Upper Paleolithic peoples in turn expanded the range of subsistence resources further, while at the same time diversity in faunal size decreases. This is attributed to more intensive use of certain types of animals. Seasonal cropping of especially productive resources, which Freeman terms wild-harvesting, becomes important in the early Upper Paleolithic. However, he stresses that subsistence behavior even in a single region such as the Iberian Peninsula was varied and diverse and appears to have become more so through the Paleolithic.

New or more intensive exploitation of nonhunted animal resources played an important part in the expansion of the Upper Pleistocene resource base. Marine foods, including shellfish, fish, and marine mammals rarely figure very significantly in Middle and early Upper Pleistocene site remains. This is true even of shoreline sites like Terra Amata (de Lumley, 1969). By Middle Stone Age times in southern Africa however, Klein finds abundant evidence of shellfish collecting and aquatic mammal and bird remains [Klein, 1977]. Later sites show that fish and nonaquatic birds were added to the diet, presumably because of improved methods for taking these items. By later Upper Paleolithic times in Europe too, Magdalenian peoples were gathering quantities of shellfish, and cropping of molluscs appears to have intensified worldwide, as in both Iberia and Southern Africa mollusc size decreases markedly through time toward the end of the Pleistocene. Intensive shellfish harvesting is also known in the North American Archaic period, from sites of the Shell Mound Tradition such as Indian Knoll [Cassidy, 1980].

Although meat consumption in the Middle and Upper Pleistocene was almost certainly higher than it had been in the Pliocene/Lower Pleistocene, it is not necessarily true that increased hunting success translated into greater meat consumption per capita than is true of modern hunter-gatherers. If the levels of consumption of hunted animal protein in modern hunting populations are an accurate analogy for Pleistocene hunters, then it is a reasonable assumption that plant foods continued to contribute a major portion of the diet in most tropical and temperate regions.

As always, the picture of Middle to Upper Paleolithic plant utilization is almost invisible in comparison to the record of faunal debris. However, some direct evidence is available. Actual remains of great quantities of hackberry seeds have been found in deposits at Zhoukoudian [Wu and Lin, 1983], which the inhabitants gathered and apparently roasted. Pollen in the deposits shows the presence of other nut species such as walnut, hazelnut, and pine, along with elm and rose, which may also have been part of the diet. In Europe, both pollen and coprolites are available from Terra Amata, but neither has yielded information about food plants or diet [de Lumley, 1969]. Plant food evidence from Iberian sites is sparse [Freeman, 1981]. Flotation of samples from Mousterian levels at Abric Agut yielded some fragmentary seeds of legumes and chenopods, among others. From Gorham's Cave, also in Mousterian levels, comes evidence of pine charcoal and broken pine cones. Whether these were collected for fuel or for the pine nuts within is unknown, however. An Upper Paleolithic site, Cueva Morin, yielded hazelnut shells, along with hammer-grindstones. LSA sites in South Africa [Klein, 1977; Deacon, 1976] provide evidence of large-scale gathering of plant staples, such as corms of various species and also preserve pits apparently used for storing fruits and seeds. Abundant archeological evidence from the Levant documents that preagricultural populations made intensive use of natural stands of Old World grains [Lamberg-Karlovsky and Sabloff, 1979]. It is possible to speculate that late Pleistocene hunter-gatherers, in keeping with a general trend toward more specialized utilization of diverse animal resources, may have invested more time and effort in collecting and preparing certain vegetable foods as well. The critical change here, however, may be more one of visibility than of degree of utilization. Preserved clues of storage facilities or of specialized implements to harvest or prepare plant foods make their presence better known, but they may only indicate relative technological advances in dealing with plant materials, rather than in dietary change itself.

Climatic fluctuations during the Middle and Later Pleistocene must have had a significant impact not only on the composition of hominid diet but also on its variability. From at least the Middle Pleistocene on, *Homo erectus* and his descendants inhabited cool temperate regions as well as more tropical ones and were clearly able to exist in the harsh cold of periglacial regions as well. While the little known about the earliest European sites, Escale cave, Vértesszöllös, and Torralba-Ambrona [Bonifay and Bonifay 1963; Freeman, 1981; Howell, 1966; Howell and Freeman, 1982; Kretzoi and Vertes, 1965] indicates that these might have been occupied mainly during warmer portions of glacial periods or during interglacials, increasing amounts of archaeological material and human remains in both western and eastern Europe during the late Middle and Upper Pleistocene attest to the ability of Pleistocene populations to adapt to harsh environmental conditions. The implications of this ecological expansion for diet are primarily inferential. Some occupation sites, such as those in the Ukraine [Klein, 1973] appear to have been primarily winter encampments inhabited during very cold periods and based on intensive hunting of reindeer and horse. By analogy with modern subarctic environments (the Ukraine in the Late Pleistocene was somewhat similar to Northern Finland), few edible plant foods would have been available for humans, and as with modern high latitude hunters, meat probably comprised all or most of the diet at these winter camps. As human populations moved into more diverse habitats throughout the Middle and Upper Pleistocene, the degree of seasonal variation in diet probably intensified and would have been more extreme for populations exploiting periglacial environments than for those groups which stayed in more temperate regions year-round. Seasonality in diets would also have increased everywhere during the more marked climatic fluctuations which were probably characteristic of interstadial and interglacial periods.

Use or control of fire is another aspect of hominid behavior which might have had significance for hominid diets in the Middle and Upper Pleistocene. Apart from controversial claims of hominid involvement with fire in archaeological deposits at Chesowanja, Kenya, at 1.4 myrs [Gowlett et al., 1981; Isaac, 1982], the earliest secure evidence for the use of fire comes much later in the archaeological record, from Escale cave, at about 750,000 yrs BP [Bonifay and Bonifay, 1963; Howell, 1966; Klein, 1979]. Evidence of fire occurs at several other Middle Pleistocene sites as well: Torralba-Ambrona (Freeman, 1981); Vértesszöllös [Kretzoi and Vertes, 1965], Terra Amata [de Lumley, 1969], and Zhoukoudian [Wu and Lin, 1983]. It is uncertain what the initial motivation or circumstances surrounding the control of fire might have been. Fire can be used as either a defensive or offensive strategy vis-a-vis other animals (to drive game or to keep predators at bay). It can also be used as a means of controlling or altering microclimates, which may have been necessary to permit the expansion of an essentially tropical primate into cold temperate regions. Fire is also important in food preparation. Heat is often necessary to make the inedible edible, by breaking down physical barriers to nutrients or by removing toxins [Peters and O'Brien, 1981a,b]. Heat may make storage and preservation of some abundant food items possible, as Freeman has speculated for the immense quantity of meat represented by the Torralba-Ambrona kills. And, by breaking down structure or consolidating matter, heat may make some food items easier to process orally, for instance, by tenderizing meat or converting grains to porridge. It is commonly assumed that using fire to cook food would decrease masticatory load and that this should result in more gracile facial and dental anatomy. However, the fossil record shows relatively little change in hominid teeth and jaws during Middle to Upper Pleistocene times, even though fire is clearly present. Reductions in tooth and jaw size come much later, with the appearance of anatomically modern *Homo sapiens* (whose appearance varies from perhaps as early as 150,000 yrs BP in Africa, to about 30,000 years BP in Europe), though Trinkaus [1982] detects some signs of change in chewing patterns in European and Asian Neanderthals about 10,000 years or so previous to the appearance of modern man. Since apparent meat consumption predates the first certain evidence of fire in hominid occupation sites by at least 1 million years, cooking was clearly not instrumental in the developing reliance on meat. It is also possible to conclude that either cooking did not in fact do much to reduce masticatory load in Middle Pleistocene hominids, or perhaps fire was not used primarily for food preparation until relatively late in the Pleistocene. Since fire is first confirmed in the prehistoric record at the same time that humans are first found in colder climate occupations in Europe and Asia, control of fire may have been a central factor in this ecological expansion. Whether its first use was related to diet and food preparation, to atmospheric considerations, or to hunting strategy, all these factors clearly come into play in later human culture. The use of heat in preparing foods is very likely to have had a long history, but the dietary implications are unclear. In the early phases, cooking may have merely maximized the extent to which meat or other foods could be utilized, instead of permitting exploitation of qualitatively new food resources.

Although major biological changes occurred during the Middle and Upper Pleistocene which resulted in the transition from *Homo erectus* to fully modern *Homo sapiens*, no corresponding quantum leaps in subsistence behavior have been found [Schoeninger, 1981, 1982]. On the other hand, subsistence patterns were not static. Change is apparent throughout this period, but it is primarily found in the degree of success hominids enjoyed in exploiting the same resources, as well as in the degree of local selectivity and specialization they exercised. Only in the very final phases of the Upper Pleistocene does the record reveal changes toward incipient sedentism and intensive resource use which made possible (or necessary) the transition to agriculture.

THE POST-PLEISTOCENE ERA: THE BEGINNINGS OF FOOD PRODUCTION

The Post-Pleistocene era, beginning at about 12,000 BP, saw enormous changes in human subsistence behavior. In the Old World, the beginnings of agriculture and animal husbandry are apparent in the prehistoric record by about 10,000 BP, and by 7,000 BP the shift to an agrarian-based economy seems well-established [Braidwood and Howe, 1960; Lamberg-Karlovsky and Sabloff, 1979]. Agriculture spread into Europe from the Near East, while other centers of domestication developed separately in Africa and Asia [Reed, 1977]. In the New World at least two and possibly three centers were involved in establishing food production. Important as this widespread phenomenon was for social and political organization, there is reason to think that at least in the earlier phases, the shift from hunting and gathering to food production involved less immediate difference in human diet than might naturally be assumed.

There is now fairly abundant evidence from many regions that humans had considerable experience with intensive collecting of grains and other high carbohydrate foods for some time before any of these begin to show signs of domestication [Flannery, 1986]. In the Near East, ancestors of many cereal grains grow in thick wild stands even today (Harlan, 1967). That human populations exploited such resources even in the late Paleolithic is suggested by the cereal grains found at Nahal Oren, Israel, a pre-Natufian site on the coast, dated at about 20,000 BP [Lamberg-Karlovsky and Sabloff, 1979; Whitehouse and Whitehouse, 1975]. By Natufian times (12,000 to 10,000 BP), sickles, scythes, querns, mortars and pestles, and storage pits are known from various sites, including Mount Carmel and Ain Mallaha, and attest to the specialized harvesting and processing of these abundant natural food sources. Wild legumes were also collected in quantity as shown by sites such as Ali Kosh (Bus Mordeh phase) [Flannery, 1965; Hole et al., 1969]. By about 10,000 BP cereals are clearly being farmed at some sites in Anatolia (Murey-bit, Cayönü Tepesi) and also at Ali Kosh in the Zagros region of Iraq [Lamberg-Karlovsky and Sabloff, 1979; Mellaart, 1975].

In the New World, despite the more complex genetic history of maize, the same general pattern seems to have occurred. Usage of at least some of the putative wild ancestors of maize intensifies long before maize is finally present in domesticated form [MacNeish, 1964a,b, 1969, 1972]. Similarly, populations in the Brazilian Archaic may have eaten wild manioc in large quantities, before any archaeological evidence of its cultivation or preparation exists [Turner and Machado, 1983]. In North America a variety of seed plants were domesticated from groups known only by wild varieties today [Smith, 1984]. Even as late as the 19th century, hunter-gatherers in California utilized a variety of wild nuts and seeds as staples, especially acorns, of which enormous quantities were gathered and ground into meal [Kroeber, 1953]. Kraybill [1977] has detailed the varieties, uses, and preagricultural occurrences of ground stone milling equipment which documents the consumption of cereals, nuts, and other plant materials that were processed and consumed in appreciable quantities long before domestication.

The domestication of animals probably began at about the same time as incipient agriculture in the Near East. Here again, the earliest stages are difficult to detect, because the species eventually domesticated were present and heavily used before any morphological evidence of domestication appears. The Karim Shahir culture of the Zagros [Braidwood, 1960; Braidwood and Howe, 1960] seems to document an early stage of proto-animal-domestication, with very abundant remains of sheep, goats, cattle, horses, and wolves. The site of Ganj-dareh in Iran also probably documents early domestication. In Mesoamerica, animal domestication did not have the same importance that it assumed in the Old World, just as intensive big-game hunting never seems to have been a major subsistence strategy in earlier times there.

For several thousand years after the beginnings of food production, the older subsistence strategies of hunting and gathering wild foods continued to coexist along with the new patterns. Thus at Jarmo, a Zagros farming village (9000-7500 BP) and the larger cities of Jericho (9300-8000 BP) and Catal Hüyük (8500-7400), wild plants, nuts, and wild game continue to make significant contributions to the diet [Braidwood, 1960; Braidwood and Howe, 1960; Kenyon, 1957; Mellaart, 1967]. As Schoeninger has demonstrated for both the Levant and Iran, on the basis of strontium levels in human bone [Schoeninger, 1981, 1982], the major changes in subsistence in the late Upper Pleistocene/Holocene era seem to be primarily economic or resource management solutions, rather than qualitative differences in the types of food utilized.

The immediate motivation for domestication and agriculture are controversial [Boserup, 1965; Cohen, 1977; Flannery, 1973; Rindos, 1980]. Theories of population pressure and inadequate natural food resources have been the most widely accepted, though as Flannery points out, the first domesticates might not have been food items at all [Flannery, 1986]. The most immediate dietary implications of food production might have been a leveling-out of food shortages caused by unpredictable annual fluctuations in natural productivity through the accumulation and storage of surplus food [Flannery, 1986]. However, there is reason to believe that in the long run, agriculturalists were then and continue to be more disadvantaged by adverse climatic conditions than would be true of more mobile hunters and gatherers in the same environment [Cassidy, 1980].

While food production may have solved short-term problems of demographic pressure, the solution in turn created new problems and dilemmas for human populations. As the intensity of food production rises, the record for the first time shows the development of consistent and significant intragroup variation in diet which appears to follow along the lines of sex and status differentiation. The Sumerian civilization of Mesopotamia has provided researchers with detailed records of the food rations accorded various classes in Sumerian society, as well as pictorial evidence of the foodstuffs available. From these sources, it is clear that although a wide variety of foods high in protein and calories was produced and available, the diet of the lower strata of society was heavily biased towards barley, while higher classes enjoyed a richer, more varied diet [Braidwood and Reed, 1957]. Middle Formative Period burials at Chalcatzingo, Mexico, (1150–550 BC) showed differential levels of bone strontium which correlated with the amount and type of grave goods associated with each skeleton [Schoeninger, 1979]. It was concluded that high-status individuals showed lower bone strontium levels because they consumed more meat in life, while lower-status individuals showed the high levels of strontium expected with a more vegetarian diet.

Evidence from several prehistoric North American populations sampled across the transition to agriculture showed that the sexes tended to be differentially affected by the new dependence on maize [Cohen and Armelagos, 1984]. In coastal Georgia [Larsen, 1981, 1983, 1984] females show greater caries incidence and more reduction in body size and tooth size after the agricultural shift than did males, implying that female diets may have been higher in carbohydrates and lower in protein than in the previous hunting/gathering phase, while male diets remained more similar in the two phases. Studies of isotopic carbon in human collagen samples from a variety of Woodland populations [Van Der Merwe and Vogel, 1978] revealed some significant sex differences which suggest that even after the introduction of maize (a C4-type plant), females consumed more wild C3-type plants than did males, while carbon isotope values were similar for both sexes in pre-maize populations. It is very likely that some sex differences in diet may always have been present in hunter-gatherer populations [Rosenberg, 1980], because of the differential access to plants and meat each sex has while foraging, as is seen in the Hadza today [Woodburne, 1968]. The division of meat is very often a source of general complaint and dissatisfaction in San bands, indicating that even in egalitarian societies access to favored foods is not perfectly uniform [Lee, 1979]. However, in the absence of any real social stratification and with most adult individuals responsible to a very large degree for procuring their own food, pre-agricultural peoples probably did not experience any consistent inequities in the distribution of food. Domestication and food production, which make possible the accumulation of food surpluses and free some individuals from the labor of food procurement, also necessitate the appearance of central authority and control over food resources, which in turn sets up a system by which food surpluses can be differentially distributed, resulting in unequal access to food.

The transition to food production also had a major effect on the general health levels of producer populations [Cohen and Armelagos, 1984]. The adoption of high-carbohydrate diets has almost everywhere coincided with marked increases in dental caries [Cook and Buikstra, 1979; Larsen, 1981, 1984; Powell, 1985; Turner and Machado, 1983]. Rises in the general level of infectious disease are also characteristic of agricultural populations, though this may be due as much to patterns of large permanent settlement as well as to nutritional stress per se [Buikstra, 1976, 1977; Ubelaker, 1980]. Evidence of systemic disease during pregnancy and in the early post-natal period affects the structure of enamel formation and contributes to increased susceptibility to dental disease and other forms of morbidity [Cook and Buikstra, 1979]. Stature and general robusticity may also decline [Angel, 1984; Larsen, 1981, 1983; Ruff et al., 1984], either as a result of lowered activity levels or possibly in response to nutritional stress and lower protein levels. Nutritional deficiency diseases, which appear to have been rare in Paleolithic populations, have been common since the adoption of agriculture [Yudkin, 1969]. Some have been particularly associated with the adoption of corn-based diets in the New World [Lallo et al., 1977]. Yudkin also points out that grain and dairy product allergies are common modern health problems, which indicates that humans are still in the process of adapting to the intensive dependence on these food items which resulted from the shift to food production.

Although prehistorians traditionally have viewed the shift to agriculture as a progressive step for human populations, more recent studies, such as those cited above and numerous others, have demonstrated that reliance on food production frequently resulted in inadequate or unbalanced diets and deterioration in the general health of prehistoric food-producing populations.

CONCLUSIONS

The picture of human subsistence behavior that can be reconstructed from the prehistoric record is one set off initially by a shift into a novel food niche in the terminal Miocene or Plio-Pleistocene, followed by progressive refinement in food procurement strategies coupled with growing diversification and specialization in food resources throughout the Middle and Upper Pleistocene, and capped by a Post-Pleistocene shift to domestication and food production which grew out of the intensive exploitation of wild foods in the late Pleistocene. Although many primates include some animal protein in their diets, hominids came to adopt a diet which was unusual not only in its high amount of meat but also for the way in which it was obtained. At first this may have been through occasional hunting with more common scavenging, but this was eventually replaced by organized persistent hunting. Plant foods have very likely always been more important components of the hominid diet, with a few special exceptions, but even here novel methods of procuring and processing plant foods have dramatically increased the range and efficiency of human feeding over that of other primates. At least since the Middle Pleistocene, humans have been able to alter the basic physical properties of many foodstuffs to enhance their edibility through cooking, grinding or milling, and through chemical treatments (such as the alkali enrichment of maize in Mesoamerica or the removal of harmful or noxious compounds in manioc and acorns).

The causes that led Upper and Post-Pleistocene human populations everywhere to intensify their efforts first to procure food from the wild and later to actively control its production may never be fully known, but increasing population pressure seems to be the most convincing explanation. Throughout the Pleistocene, the evidence suggests a constant push to increase technological mastery over the food supply. Ironically, the dependence on agriculture and domestication meant that although in the short-term, food resources were controlled and somewhat more predictable, it is also true that for the first time adverse climatic conditions or simply uneven distribution systems could leave large numbers of individuals without adequate diets, often resulting in chronic shortages. The greater mobility and more diverse diet of the Pleistocene hunter-gatherers might have enabled earlier populations to minimize losses due to natural fluctuations in the food supply more easily than sedentary food producers are able to do.

With agriculture have come a variety of deficiency and infectious diseases and often a deterioration in general levels of health. Eaton and Konner (1985) have compared contemporary diets of industrialized countries to several hypothetical models of preagricultural diets, based on those of various living hunter/gatherer populations, and concluded that whatever the relative percentages of meat and vegetable food in prehistoric diets, the modern diet is deficient or inadequate in several fundamental ways. Protein, fiber, vitamin C, and calcium are, on the one hand, all much lower in the average American diet than the hypothetical Paleolithic diet, even with only 35% of the diet derived from meat. On the other hand, levels of sodium and fat, particularly saturated fats, are much higher. Evidence of the relationship of these imbalances to major chronic diseases of the developed world is so far controversial but continues to accumulate.

Not only was the agricultural "revolution" not really so revolutionary at its inception, it has also come to represent something of a nutritional "devolution" for much of mankind. The process of adapting to these changes in diet is clearly not complete, but further progress will have to involve not only advances in food technology but must encompass global political and economic developments as well.

ACKNOWLEDGMENTS

I would like to thank Teri Silvio for her help in the preparation of this manuscript.

REFERENCES

Ambrose SH, DeNiro MJ (1986): Reconstruction of African human diet using bone collagen carbon and nitrogen isotope ratios. Nature 319:321-324.

Angel JL (1984): Health as a crucial factor in the changes from hunting to developed farming in the Eastern Mediterranean. In Cohen MN, Armelagos GJ (eds): "Paleopathology at the Origins of Agriculture." New York: Academic Press, pp 51-73.

Ardrey R (1961): "African Genesis: A Personal Investigation into the Animal Origins and Nature of Man." New York: Atheneum.

Ardrey R (1976): "The Hunting Hypothesis." New York: Atheneum.

Arnott ML (1975): "The Anthropology of Food and Food Habits." The Hague: Mouton.

Behrensmeyer AK (1978): The habitat of Plio-Pleistocene hominids in East Africa: taphonomic and microstratigraphic evidence. In Jolly CJ (ed): "Early Hominids of Africa." New York: St. Martin's Press, pp 165-189.

Behrensmeyer AK, Cooke HBS (1985): Paleoenvironments, stratigraphy, and taphonomy in the African Pliocene and early Pleistocene. In Delson E (ed): "Ancestors: The Hard Evidence." New York: Alan R. Liss, Inc., pp 60-62.

Behrensmeyer AK, Gordon KD, Yanagi GT (1986): "Trampling as a cause of bone surface damage and pseudo-cutmarks." Nature 319:768-771.

Binford LR (1977): Olorgesailie deserves more than the usual book review. J Anthropol Res 33:493-502.

Binford LR (1981): "Bones: Ancient Men and Modern Myths." New York: Academic Press.

Binford S (1968): Early upper Pleistocene adaptations in the Levant. Am Anthropol 70:707-717.

Blumenschine R (1986): What lions leave behind—scavenging versus hunting in the human past. Paper presented to the Anthropological Society of Washington, January 18, 1986.

Boaz NT, Gauld SC (1979): Coprolite analysis and early hominid paleobiology. Am J Phys Anthropol 50:420.

Boaz NT, Hample J (1978): Strontium content of fossil tooth enamel and diet of early hominids. J Paleontol 52:928-933.

Boesch C, Boesch H (1981): Sex differences in the use of natural hammers by wild chimpanzees: a preliminary report. J Hum Evol 10:585-593.

Bonifay MF, Bonifay E (1963): Un gisement à faune épi-villafranchienne a Saint-Estève-Janson (Bouches-du-Rhône). C R Acad Sci Paris 256:1136-1138.

Boserup E (1965): "The Conditions of Agricultural Growth." Chicago: Aldine.

Bower B (1985): Hunting ancient scavengers. Sci News 127:155-157.

Brace CL (1967): "The Stages of Human Evolution." Englewood Cliffs, NJ: Prentice-Hall.

Brace CL (1969): The australopithecine range of variation. Am J Phys Anthropol 31:255.

Brace CL (1973): Sexual dimorphism in human evolution. Yrbk Phys Anthropol 16:50-68.

Braidwood RJ (1960): The agricultural revolution. Sci Am 203:130-148.

Braidwood RJ, Howe B (1960): "Prehistoric Investigations in Iraqi Kurdistan." Studies in Ancient Oriental Civilization, No. 31. Chicago: University of Chicago Press.

Braidwood RJ, Reed CA (1957): The achievement and early consequences of food-production: a consideration of the archeological and natural-historical evidence. Cold Spr Hrbr, Symp Quant Biol 22:19-31.

Brain CK (1969): The contribution of Namib Desert Hottentots to an understanding of australopithecine bone accumulations. Sci Pap Namib Desert Res Stn 39:13-22.

Brain CK (1970): New finds at Swartkrans australopithecine site. Nature 225:1112-1118.

Brain CK (1972): An attempt to reconstruct the behaviour of *Australopithecus*: the evidence for interpersonal violence. S. Afr Mus Assn Bull 9:127-139.

Brain CK (1978): Some aspects of the South African australopithecine sites and their bone accumulations. In Jolly C (ed): "Early Hominids of Africa." New York: St. Martin's Press, pp 131-164.

Brain CK (1981): "The Australopithecines: The Hunters or the Hunted?" Chicago: University of Chicago Press.

Brain CK (1984): The evidence for bone modification by hominids in southern Africa. In: "Abstracts of the First International Conference on Bone Modification." Orono, Maine: Center for the Study of Early Man, pp 5-6.

Brain CK (1985): Cultural and taphonomic comparisons of hominids from Swartkrans and Sterkfontein. In Delson E (ed): "Ancestors: The Hard Evidence." New York: Alan R. Liss, Inc., pp 72-75.

Brooks AS (1984): San land-use patterns, past and present. In Hall M, Avery G, Avery DM, Wilson ML, Humphreys AJB (eds): "Frontiers: Southern African Archaeology Today." Cambridge Monographs in African Archaeology, 10. Oxford: B.A.R., pp 40-52.

Broom R (1950): The genera and species of the South African fossil ape-men. Am J Phys Anthropol 8:1-13.

Brothwell D, Brothwell P (1969): "Food in Antiquity." London: Thames and Hudson.

Brown F, Harris J, Leakey R, Walker A (1985): Early *Homo erectus* skeleton from west Lake Turkana, Kenya. Nature 316:788-792.

Buikstra JE (1976): "Hopewell in the Lower Illinois Valley." Northwestern Archeological Program Scientific Papers, Vol 2. Chicago: Northwestern University.

Buikstra JE (1977): Biocultural dimensions of archeological study: a regional perspective. In Blakely RL (ed): "Biocultural Adaptation in Prehistoric America." Athens, GA: University of Georgia Press, pp 67-84.

Bunn H (1981): Archaeological evidence for meat-eating by Plio-Pleistocene hominids from Koobi Fora and Olduvai Gorge. Nature 291:574-577.

Bunn H (1983): Evidence on the diet and subsistence patterns of Plio-Pleistocene hominids at Koobi Fora, Kenya, and at Olduvai Gorge, Tanzania. In Clutton-Brock J, Grigson C (eds): "Animals and Archaeology." London: British Archaeological Reports, pp 21-30.

Butzer KW (1975): Geological and ecological perspectives on the middle Pleistocene. In Butzer KW, Isaac GL (eds): "After the Australopithecines." The Hague: Mouton, pp 857-873.

Cachel S (1975): A new view of speciation in *Australopithecus*. In Tuttle, RH (ed): "Paleoanthropology, Morphology and Paleoecology." The Hague: Mouton, pp 183-201.

Campbell BG (1966): "Human Evolution." Chicago: Aldine.

Cassidy CM (1980): Nutrition and health in agriculturalists and hunter-gatherers. In Jerome NW, Kandel RF, Pelto GH: "Nutritional Anthropology." Pleasantville, New York: Redgrave Publ. Co., pp 117-145.

Chisholm BS, Nelson DE, Schwarcz HP (1983): Marine and terrestrial protein in prehistoric diets on the British Columbia coast. Curr Anthropol 24:396-398.

Clarke RJ (1985): *Australopithecus* and early *Homo* in southern Africa. In Delson E (ed): "Ancestors: The Hard Evidence." New York: Alan R. Liss, Inc., pp 171-177.

Cohen MN (1977): "The Food Crisis in Prehistory." New Haven: Yale University Press.

Cohen MN, Armelagos GJ (1984): "Paleopathology at the Origins of Agriculture." New York: Academic Press.

Cook DC, Buikstra JE (1979): Health and differential survival in prehistoric populations: prenatal dental defects. Am J Phys Anthropol 51:649-664.

Corrucini RS, Henderson AM (1978): Multivariate dental allometry in primates. Am J Phys Anthropol 48:203-208.

Creighton GK (1980): Static allometry of mammalian teeth and the correlation of tooth size and body size in contemporary mammals. J Zool Lond 191:435-443.

Dart RA (1940): The status of *Australopithecus*. Am J Phys Anthropol 26:167-186.

Dart RA (1949): The predatory implemental technique of *Australopithecus*. Am J Phys Anthropol 7:1-38.

Dart RA (1953): The predatory transition from ape to man. Int Anthropol Ling Rev 1:201-217.

Dart RA (1957): "The osteodontokeratic culture of *Australopithecus prometheus*." Memoir 10. Pretoria: Transvaal Museum.

Dart RA (1962): A cleft adult mandible and nine other lower jaw fragments from Makapansgat. Am J Phys Anthropol 20:267-286.

Deacon HJ (1976): Where hunters gathered. S Afr Archaeol Soc Monogr Ser 1:1-231.

Dennell RW (1979): Prehistoric diet and nutrition: some food for thought. World Arch 2(2):121-135.

DeNiro MJ (1985): Postmortem preservation and alteration of in vivo bone collagen isotope ratios in relation to palaeodietary reconstruction. Nature 317:806-809.

DeNiro MJ, Epstein S (1978): Carbon isotopic evidence for different feeding habits in two hyrax species occupying the same habitat. Science 201:906-908.

Dunbar RIM (1976): Australopithecine diet based on a baboon analogy. J Hum Evol 5:161-167.

Eaton SB, Konner M (1985): Paleolithic nutrition. New Eng J Med 312:283-289.

Farb P, Armelagos G (1980): "Consuming Passions." New York: Washington Square Press.

Flannery KV (1965): The ecology of early food production in Mesopotamia. Science 147:1247-1256.

Flannery KV (1973): The origins of agriculture. Ann Rev Anthropol 2:271-310.

Flannery KV (1986): "Guila Naquitz: Archaic Foraging." New York: Academic Press.

Freeman L (1981): The fat of the land: notes on Paleolithic diet in Iberia. In Harding, RS, Teleki, G (eds): "Omnivorous Primates." New York: Columbia University Press, pp 104-165.

Freeman LG, Howell FC (1981): Acheulian occupation at Ambrona (Spain). 46th Annual SAA Meetings Abstract, San Diego.

Freeman LG, Howell FC (1982): Acheulian hunters on the Spanish Meseta: Torralba and Ambrona reconsidered. AAA Meetings Abstracts, Washington, D.C.

Gilbert RI, Mielke JH (1985): "The Analysis of Prehistoric Diets." New York: Academic Press.

Glob PV (1969): "The Bog People." Ithaca: Cornell University Press.

Goldstein S, Post D, Melnick D (1978): An analysis of cercopithecoid odontometrics. Am J Phys Anthropol 49:517-532.

Gowlett JAJ, Harris JWK, Walton D, Wood BA (1981): Early archaeological sites, hominid remains and traces of fire from Chesowanja, Kenya. Nature 294:125-129.

Grine FE (1981): Trophic differences between 'gracile' and 'robust' australopithecines: a scanning electron microscope analysis of occlusal events. S Afr J Sci 77:203-230.

Grine FE (1986): Quantitative analysis of occlusal microwear in *Australopithecus* and *Paranthropus*. In Johari O (ed): "SEM/1986." Chicago: SEM, Inc. (in press).

Harding RS (1981): An order of omnivores: nonhuman primate diets in the wild. In Harding, RS, Teleki, G (eds): "Omnivorous Primates." New York: Columbia University Press, pp 191-214.

Harlan JR (1967): A wild wheat harvest in Turkey. Archaeology 20:187-201.

Hasegawa T, Hiraiwa M, Nishida T, Takasaki H (1983): New evidence of scavenging behavior in wild chimpanzees. Curr Anthropol 24:231-232.

Hayden B (1979): "Lithic Use-Wear Analysis." New York: Academic Press.

Hayden B (1981): Subsistence and ecological adaptations of modern hunter/gatherers. In Harding, RS, Teleki G (eds): "Omnivorous Primates." New York: Columbia University Press, pp 344-421.

Hole F, Flannery KV, Neely JA (1969): "Prehistory and Human Ecology of the Deh Luran Plain." Museum of Anthropology, Memoirs, No. 1. Ann Arbor: University of Michigan.

Horowitz A, Siedner G, Bar Yosef O (1973): Radiometric dating of the Ubeidiya Formation, Jordan Valley, Israel. Nature 242:186-187.

Howell FC (1966): Observations on the earlier phases of the European lower paleolithic. Am Anthropol 68:88-201.

Howell FC (1970): "Early Man." New York: Time-Life.

Howell FC, Freeman LG (1982): Ambrona: an early Stone Age site on Spanish Meseta. The LSB Leakey Foundation News 22(1):11-13.

Isaac GL (1971): The diet of early man: aspects of archaeological evidence from lower and middle Pleistocene sites in Africa. World Arch 2:278-299.

Isaac GL (1977): "Olorgesailie: Archaeological Studies of a Middle Pleistocene Lake Basin in Kenya." Chicago: University of Chicago Press.

Isaac GL (1978a): The archaeological evidence for the activities of early African hominids. In Jolly C (ed): "Early Hominids of Africa." New York: St. Martin's Press, pp 219-254.

Isaac GL (1978b): The food-sharing behavior of protohuman hominids. Sci Am 238(4):90-108.

Isaac GL (1981): Archaeological tests of alternative models of early hominid behaviour: excavation and experiments. Phil Trans R Soc Lond B 292:177-188.

Isaac GL (1982): Early hominids and fire at Chesowanja, Kenya. Nature 296:870.

Isaac GL, Crader D (1981): To what extent were early hominids carnivorous? an archaeological perspective. In Harding, RS, Teleki, G (eds): "Omnivorous Primates." New York: Columbia University Press, pp 37-103.

Jolly CJ (1970): The seed-eaters: a new model of hominid differentiation based on a baboon analogy. Man 5:5-26.

Kay RF (1975a): Allometry and early hominids. Science 189:63.

Kay RF (1975b): The functional adaptations of primate molar teeth. Am J Phys Anthropol 43:195-216.

Kay RF (1981): The nut-crackers—a new theory of the adaptations of the Ramapithecinae. Am J Phys Anthropol 55:141-151.

Keeley LH (1980): "Experimental Determination of Stone Tool Uses: a Microwear Analysis." Chicago: University of Chicago Press.

Keeley LH, Toth N (1981): Microwear polishes on early stone tools from Koobi Fora, Kenya. Nature 293:464-465.

Kenyon K (1957): "Digging Up Jericho." London: Benn.

King GE (1975): Socioterritorial units among carnivores and early hominids. J Anthropol Res 31:69-87.

Klein RG (1973): "Ice-Age Hunters of the Ukraine." Chicago: University of Chicago Press.

Klein RG (1975): Paleoanthropological implications of the non-archeological bone assemblages from Swartklip I, southwestern Cape Province, South Africa. Quatern Res 5:257-288.

Klein RG (1977): The ecology of early man in southern Africa. Science 197:115-126.

Klein RG (1979): Stone Age exploitation of animals in southern Africa. Am Sci 67:151-160.

Klein RG (1982): Age (mortality) profiles as a means of distinguishing hunted species from scavenged ones in Stone Age archeological sites. Paleobiology 8:151-158.

Klein RG (1983): The Stone Age prehistory of southern Africa. Ann Rev Anthropol 12:25-48.

Kraybill N (1977): Pre-agricultural tools for the preparation of foods in the Old World. In Reed CA: "The Origins of Agriculture." The Hague: Mouton, pp 485-519.

Kretzoi M, and Vertés L (1965): Upper Biharian (Intermindel) pebble-industry occupational site in western Hungary. Curr Anthropol 6:74-87.

Kroeber AL (1953): "Handbook of the Indians of California." Reprint of 1925 edition, Berkeley: California Book Co.

Lallo JW, Armelagos GJ, Mensforth RP (1977): The role of diet, disease, and physiology in the origin of porotic hyperostosis. Hum Biol 49:471-83.

Lamberg-Karlovsky CC, Sabloff JA (1979): "Ancient Civilizations." Menlo Park, Ca: Benjamin Cummings.

Larsen CS (1981): Skeletal and dental adaptations to the shift to agriculture on the Georgia coast. Curr Anthropol 22:422-423.

Larsen CS (1983): Deciduous tooth size and subsistence change in prehistoric Georgia coast populations. Curr Anthropol 24:225-226.

Larsen CS (1984): Health and disease in prehistoric Georgia: the transition to agriculture. In Cohen MN, Armelagos GJ (eds): "Paleopathology at the Origins of Agriculture." New York: Academic Press, pp 367-392.

Leakey MD (1971): "Olduvai Gorge, Vol 3." Cambridge: Cambridge University Press.

Leakey REF, Walker AC (1985): *Homo erectus* unearthed. Nat Geogr 168:624-629.

Lee RB (1968): What hunters do for a living, or how to make out on scarce resources. In Lee RB, De Vore I (eds): "Man the Hunter." Chicago: Aldine, pp 30-48.

Lee RB (1979): "The !Kung San." Cambridge: Cambridge University Press.

Lee RB, De Vore I (eds) (1968): "Man the Hunter." Chicago: Aldine.

Lewin R (1984): Archeology briefing. Science 226:428-429.

Lewin R (1986): When stones can be deceptive. Science 231:113-115.

de Lumley H (1969): A paleolithic camp at Nice. Sci Am 220:42-50.

MacNeish RS (1964a): Ancient Mesoamerican civilization. Science 143:531-537.

MacNeish RS (1964b): The food gathering and incipient agriculture stage of prehistoric Middle America. In West RC (ed): "Natural Environments and Early Cultures." Austin: University of Texas Press, pp 413-426.

MacNeish RS (1969): Speculation about how and why food production and village life developed in the Tehuacan Valley, Mexico. Archaeology 24:307-315.

MacNeish RS (1972): The evolution of community patterns in the Tehuacan Valley of Mexico and speculations about the cultural process. In Ucko PJ, Tringham R, Dimbleby GW (eds): "Man, Settlement, and Urbanism." London: Duckworth, pp 67-93.

Martin PS (1967): Prehistoric overkill. In Martin PS, Wright HE: "Pleistocene Extinctions." New Haven: Yale University Press, pp 75-120.

Martin PS, Wright HE (1967): "Pleistocene Extinctions." New Haven: Yale University Press.

Martin RD (1983): "Human brain evolution in an ecological context." Fifty-second James Arthur Lecture on the Evolution of the Human Brain, 1982. New York: American Museum of Natural History.

McGrew W, Tutin C, Baldwin P (1979): Chimpanzees, tools and termites: cross-cultural comparisons of Senegal, Tanzania and Rio Muni. Man 14:185-214.

Meggitt MJ (1962): "Desert People: a Study of the Walbiri Aborigines of Central Australia." Sydney: Angus and Robertson.

Mellaart J (1967): "Çatal Hüyük: A Neolithic Town in Anatolia." London: Thames and Hudson Ltd.

Mellaart J (1975): "The Neolithic of the Near East." London: Thames and Hudson.

Peters CR, Maguire B (1981): Wild plant foods of the Makapansgat area: a modern ecosystems analogue for *Australopithecus africanus* adaptations. J Hum Evol 10:565-583.

Peters CR, O'Brien EM (1981a): The early hominid plant-food niche: insights from an analysis of human, chimpanzee, and baboon plant exploitation in eastern and southern Africa. Curr Anthropol 22:127-140.

Peters CR, O'Brien EM (1981b): Wild plant genera exploited for food by humans, chimpanzees, and baboons in eastern and southern Africa: Master Table 1980. Athens, GA: published by the authors.

Peters CR, O'Brien EM (1982): Reply. Curr Anthropol 23:214-218.

Peters CR, O'Brien EM, Box EO (1984): Plant types and seasonality of wild-plant foods, Tanzania to Southwestern Africa: resources for models of the natural environment. J Hum Evol 13:397-414.

Peters R, Mech L (1975): Behavioral and intellectual adaptations of selected mammalian predators to the problem of hunting large animals. In Tuttle, RH (ed): "Socioecology and Psychology of Primates." The Hague: Mouton, pp 279-300.

Pilbeam DR, Gould SJ (1974): Size and scaling in human evolution. Science 186:892-901.

Potts R (1982): "Lower Pleistocene Site Formation and Hominid Activities at Olduvai Gorge, Tanzania." Ph.D. dissertation, Harvard University.

Potts R (1983): Foraging for faunal resources by early hominids at Olduvai Gorge, Tanzania. In Clutton-Brock J, Grigson C (eds): "Animals and Archaeology, Vol. 1." Oxford: Brit Arch Reps, pp 51-62.

Potts R (1984): Hominid hunters? Problems of identifying the earliest hunter/gatherers. In Foley R (ed): "Community Ecology and Human Adaptation in the Pleistocene." London: Academic Press, pp 129-166.

Potts R (1986): Reconstructions of early hominid socioecology: a critique of primate models. In Kinzey W (ed): "Primate Models for the Evolution of Human Behavior." New York: SUNY Press (in press).

Potts R, Shipman P (1981): Cutmarks made by stone tools on bones from Olduvai Gorge, Tanzania. Nature 291:577-580.

Powell ML (1985): The analysis of dental wear and caries for dietary reconstruction. In Gilbert RI, Mielke JH (eds): "The Analysis of Prehistoric Diets." New York: Academic Press, pp 307-338.

Puech P-F (1984): Acidic-food choice in *Homo habilis* at Olduvai. Curr Anthropol 25:349-350.

Puech P-F, Albertini H, Serratrice C (1983): Tooth microwear and dietary patterns in early hominids from Laetoli, Hadar and Olduvai. J Hum Evol 12:721-729.

Read-Martin CE, Read DW (1975): Australopithecine scavenging and human evolution: an approach from faunal analysis. Curr Anthropol 16:359-368.

Reed CA (1977): "Origins of Agriculture." The Hague: Mouton.

Rindos D (1980): "The Origins of Agriculture." New York: Academic Press.

Robinson JT (1954a): Prehominid dentition and hominid evolution. Evolution 8:324-334.

Robinson JT (1954b): The genera and species of the Australopithecinae. Am J Phys Anthropol 12:181-200.

Robinson JT (1956): The dentition of the Australopithecinae. Mem Transv Mus 9:1-179.

Robinson JT (1961): The australopithecines and their bearing on the origin of man and of stone tool making. S Afr J Sci 57:3-16.

Robinson JT (1963): Adaptive radiation in the australopithecines and the origin of man. In Howell FC, Bourliere F (eds): "African Ecology and Human Evolution." Chicago: Aldine, pp 385-416.

Rosenberg EM (1980): Demographic effects of sex-differential nutrition. In Jerome NW, Kandel RF, Pelto GH (eds): "Nutritional Anthropology." Pleasantville, New York: Redgrave Publ. Co., pp 181-203.

Ruff CB, Larsen CS, Hayes WC (1984): Structural changes in the femur with the transition to agriculture on the Georgia coast. Am J Phys Anthropol 64:125-136.

Schaller GB, Lowther GR (1969): The relevance of carnivore behavior to the study of early hominids. Southwest J Anthropol 25:307-341.

Schoeninger MJ (1979): Diet and status at Chalcatzingo: some empirical and technical aspects of strontium analysis. Am J Phys Anthropol 51:295-310.

Schoeninger MJ (1981): The agricultural "revolution": its effect on human diet in prehistoric Iran and Israel. Paléorient 7:73-91.

Schoeninger MJ (1982): Diet and the evolution of modern human form in the Middle East. Am J Phys Anthropol 58:37-52.

Schoeninger MJ, DeNiro MJ (1984): Nitrogen and carbon isotopic composition of bone collagen from marine and terrestrial animals. Geochim Cosmochim Acta 48:625-639.

Schoeninger MJ, DeNiro MJ, Tauber H (1983): Stable nitrogen isotope ratios of bone collagen reflect marine and terrestrial components of prehistoric human diet. Science 220:1381-1383.

Sept J (1986): In search of our roots: East African wild plant foods and ancient gatherers. Paper presented to the Anthropological Society of Washington, January 18, 1986.

Shipman PL (1983): Early hominid lifestyle: hunting and gathering or foraging and scavenging? In Clutton-Brock, J, Grigson, C (eds): "Animals and Archaeology: 1. Hunters and their Prey." Oxford: British Archaeological Reports, pp 31-49.

Shipman PL (1984): Altered bones from Olduvai Gorge, Tanzania: techniques, problems and implications of their recognition. In: Abstracts of the First International Conference on Bone Modification. Orono, Maine: Center for the Study of Early Man, pp 32-33.

Shipman PL (1986): Scavenging or hunting in early hominids: theoretical framework and tests. Am Anthropol 88:27-43.

Shipman P, Bosler W, Davis KL (1981): Butchering of giant geladas at an Acheulian Site. Curr Anthropol 22:257-268.

Shipman P, Rose J (1983): Evidence of butchery and hominid activities at Torralba and Ambrona: an evaluation using microscopic techniques. J Arch Sci 10:465-474.

Sillen A (1981): Strontium and diet at Hayonim Cave. Am J Phys Anthropol 56:131-137.

Sillen A (1985): Diagenesis of the inorganic phase of vertebrate cortical bone. Paper presented to Carnegie Institution of Washington, Conference on Biomineralization Processes and the Fossil Record, Warrenton, Virginia, April 14, 1985.

Sillen A, Kavanaugh M (1982): Strontium and paleodietary research: a review. Yrbk Phys Anthropol 25:67-90.

Smith BD (1984): *Chenopodium* as a prehistoric domesticate in eastern North American: evidence from Russell Cave, Alabama. Science 226:165-167.

Speth JD, Davis DD (1976): Seasonal variability in early hominid predation. Science 192:441-445.

Strum SC (1981): Processes and products of change: baboon predatory behavior at Gilgil, Kenya. In Hardin RS, Teleki G: "Omnivorous Primates." New York: Columbia University Press, pp 255-302.

Sugardjito J, Nurhuda N (1981): Meat-eating behavior in orangutans, *Pongo pygmaeus*. Primates 22:414-416.

Sutcliffe AJ (1972): Spotted hyaena: crusher, gnawer, digestor and collector of bones. In Washburn, SL, Dolhinow, P (eds): "Perspectives on Human Evolution." New York: Holt, Rinehart and Winston, pp 141-150.

Szalay FS (1975): Hunting-scavenging protohominids: a model for hominid origins. Man 10:420-429.

Teleki G (1973): The omnivorous chimpanzee. Sci Am 228(1):32-42.

Teleki G (1981): The omnivorous diet and eclectic feeding habits of chimpanzees in Gombe National Park, Tanzania. In Harding, RS, Teleki, G (eds): "Omnivorous Primates." New York: Columbia University Press, pp 303-343.

Thackeray F (1981): Comment. Curr Anthropol 22:265-266.

Thompson PR (1975): A cross species analysis of carnivore, primate and hominid behavior. J Hum Evol 4:113-124.

Thompson PR (1976): A behavior model for *Australopithecus africanus*. J Hum Evol 5:547-558.

Tobias PV (1967): "The Cranium and Maxillary Dentition of *Australopithecus (Zinjanthropus) boisei*. Olduvai Gorge, Vol 2." Cambridge: Cambridge University Press.

Toth N (1985): The Oldowan reassessed: a closer look at early stone artifacts. J Arch Sci 12:101-120.

Trinkaus E (1982): Evolutionary trends in the Shanidar Neandertal sample. Am J Phys Anthropol 57:237.

Turner CG, Machado LMC (1983): A new dental wear pattern and evidence for high carbohydrate consumption in a Brazailian Archaic skeletal population. Am J Phys Anthropol 61:125-130.

Ubelaker DH (1980): "Human Bones and Archeology." Washington: US Dept of the Interior.

Van Couvering JAH, Stucky RK (1981): Comment. Curr Anthropol 22:266.

Van Der Merwe NJ, Vogel JC (1978): 13-C Content of human collagen as a measure of prehistoric diet in woodland North America. Nature 276:815-816.

Vrba ES (1975): Some evidence of chronology and paleoecology of Sterkfontein, Swartkrans and Kromdraai from the fossil Bovidae. Nature 254:301-304.

Vrba ES (1985): Ecological and adaptive changes associated with early hominid evolution. In Delson E (ed): "Ancestors: The Hard Evidence." New York: Alan R. Liss, Inc., pp 63-71.

Walker AC (1980): Functional anatomy and taphonomy. In Behrensmeyer AK, Hill AP (eds): "Fossils in the Making." Chicago: University of Chicago Press, pp 182-196.

Walker AC (1981): Dietary hypotheses and human evolution. Phil Trans R Soc Lond B292:57-64

Walker AC, Leakey REF (1978): The hominids of East Turkana. Sci Am 239:54-66.

Walker AC, Hoeck H, Perez L (1978): Microwear of mammalian teeth as an indicator of diet. Science 201:908-910.

Walker AC, Zimmerman MR, Leakey REF (1982): A possible case of hypervitaminosis A in *Homo erectus*. Nature 296:248-250.

Wallace JA (1973): Tooth chipping in the australopithecines. Nature 244:117-118.

Wallace JA (1975): Dietary adaptations of *Australopithecus* and early *Homo*. In Tuttle R (ed): "Paleoanthropology, Morphology and Paleoecology." The Hague: Mouton, pp 203-223.

Washburn SL, Lancaster CS (1968): The evolution of hunting. In Lee RB, De Vore I (eds): "Man the Hunter." Chicago: Aldine, pp 293-303.

Webster D (1981): Late pleistocene extinction and human predation: a critical overview. In Harding, RS, Teleki, G (eds): "Omnivorous Primates." New York: Columbia University Press, pp 556-594.

Whitehouse D, Whitehouse R (1975): "Archaeological Atlas of the World." London: Thames and Hudson Ltd.

Wing E, Brown A (1979): "Paleonutrition." New York: Academic Press.

Wolpoff MH (1971): Competitive exclusion among lower Pleistocene hominids: the single species hypothesis. Man 6:601-614.

Wolpoff MH (1973): Posterior tooth size, body size, and diet in South African gracile australopithecines. Am J Phys Anthropol 39:375-394.

Wolpoff MH (1974): The evidence for two australopithecine lineages in South Africa. Yrbk Phys Anthropol 17:113-139.

Wolpoff MH (1976): Primate models for australopithecine sexual dimorphism. Am J Phys Anthropol 45:497-510.

Wolpoff MH (1978): Some aspects of canine size in the australopithecines. J Hum Evol 7:115-126.

Wood BA (1985): Early *Homo* in Kenya, and its systematic relationships. n Delson E (ed): "Ancestors: The Hard Evidence." New York: Alan R. Liss, Inc., pp 206-214.

Wood BA, Stack CG (1980): Does allometry explain the differences between "gracile" and "robust" australopithecines? Am J Phys Anthropol 52:55-62.

Woodburne J (1968): An introduction to Hadza ecology. In Lee RB, DeVore I (eds): "Man the Hunter." Chicago: Aldine, pp 49-55.

Wu R, Lin S (1983): Peking Man. Sci Am 226(6):86-94.

Yengoyan AA (1968): Demographic and ecological influences on aboriginal Australian marriage sections. In Lee RB, De Vore I (eds): "Man the Hunter." Chicago: Aldine, pp 185-199.

Yudkin J (1969): Archaeology and the nutritionist. In Ucko PJ, Dimbleby GW (eds): "The Domestication and Exploitation of Plants and Animals." Chicago: Aldine, pp 547-552.

Nutritional Anthropology, pages 41-63
© 1987 Alan R. Liss, Inc.

Food and Bicultural Evolution:
A Model for the Investigation of Modern
Nutritional Problems

Solomon H. Katz

Krogman Growth Center, University of Pennsylvania, Philadelphia,
Pennsylvania 19103

INTRODUCTION

Contrary to the popular belief that current technology can solve the food problems of modern humanity, there is other evidence suggesting that new problems associated with food and nutrition are occurring [Brown and Wolf, 1985; Katz et al., 1985; Eaton and Konner, 1985]. Available solutions related to the economics of food production, storage, and distribution are not keeping up with the worldwide growth of human population. Besides the obvious and massive current famine in Africa, there are also less evident nutritional problems elsewhere. For example, the diets of infants of working mothers in urban environments, specific nutrient deficiencies in migrants to new countries, food sensitivities from the introduction of food sources from other regions, and the excessive consumption of high caloric foods [Ames, 1983] represent important nutritional challenges to various segments of populations that may otherwise appear as a whole to have few nutritional problems.

As a result of various problems with nutritional deficiencies and excesses, there is an increasing awareness throughout the world of the need for a more integrated approach to solving problems of food and nutrition in order to achieve an improved balance between our nutritional needs and food resources. This chapter attempts to address this problem by using a holistic anthropological approach to develop a framework with which we can begin to explore in depth some of the broad and specific as well as past and present constraints underlying patterns of human food consumption. The framework of such an anthropological approach involves both a concern with the processes underlying the evolution of our diet at the species level as well as an accounting for the diversity of the diets of human societies that currently populate the world.

EVOLUTIONARY MODELS OF NUTRITIONAL ADAPTATION
Diet and Evolution

The evolution of hominid capacity for culture-bearing, as currently conceptualized, involved a complex interplay among biology, behavior, and environment. In fact, a body of evidence suggests that the success of Homo sapiens had a great deal to do with how well humans exploited the dietary resources of their environments. For example, the proliferation of a tool-using culture complex appears related to the decrease in tooth size and masticatory apparatus [McKee, 1984]. Evidence from the comparative phylogeny of digestive systems of nonhuman primates suggests that, in humans, culturally mediated predigestive processing (cooking, etc.) of foods favored decreased elaboration of specialized digestive mechanisms required for the detoxification of certain foods. In nonhuman primates this problem was solved by symbiotic microorganisms resident within the lower gut [Parra, 1978]. The net effect of these changes implies a coevolution of the genetic factors underlying the expression of the structures and functions of the entire digestive system (including not only the teeth, jaws, and face, but also the entire gastroenteric system) with the universal cultural practices involved in the conversion of raw produce into cooked food. Thus when we study the human food chain of contemporary populations, we need to recognize that it represents the product of a series of highly diverse, complex, and continuing evolutionary processes unique to the various raw products that are found in the different environments in which human populations have evolved and are evolving.

Biocultural Adaptability and Evolution

The concept that biological evolution has been supplemented, complemented, and partially directed by a wide range of cultural adaptations is becoming more widely accepted. There appears to be a reciprocal feedback process between human biology and behavior in which biological needs, cultural responses, and environmental resources tend to reach a dynamic equilibrium over time. The latter concept of a dynamic equilibrium refers to the hypothesis that the information content of the two systems tends to remain in balance even though the quantity and specificity of the information at the biological and cultural levels shift from one point in time to another (Fig. 1). Elsewhere I have defined this process of change in information content as biocultural evolution [Katz, 1973].

The basis of the heuristic biocultural evolutionary approach underlying this paper is that in every human population there is a time-dependent dynamic equilibrium among ecological, sociocultural, human biological, and demographic variables. This scheme can also be conceptualized as a population's "genetic information pool" interacting with its "cultural information pool," which is made uniquely possible by the evolved capacities of the human brain (CNS). This model leads to hypotheses about mechanisms of transmission, storage, and change within the biological and sociocultural information pools, and particularly about their integration over time.

There are advantages in using this broad model of biocultural evolution for the interface between food and nutrition because: 1) the exploitation of the nutritional aspects of the ecosystem is probably the single most important

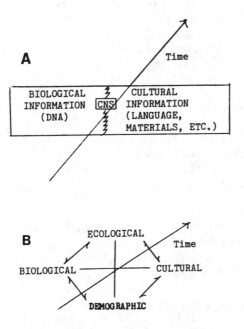

Fig. 1. Different ways in which the critical variables interact in the processes of biocultural evolution. 1A shows the evolution of the information content over time of the biological and cultural systems involving behavior and the neural substrates of the human brain (CNS/as critical). 1B shows the interaction of the different dimensions of a human population with plants they consume.

group of factors operating in the biocultural evolution of humanity; in the broadest sense the solution of food problems is necessary for the sustenance, reproduction, and growth of the population; 2) food consumption provides a clear interface between biological and cultural mechanisms of adaptation; 3) the biological effects of inappropriate and/or inadequate nutrients are becoming well enough understood so that finely tuned hypotheses about traditional food practices can be generated; 4) the range of variation in human foods is immense and, as well, the problems related to food are universal so that there are abundant archaeological and cross-cultural data available on their possible solutions; 5) there are measureable macro and micro outcomes to problems involving nutrition such as changes in population size, biology, technology, and culture; and 6) there is abundant evidence that subsistence changes from hunting and gathering economies to sedentary agricultural modes with the domestication of plants and animals which took place during the neolithic era represented the major change leading to the biocultural evolution of modern civilizations [Katz, 1982; Harlan et al, 1976; Harlan, 1985].

While this broad evolutionary model is useful, there are some obvious constraints upon the evolution of the implicit and explicit knowledge about foods and their consumption patterns within a society. Understanding the full significance of this knowledge could aid our understanding of food behaviors. We know that there is a biological component accounting for the "fit" between the food consumed and biological needs and/or processes. These needs can be divided into various categories of nutritional value, such as protein efficiency and related ratios, caloric content, trace elements, vitamins, etc. Obviously, this fit between food and nutritional value becomes more significant if the food is a staple for a particular population. There is also the ecological component associated with the relative abundance of the food and the ease with which it can be gathered or hunted, on the one hand, or cultivated and/or domesticated on the other. A wide range of environmental variables, such as rainfall, altitude, sunlight, and temperature, coupled with soil conditions, all play important roles.

Another component is the pharmacological properties of the food. Many edible plants contain highly active toxins, psychoactive drugs, and a wide variety of other compounds whose influence can supplement or even replace the full range of artificially synthesized drugs [Katz, 1982; Katz, 1979]. Clearly, the effects of psychoactive drugs synthesized and/or extracted from plants, such as alcohol and coca, take on exceptional qualities well beyond their nutritional value and must be taken into special consideration for their specific effects, e.g., their addictive properties. Related to the pharmacological variable is a genetic component which can limit the "fit" between populations of consumers and the metabolism and digestibility of the foods they eat. Often the natural constituents of foods may contain a factor(s) which may be specifically compatible or incompatible with the genetic constitutions of the individuals within the population [Simoons, 1969a; Simoons, 1969b; Menozzi et al., 1978].

Over the last 20 years a group of coworkers and I have attempted to integrate factors related to those mentioned above in order to build an empirically grounded conceptual framework that was based on important nutritional problems involving the human food chain (Fig. 2) in which biocultural evolutionary hypotheses could be assessed and tested [e.g., Katz and Foulks, 1970; Katz et al., 1974; Katz and Schall, 1979]. Much of our recent work has focused on foods from the major domesticated plants including, among others: maize, cereal grains, rice, bitter manioc, potatoes, fava beans, and soybeans, as well as various spices, garlic, and xanthine-based drinks. Several important principles have emerged from these studies that have direct bearing on the human food chain. Briefly, they are: 1) all of the major foods require transformations between the "raw and cooked" states before being finally consumed; 2) with the increasing dependence on the productivity of the major plants the importance of these transformations increases since most crops or plants have specific limitations in the availability of essential nutrients and/or toxic constituents; 3) the efficiency of the behavioral and biological adaptations controlling their transformations appear to have strong advantages, particularly with regard to minimizing loss of raw product, maximizing the efficiency of the energy consumed for transformation and optimizing the nutritient qualities of the food; 4) feedback relations involving biocultural adaptation and evolution can exist all the way up and down the human food chain from metabolism to production; 5) generally, cultural traditions in each step from production to cuisine are represented by slow rates of change over long time intervals in regions where the plant was first domesticated.

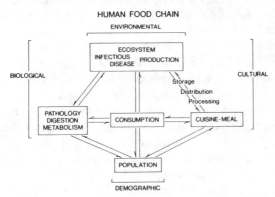

Fig. 2. Interactions and various steps of the human food chain from both biological and cultural perspectives.

SPECIFIC NUTRITIONAL ADAPTATIONS TO MAJOR CULTIGENS

We have been investigating this interface between human nutritional needs and the traditional cultural food practices that satisfy these nutrient needs of the individual and the population as a whole in order to demonstrate the ways in which this biocultural evolutionary framework can be used. Specifically, I have selected several principal examples from our analyses: maize, soybeans, fava beans, and manioc.

Maize

Maize was the staple crop providing the agroeconomic basis of the great Mesoamerican civilizations despite the fact that raw maize has serious nutritional limitations. However, it has been demonstrated that if maize is first treated with an alkali solution before consumption, the alkali liberates niacin from an undigestible complex and significantly improves the amino acid quality of the digestible protein fraction of the zein and germ [Katz et al., 1974; Katz et al., 1975]. Since the presence or absence of this alkali processing technique may therefore have provided an important limitation in the nutritional efficacy of maize diets, we attempted to determine the degree to which native American societies traditionally depended upon this technique in their consumption of maize. Specifically, we hypothesized that the use of alkali processing techniques would significantly increase the nutritional advantages to those native American societies that depended upon this food resource. In order to test this hypothesis we assessed both consumption and production among traditional native American populations that used alkali and those that did not, in the traditional preparation and processing of maize into specific foods. Figure 3 presents a histogram comparing the production and consumption data from those societies that did and did not use alkali. This sample was derived from cross-cultural data from a study over 50 native American societies in which we determined the relations among the use of alkali processing techniques and the degree of production and consumption of maize in areas where it was ecologically feasible for this kind of agriculture. The results of this study demonstrated a highly significant relationship between the degree of dietary and agricultural dependence on maize and the use of alkali processing. Figure 4 indicates the geographic distribution of alkali use.

These striking results allowed us to conclude that cuisine plays a highly significant role in optimizing of maize diets. They also emphasize the significance of this step in the food chain. In fact, it is possible to suggest that alkali treatment became the basis for optimizing the nutritional quality of maize, which became the major food supporting the growth of Mesoamerican civilization. More specifically, this food processing technique was almost certainly

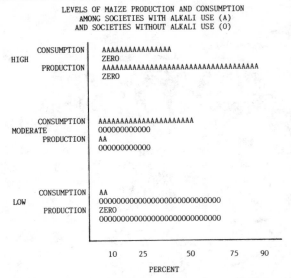

LEVELS OF MAIZE PRODUCTION AND CONSUMPTION
AMONG SOCIETIES WITH ALKALI USE (A)
AND SOCIETIES WITHOUT ALKALI USE (0)

Fig. 3. Relations between consumption and production of maize by Native American populations who traditionally use alkali processing and by those who do not use it for their preparation of maize. Adapted from Katz et al. [1974].

involved in facilitating the intensification of maize agriculture, which in turn led to substantial modifications in the organization and structure of Meso-American society [Katz et al, 1975]. Furthermore, these social modifications ultimately had effects on the demography and the ecology of the populations and hence even influenced their genetic composition. Thus, over many centuries there was an indirect link between the cultural processes underlying the development of this technology and the biological adaptability and evolution within these societies [Katz et al., 1974].

Soybeans in China

Although soybeans (glycine max) are probably the most important dietary legume in the world today, they contain a potent antitrypsin factor (ATF) which can produce serious gastric distress after consumption, reduced protein digestion, and chronic deficiencies in amino acid uptake [Rackis et al., 1962]. This ATF is not deactivated by ordinary cooking, yet evidence for the use and origin of soybeans in China extend back to the Neolithic [Chang, 1977]. By the mid 1940s western food scientists were already experimenting to optimize the nutritional quality of soybeans for human consumption. They found that grinding the beans, heating them to boil for a relatively short period of time (10-15 min vs. several h) followed by the use of a divalent cation, such as one found in a calcium or magnesium salt, to precipitate the nutritious protein,

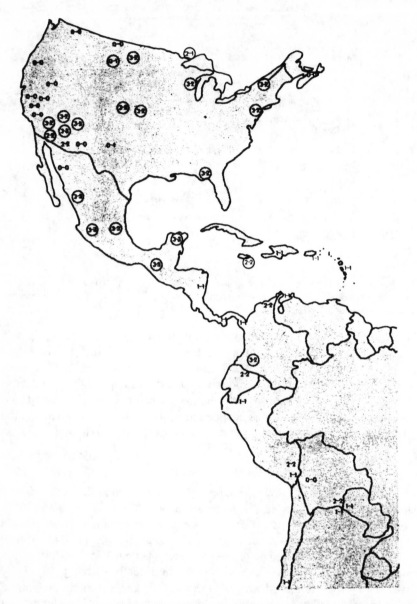

Fig. 4. Ratings given to each society for maize cultivation and consumption and the use of alkali for cooking corn. For each society, two numbers are shown. The first number indicates the rating for maize cultivation. The second number indicates the rating for maize consumption. Societies utilizing alkali processing techniques have circled numbers.

would leave the ATF in the supernatant [Morse, 1950]. The curd thus produced was a completely digestible high quality protein that, if consumed with rice which has ample quantities of methionine, provided a well-balanced diet.

Given these basic facts on the nutritional qualities of soybean and, particularly, ATF, we conducted a survey of all food data on 60 societies from Southeast Asia, Asia, and the Pacific listed in the Human Resources Area Files (HRAF) as well as expanding this source with data from all nutritional sources that we could locate to determine the degree to which traditional processing of soybeans deactivated the ATF and followed the optimal procedure for precipitating the protein outlined above. Finally, if deactivation of ATF was achieved and optimal procedures were practiced, we would attempt to document how these culinary practices evolved [Katz and Ricci, 1978].

First, in testing the initial hypothesis, we found a one-to-one relationship between traditional practices that deactivate the ATF and the tradiational use of soybeans by those populations as a human food resource. Secondly, we found that not all recipes followed the optimum procedure (Fig. 5). Nevertheless, approximately 90% of the processed soybeans consumed in Asia today are eaten as a calcium and/or magnesium curd. This led us into an examination of the third question about the evolution of these transformations.

In this case we were fortunate in being able to consult the extensive documentation within Chinese history to help sort out the sequence leading to the efficient deactivation of soybean ATF. Basically, we found evidence that roasting was first practiced in Neolithic times and that the earliest written mention of them was in the *Materia Medica* (2838 BC) in which they were prescribed as a medicine. The next clear evidence for the deactivation of ATF

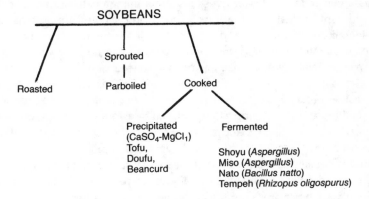

Fig. 5. This flow chart shows the different approaches to cuisine employed traditionally by Asian societies to deactivate the antitrypsin factor in soybeans.

was using fermentation, practiced as early as the Chou Dynasty (1134–246 BC), when the beans were apparently first designated as the fifth sacred grain along with barley, wheat, millet, and rice. However, it was not until the later Han dynasty that the bean curd processing techniques were first mentioned. Initially it was striking to find that the bean became designated as sacred before an efficient technique evolved to extract its high-quality proteins. However, an analysis of the ancient Chinese characters in use in the Chou Dynasty yielded a potential clue to this discrepancy. In each case the pictograph for the sacred cereal grains clearly stresses the seed and stem structure of the plant, whereas in the case of soybeans it is the root structure, particularly the part that deals with the nitrogen-fixing bacterial nodules on the roots. Also, the most detailed mention of soybeans is in the agricultural literature of this period (soybeans and millet rotation was widely practiced in the fifth to the third century BC; [Chang, 1978]). This is significant because Chinese agriculture was already known to be strained by a lack of sufficient nitrogen-based fertilizer [Ho, 1975]. Hence, our investigation supports the hypothesis that the spread of soybeans was initially more closely related to the agricultural end of the food chain until optimum methods for extracting their proteins evolved, whereupon soybeans in combination with rice evolved into the major source of protein in the diets of most Asian populations. Thus, in this case, the relationship between consumption and production on the food chain was reversed apparently due to the so-called "green manure" effect of soybeans.

These remarkable sequences raise other new questions about this biocultural evolutionary process as it pertains to human subsistence. Most importantly, they suggest that an examination of the entire human food chain is necessary in order to answer questions about human behavior and food. It is not sufficient to deal with the topic of food production without relating it to considerations of nutrition and vice versa. Under traditional circumstances, there are many intervening steps and processes that have evolved over time and play crucial roles in maintaining a balanced equilibrium between the biological needs and the cultural prescriptions for their fulfillment. For example, realizing that soybeans are highly limited as a source of food because of their antitrypsin factor is important, but that does not completely account for their early use in China. Likewise, to generalize on the specific limitations of maize without taking into account the nutritional complementarity that exists when it is consumed with lysine-rich beans, or similarly, the consumption of methionine-deficient soybean curd without reference to the consumption of methionine-rich rice limits our understanding of the traditionally role of cuisine in the regulation of the balance of dietary nutrients. Hence, on the basis of these and other data, we have concluded that over the past 10,000 years those populations that became increasingly dependent on an agricultural subsistence pattern developed a series of biocultural evolutionary equilibria with plant foods. These equilibria probably became stabilized along each step of the human food chain spanning transformations from alterations of the environment to cuisines and from patterns of consumptions to the genes controlling enzymatic pathways in the metabolism of the food (Fig. 2).

An examination of these food preparation methods for maize and soybeans offers considerable insight into the evolution of cultural practices linked to the supply of essential nutrients. However, the connection between those cultural practices surrounding food preparation and their direct effects on any specific changes in the genetic composition of the population and, hence, its biological evolution is not amenable to further quantitative analyses. To take this biocultural evolutionary approach further, we have been attempting to develop models and hypotheses about how food practices influence specific genetic characteristics. Accordingly, this paper considers and extends our work [Katz and Schall, 1979; Mihalik and Katz, unpublished manuscript] on the interrelations among cultural factors underlying the continued consumption of fava beans in the circum-Mediterranean region, where they produce a severe and often deadly hemolytic anemia, and bitter manioc consumption as a possible ecogenetic factor in the evolution of resistance to malaria. Since the genetic condition underlying favism is already documented, the test cases presented in this chapter allow for the development of more comprehensive heuristic models to evaluate quantitatively the coevolutionary interactions between biologically based genetic adaptation and traditional cultural practices.

Fava Beans, G-6PD Deficiency, and Malaria

The use of fava beans as a major source of food in the circum-Mediterranean region can be traced archaeologically all the way back to Neolithic times. However, it is well documented that fava bean consumption is particularly toxic to G-6PD- (glucose-6-phosphate dehydrogenase)-deficient individuals. Given their toxicity it is paradoxical that fava beans continued to form a major part of the diet throughout this region. The ethnographic history and folklore concerning their consumption reveal very strong prescriptive and proscriptive behavior. In fact, Andrews (1949) has reported that the folklore surrounding their use and consumption is the most extensive of any food in Indo-European history. However, in a geographic survey conducted much like that for maize, we found an unusual overlap, depicted on Figure 6, between fava bean consumption, the occurrence of malaria, and the gene for G-6PD deficiency [Katz and Schall, 1979]. The latter is an X-linked genetic trait that renders the red blood cells of the hemizygous males and homozygous-deficient females

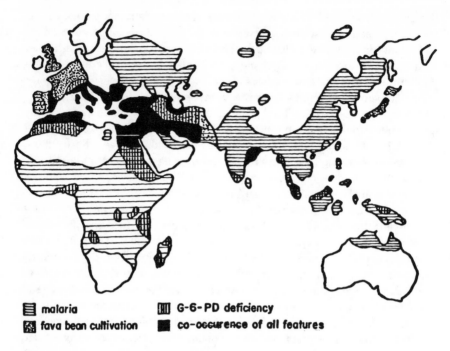

☰ malaria   ▥ G-6-PD deficiency

▩ fava bean cultivation   ■ co-occurence of all features

Fig. 6. This map shows the overlapping and non-overlapping distributions of glucose-6-phospate dehydrogenase (G-6PD) deficiency with malaria and fava bean consumption throughout the Eurasian, African, and Australian continents.

highly sensitive to the powerful hemolytic effects of the strong oxidant compounds found in the beans. When consumed by these highly sensitive individuals, the beans lead to a rapid toxic episode resulting in very serious illness or death [Katz and Schall, 1986].

While it was known that frequency of the G-6PD-deficient gene was closely and positively associated with the occurrence of malaria, it was not recognized that the geographic occurrence of fava bean consumption matched in many regions of the world the occurrence of many of the more severe forms of G-6PD deficiency and the occurrence of malaria. Generally, it was accepted that the gene, through some unknown mechanism, was associated with resistance to this very important disease. Finally, it was also known that the ingestion of antimalarial drugs by these G-6PD-deficient individuals also produced a profound hemolytic anemia which was just like that produced by the consumption of fava beans [Katz, 1979]. This and other data we developed in our laboratory led us to hypothesize that by the consumption of fava beans heterozygous females, who were carriers of the gene but not sensitive to the toxic effects of the bean, were rendered more resistant to malaria via the pharmacological constituents of the beans. After presenting our hypothesis to the Center for Tropical Diseases in Jerusalem, Golenser et al. [1983] conducted experiments in in vitro cultures of malaria-infected normal and G-6PD-deficient erythrocytes and demonstrated that with the addition of isouramil (one of the strong oxidant compounds present in fava beans), there was a significant decrease in malarial parasitic growth rates in the G-6PD-deficient as opposed to the normal control cells. Moreover, in parasitized erythrocytes, the addition of isouramil also had direct antimalarial effects in both normal and G-6PD-deficient cells during two of the stages of parasitic development.

Although it is important to point out that these data only confirm the role in vitro and not in vivo that these strong oxidant constituents of the beans play in altering the advantages of both G-6PD-deficient and normal cells, the in vitro system is very well understood and it is very likely that this evidence will be confirmed in vivo. Overall, we suggested [Katz and Schall, 1979] that although normal individuals also benefitted from fava bean consumption, selection favored the G-6PD-deficient gene in the heterozygous females. Hence, a balance was established between the gene for deficiency and the continued use of a bean that was, on the one hand, deadly and, on the other, lifesaving. In this case, a food influences metabolic pathways to enhance the resistance to one disease, i.e., malaria, while increasing the risk of another, favism, which is likely to be associated with many of the prescriptive and proscriptive behaviors recorded throughout Indo-European history. From the biocultural evolutionary perspective this suggested for the first time that the cultural support mechanisms for the continued consumption and selective avoidance of the beans were intricately involved in the biological evolution of a gene that is implicated in one of the most common genetic disorders in the world [Katz, 1986].

Bitter Manioc

The biological findings on the relations of genetics, food, pharmacology, and disease led to an investigation of bitter manioc, another food with potent pharmacological effects. This extraordinarily productive and hearty root crop (*Manihot esculenta*) contains cyanate, which is bound to glycosides distributed throughout the tuber pulp. Any physical damage to bitter manioc releases a potent glycosidase which immediately acts to free small amounts of cyanide (HCN). Hence bruising the pulp and squeezing it releases glycosidases, which in turn break the glycosidic bonds. This process frees the HCN, and cooking the juice and pulp volatilizes the HCN into the air. In the event the bitter manioc is consumed without first squeezing and subsequently cooking the root, the probability of deadly toxic effects remains very high [Mihalik and Katz, unpublished manuscript]. In experiments with the traditional South American Indian (Amerindian) preparation, cassareep (a pepperpot-like stew), we found most of the cyanate was liberated. However, a significant but not toxic quantity remained in the glycosidic form. In our experiments, we found that the sodium cyanide levels averaged 235 mg/100 g of cassareep. During digestion this HCN is slowly liberated and the cyanate fraction presumably is absorbed by the body.

It has been demonstrated that the cyanate (CN−) carbamylates hemoglobin S (HbS) in sickle cell anemia (SSA) and acts as an antisickling agent (Cerami, 1974). The consumption of bitter manioc may be associated with sufficient intake of cyanate to ameliorate the effects of SSA crises. For example, Cerami (1974) reports that 10–35 mg/kg body weight/day was sufficient to achieve an antisickling effect, with the lower dose as the most effective in terms of minimum neurologic side effects. Hence, a 100 g portion of cassareep consumed over an entire day would provide sufficient cyanate to treat effectively a 10–12 kg child with SSA. However, this theoretical estimate needs to be confirmed under normal field conditions, since it assumes that all of the estimated dose of cyanate is taken up during digestion.

Another intriguing aspect of bitter manioc consumption is that cyanate inhibits erythrocyte G-6PD activity [Glader and Conrad, 1972]. Jackson et al. [1986], in tests to determine the antisickling effects of the traditional Liberian recipe for bitter manioc, fed it to normal pigs and demonstrated that G-6PD activity was inhibited. Also Glader and Conrad [1972] demonstrated in in vitro experiments that G-6PD activity was inhibited in human erythrocytes at the same levels that we found would theoretically be present in the experiments with the cassareep. Since the inhibition of G-6PD activity would lead to an increased fragility of erythrocytes infected with malaria (due to their inability to withstand the high levels of malarial parasite-produced oxidants), it is possible that the quantity of cyanate from bitter manioc consumption is sufficient to potentiate an antimalarial effect on the African type of G-6PD deficiency variant. This hypothesis is very analogous to the effect that fava oxidants have on the Mediterranean type of G-6PD deficiency. Hence, the presence of cyanate-like fava bean consumption elsewhere may have a direct effect on the evolution of the G-6PD gene in West African populations by protecting the deficient individuals from malarial infection.

Further laboratory, clinical, and epidemiological studies need to be conducted in vitro and in vivo to confirm these two genetic hypotheses. It is possible that one or both effects occur, i.e., protection against life-threatening SSA crises and enhancement of the G-6PD-deficient resistance to malaria.

However, at this stage it is nevertheless striking to note the rapid rate at which, over the last 400 years, this crops has spread throughout sub-Saharan Africa in a broad band that is similar to the distribution of SSA, G-6PD deficiency, and malaria [Mihalik and Katz, unpublished manuscript]. It is entirely possible that if this food lowered mortality rates due to SSA crises, then it follows that the very rapid rise in the postulated gene frequency of HbS in Africa may in part be due to the enhanced selective advantage of recessive SSA provided by this food mechanism. In addition, it is also possible that the consumption of bitter manioc has separately enhanced the frequency of the African G-6PD gene by potentiating the oxidant senstivity of the malarial parasitized erythrocyte leading to their early sequestration and destruction by the spleen, thus interrupting the parasitic life cycle and thereby decreasing the effects of the disease.

Biocultural Evolution and Cuisine

Adding these "ecogenetic" cases to other examples of foods currently under investigation, such as the highly adaptive role of yeast in brewing and breadmaking [Katz and Brown, 1982] or the significance of spices and herbs as antioxidants and pharmacologically active agents [Katz, 1982], it becomes increasingly apparent that most human foods fit into some culturally evolved pattern where there are multiple interactions among various aspects of the ecosystem, the cultural means of exploitation, and the genetic constitutions of the individual consumers [Simons, 1983].

These genetic and physiological factors play roles in varying proportions in the development and evolution of cultural "knowledge" concerning the processes of preparation of food from the raw state to a "cooked" state. The actual degree to which these biological factors do play a role leads to several questions about the "fit" between biological and cultural factors: 1) How close is the fit between how knowlege or information accumulates in traditional societies over time and what we now know from scientific evidence about optimal patterns of preparation and consumption from the point of view of the biological dimensions discussed above? For example, to what degree are culturally prescribed food combinations during the same meal or time period nutritionally compatible with one another? 2) What are the principles by which societies invent, maintain, and distribute this knowledge of foods? 3) To what degree is this knowledge about foods linked to other food-related and -unrelated practices within society and to what extent does it provide an adaptive basis for integrating other aspects of traditional practices, beliefs, myths, and symbols within a society? 4) What are the conditions under which the probabilities favor experimentation and/or nonadaptive preparations in the use of foods, whether traditional or nontraditional? 5) What is the nutritional significance of the technologies underlying the various processing traditions such as heating, fermentation (yeasts, molds, bacteria, etc.), soaking, sprouting, peeling, drying, mashing, spicing, and combinations with other foods and chemicals associated with the transformation of raw produce into foods? 6) What governs the degree of explicit versus implicit knowledge a society might accrue about specific foods or food in general?

While answers to these and other questions could provide the basis for more cogent theoretical developments on the relation of food and biocultural evolution, they could also have a more immediate impact upon our specific understanding of human food behavior throughout the contemporary world. At a theoretical level we must also begin to conceive of the evolutionary feedback relations between and among the various elements of the entire human food chain for any particular population. One conceptualization of the important variables and their relations is presented on Figure 2. As our knowledge about any particular food source increases we can use this kind of heuristic model as a potential resource for formulating additional questions not covered above. The remainder of this paper addresses issues that exemplify the utility of this approach toward examining the interface between biological evolution and adaptation and cultural beliefs and practices that shape human food behaviors in modern scientists and underlie the development of various pathological and nonpathological conditions.

The "Lock and Key" Hypothesis

It is evident that, although the process of domestication brought about considerable increases in plant productivity [Harlon et al., 1976], it had a much smaller influence on the degree to which the plants retained various toxic and antinutritive defenses against insect and animal predation. Although it was possible to selectively breed plants with lowered levels of toxin to make them more attractive for human consumption, the cultigens would have been left vulnerable to predation by a wide range of organisms. Instead, what appears to have evolved is the cultural knowledge on how to exploit the plant nutrients either by removing the offending compound(s) or by detoxifying them through some other reaction and/or combination with another food. For example, plant seeds contain a variety of important nutrients, but they have evolved various defense mechanisms. Harborne [1982] classifies three types of predatory protection: lectins, protease inhibitors, and alkaloids. In their raw form these toxicants can be lethal, but heating and other preparatory techniques can denature lectins and protease inhibitors and increase the solubility of alkaloids which can then be washed out. Similarly, phytates and oxalates from cereal grains and tuber crops which bind important minerals and limit their bio-availability can be deactivated by processes of fermentation, such as those used in brewing and breadmaking [Katz and Brown, 1982]. Obviously, such knowledge was not accessible to other organisms and therefore human populations who retained this knowledge at a cultural level were able to transform and occupy an important econiche successfully and thus displace other species which depended mostly on the slower process of genetic adaptation to the various toxic and antinutritive qualities of these plants.

In human societies, this knowledge was stored in the form of culturally specific beliefs and practices about food and cuisine which were transferred from one generation to the next. However, like most culturally specific behaviors these food-related behaviors were inextricably woven into the language, religion, rituals, myths, symbolism, and history of the population. One means of conceptualizing this important problem is to conceive of the "raw and cooked" relationship as a "lock and key" relationship. On the one hand, the antinutritive and toxic constituents naturally present to defend against predation were kept "locked" into the plants' cultigens even though they were increasingly domesticated in the direction of higher productivity. On the other hand, the cultural knowledge, which rapidly evolved within the constraints of the biocultural evolutionary process, became the "key" to unlock the full nutritional potential of the foods. Since this knowledge about food processing is tightly integrated into the language and rituals of cuisine, we hypothesized that such knowledge is much less likely to be transferred cross-culturally than the agricultural technology and seeds for cultivating the plants.

If this "lock and key" concept is correct, it would have highly significant implications for the spread of domesticated plants around the world. Introduction of new, highly productive crops to different areas of the world could not bring about effective consumption until the appropriate information was transferred from where the crop first evolved. In extreme cases where there were genetic adaptations present, consumption of these cultigens without "key" information could potentially produce serious pathologies. Considering the complexity and the number of new plants introduced throughout the world in modern times, the potential for establishing a new equilibrium between the qualities of the newly introduced plants and the cuisine that must be evolved to exploit them may be substantially more complicated than if only one food were introduced. There are obvious benefits to the introduction of new domesticates such as the potential for new sources of calories. For example, after remaining constant for approximately 1,000 years, the population of China doubled in size within 150 years after the introduction of the potato, which allowed occupation of a previously underexploited econiche in the mountains [Ho, 1959]. In one sense there also may be benefits but they are often limited depending on the degree of dependence of a population on the new food.

Tests of The "Lock and Key" Hypothesis

It is evident that the "lock and key" concept would be particularly applicable to the time of the great voyages when there was little cultural congruity between the American Native and the European explorer. This would suggest that the "key" cultural knowledge about cuisine would be unlikely to be transferred effectively from the American Natives to the European explorers. Alternatively, knowledge about the agricultural technology was much more evident in that the rules governing planting were already understood by the Europeans and, since the transfer also involved seeds and/or roots, these were easily planted and experimented upon once the explorers returned to Europe. In order to test hypotheses derived from this "lock and key" concept, we attempted to use the knowledge we have developed on maize and alkali processing as a test case of the concept. Two questions were considered: first, was the alkali processing technique practiced all through Meso-America ever transferred back to Europe by the early explorers and secondly, if not, did it ever evolve in those societies that adopted the use of maize as an important source of nutrition? To test this hypothesis and answer these questions we used historical records, anthropological field notes, agricultural survey data, and various nutritional data bases that listed the occurrence of pellegra and various forms of malnutrition [Katz and Wolfe, 1978].

Briefly, we found clear historic evidence for the transfer of the seeds of maize by Columbus and its quick adoption in Spain as a highly productive crop but no mention of it in any context with alkali processing [Miracle, 1966]. However, there is evidence that pellegra soon developed following its use and before many years passed maize was abandoned as a major source of human nutrition and relegated to feeds for farm animals [Roe, 1977]. Next, we traced its introduction to Africa by European traders where it became an indigenous crop of some considerable significance up to the present. In a survey based upon the HRAF, and all other ethnographic data we could locate on food in more than 50 African societies that reported the use of maize over the last 50 years, no evidence emerged that it was ever treated with alkali. However, what did emerge was that maize was used, like sorghums, in brewing and although it is probably not as efficient as alkali processing, brewing does result in the growth of yeasts that have considerably better balances of amino acids and niacin, which would have been unavailable without the alkali treatment of maize. Thus, alkali processing was not transferred and nothing as efficient evolved to take its place. This is reflected by the fact that in the last decade the incidence of pellegra in Africa is highly correlated (Spearman's rho = 0.70) with the degree of consumption of maize on a country-to-country basis, irrespective of the degree to which brewing was practiced [Katz and Wolfe, 1978]. These results strongly support the lock and key hypothesis, but the question remains as to whether this result applies to other modern food practices.

Although it is beyond the scope of this paper to develop each of the examples that follow, it is evident that there are a number of important examples of disequilibria of the human food chain involving many, if not all, populations of the world participating in the modern food and agricultural economy. The balance between modern economic factors influencing food consumption and the traditional equilibrium represented by the food chain diagram presented earlier (Fig. 2), suggests that in modern times the equilibrium is shifting very quickly. In one sense, the incidence of nutritionally based diseases is a good indicator of how far out of balance the equilibrium has shifted. For example, the use of new means to alter various aspects of the food chain are associated with a number of practices which have implications for the occurrence of chronic disease. Specifically, a wide range of chemicals, introduced in foods to assure greater storage life, and insecticides, introduced to control insect predation of plant species that have had some of their protective qualities removed by selective breeding, have all been implicated in producing increased rates of cancer.

Perhaps the greatest changes in cultigens have been in the selection and introduction of new variants of plants which fit the needs of various environmental and perceived nutritional needs of indigenous populations. In some cases, however, the new cultigen does not fit the taste and/or other properties of the local cuisine as well as they fit nutritional needs of the consumers. For example, floury type high-lysine maize is known to have been rejected as inedible by the consumers to whom it was shipped and was left to rot in the local warehouses of some Latin American countries whose people are used to consuming a different type of tortilla than that which can be made with this variety of maize. In another current case, wheat is being introduced to Bangladesh which has never before consumed large quantities. Traditionally the people of this region have been rice farmers and with the introduction of a new crop, there is the risk that coeliac disease [Simoons, 1969a,b] which is associated with the gluten protein fraction of wheat, will increase significantly. Since it is known that gluten sensitivity increases diarrheal diseases and that the HLA-8 antigen, which is associated with gluten sensitivity, is present in high concentrations in Pakistan [Simoons, 1983], where the population's genetic composition is thought to be closely related to that of the population of Bangladesh, it is possible that elevated rates of gluten sensitivity will be diagnosed as gastroenteric infections, which are common in the area, and not as a gluten sensitivity. In other areas new crops such as the peanut (ground-nut) are being introduced as effective new crops without sufficient attention being paid to the fact that the peanut can develop, upon prolonged contact with the soil around the plant, one of the most potent aflotoxins known. Since aflotoxins of the kind that develop on the peanut are already associated with increases in liver cancer in African populations, it is likely that similar problems will develop in those areas of New Guinea where the crop has been introduced.

In summary, the processes of equilibration following the introduction of new plant foods may be particularly important in understanding the source of some of the major nutritional problems confronting the world today. Returning to the "lock and key" hypothesis helps clarify this issue further. When new plants were introduced, the evolution of the cultural "key" for exploiting the plant optimally did not occur immediately. Instead there was a period of equilibration of the indigenous human food chain to the new source of nutrition. While the evolution of the cultural "key" is usually much more rapid than the evolution of genetic mechanisms to optimally extract the nutritional quality of the food, cultural change in the realm of cuisine is often much less rapid than change in other areas of cultural identity. It appears that since cuisine is such an important source of cultural identity, it is very resistant to change. Thus, it is reasonable to assume that the complex problems that developed with the use of new foods throughout the world in the past still continue to provide serious problems of malnutrition throughout the world today.

This concept of disequilibrium of the food chain becomes clearer if we review the history of food over the last 500 years on a worldwide basis. Four phenomena are evident: 1) beginning with the great voyages from Europe involving Spain, Portugal, and England, food discovered in use in the Americas were spread throughout the various trade routes and were cultivated in a variety of new environments; 2) population size grew quickly in response to new sources of calories and other essential nutrients; 3) most often the large domesticated varieties spread quickly, but the highly evolved techniques for preparing the foods did not and most plant foods were treated like other similar cultigens raised in the particular habitat; and 4) a variety of nutritional problems developed in response to these less than optimal adaptations of cuisine. Taking the "lock and key" hypothesis one step further suggests that the cultural discoveries about food exploitation also take considerable time to become integrated into the cuisine of the population and that the degree of disequilibrium can be measured in terms of the degree and types of malnutrition expressed.

CONCLUSION

In conclusion, this chapter has attempted to develop the basis for demonstrating the association between consumption of major plant cultigens and their effects on the health of past and present populations. If we look more broadly at the evolutionary perspective several relevant conclusions can be reached. First, the human digestive system has gradually evolved to become dependent on the extradigestive processes provided by our cultures. In turn, there has been a biocultural evolutionary process which involves the elaboration of a human food chain that incorporates cuisine into most aspects of human existence. The result is a complex process whereby knowledge about how to extract the optimal nutrients from foods becomes a vital part of the survival of human populations once plants become domesticated. This is because plants frequently have toxic and other antinutritive properties that must be removed before consumption. With the advent of agriculture there is an increased dependence on fewer plants and, therefore, the knowledge about optimal extraction and combination with other foods becomes more highly selected. The result is the development of major cuisines with elaborately evolved rules which help to optimize various aspects of the food chain. However, in modern times the spread of new foods, new processing techniques, and new crops has shifted the traditional food chain systems out of equilibrium and the result is poor distribution and economic policies leading to massive deficiencies of calories and nutrients which influence the poor and rich populations alike, due to either a lack, an excess, or an imbalance of the foods consumed. Finally it is evident that although the kinds of approaches currently advocated in nutritional and agricultural policies are necessary, they are not sufficient to solve the health problems associated with food. What is needed also is a comprehensive analysis of the biocultural evolution of human cuisine so that data on individual societies can be modeled, in order to understand ways of reestablishing the equilibria present in the traditional food chain in a society as it undergoes the rapid changes of modern times.

REFERENCES

Ames BN (1983): Dietary carcinogens and anti-carcinogens. Science 221:256-263.
Andrews AC (1949): The bean and Indo-European totemism. Am Anthropol 51:274-292.

Brown LR, Wolf EC (1985): "Reversing Africa's Decline." Worldwatch Paper 65. Washington D.C.: Watchworld Institute.

Cerami A (1974): Review of the development of cyanate as a drug in the treatment of sickle cell anemia. Ann NY Acad Sci 241:538-544.

Chang KC (1977): "Food in Chinese Culture." New Haven: Yale University Press.

Chang TI (1978): The Origin and Early Cultures of the Cereal Grains and Food Legumes, Presented at the Origins of Chinese Civilization Conference, Berkeley.

Eaton SB, Konner M (1985): Paleolithic nutrition: A consideration of its nature and current implications. New Engl J Med 312(5):283-289.

Glader BE, Conrad ME (1972): Cyanate inhibition of erythrocyte G-6pd. Nature 237:336-337.

Golenser JJ, Miller JJ, Spiro DT, Novak T, Chevion M (1983): Inhibitory effect of a fava component on the in vitro development of Plasmodium falciparum in normal and G-6PD deficient erythrocytes. Blood 618(3):507-510.

Harborne G (1982): "Introduction of Ecological Biochemistry." New York: Academic Press.

Harlan JR, de Wet JMJ, Stemler ABL (eds) (1976): "Origins of Agriculture." The Hague: Mouton.

Harlan JR (1985): Indigenous African Agriculture in The Origins of Plant Cultivation in World Perspective. Symp Am Assoc Adv Sci, Los Angeles, May 1985.

Ho PT (1959): Studies on the population of China. Plant Sci Bull, p 59.

Ho PT (1975): "The Cradle of the East." Hong Kong: Chinese University of Hong Kong and the University of Chicago Press.

Jackson LC (1986): Dietary Cassava, Sickle Hemoglobin Fitness, and Falciparum Malaria in Liberia. Hum Biol (in press).

Jackson LC, Chandler JP, Jackson RT (1986): Inhibition and adaptation of Red Cell Glucose-6-Phosphate Dehydrogenase (G-6PD) in vivo to chronic sublethal dietary cyanide in an animal model. Hum Biol 58(1):67-77.

Katz SH, Foulks EF (1970): Calcium homeostatis and behavioral disorders. In Katz SH (ed): Symposium on Human Adaptation. Am J Phys Anthropol 32:225-316. Also republished in Y Cohen (ed): "Man in Adaptation." Chicago: Aldin Press, 1972.

Katz SH (1973): Evolutionary Perspective on Purpose and Man. Symposium on Human Purpose. Zygon 8:325-340.

Katz SH, Hediger M, Valleroy L (1974): Traditional maize processing techniques in the New World: Anthropological and nutritional significance. Science 184:765-773.

Katz SH, Hediger M, Valleroy L (1975): The anthropological and nutritional significance of traditional maize processing techniques in the New World. In Watts E, Lasker B, Johnston F (eds): "Biosocial Interrelations in Population Adaptation." The Hague: Mouton, pp 195-234.

Katz SH, Ricci JA (1978): Traditional Soybean Processing. Presented at the Intl Union of Anthropol and Ethnol Sci, New Delhi.

Katz SH, Wolfe A (1978): Maize in Africa. Presented at the Intl Union of Anthropol and Ethnol Sci, New Delhi.

Katz SH (1979): Un exemple d'evolution bioculturelle: la feve. In Fischler C (ed): "Pour une anthropologie biocultural de l'alimentation." (Fava Bean Consumption and Human Evolution) Social Communications (Paris) 31:53-69. Republished in Italian (1981): "Atti Alimentari E Atticulinari." Bologna: Documentzione Scientifica Editrice, pp 51-64.

Katz SH, Schall JI (1979): Fava bean consumption and biocultural evolution. Med Anthropol 4:459-477.

Katz S (1982): Food, behavior, and biocultural evolution. In Barker W (ed): "Nutrition and Behavior." Hartford, Connecticut: Avi Press, pp 171-188.

Katz SH, Brown S (1982): Beer and bread: An evolutionary perspective on cuisine. In Am Assoc Adv of Sci Symp on Religion and Food, Toronto.

Katz SH, Hediger ML, Zemel BS, Parks JS (1985): Adrenal androgens, body fat, and advanced skeletal age in puberty: new evidence for the relations of adrenarche and gonadarche in males. Hum Biol 57(3):401-413.

Katz SH (1986): Favism and malaria: A test case of biocultural evolution. In Harris M (ed): "Food Preferences and Aversions." Philadelphia: Temple University Press (in press).

Katz SH, Schall J (1986): Favism and Malaria: A Model of Nutrition and Biocultural Evolution. In Etkin N (ed): "Plants in Indigenous Medicine and Diet: Biobehavioral Approaches." Bedford Hills, N.Y. Bedford Hills, N.Y. Redgrave Press, pp 211-228.

McKee JK (1984): A genetic model of dental reduction through the probable mutation effect. Amer J Phys Anthropol 65:231-241.

Menozzi P, Piazza A, Cavalli-Sforza L (1978): Synthetic maps of human gene frequencies in Europeans. Science 201:786-792.

Mihalik G, Katz SH (nd): Cyanate content of cassareep: health implications. Unpublished manuscript.

Miracle MP (1966): "Maize in Tropical Africa." Madison: University of Wisconsin Press, pp 101-131.

Morse WJ (1950): History of soybean production. In Mackley et al. (eds): "The Definitive Soybean and Soybean Products." I:3-59.

Parra R (1978): Comparison of foregut and hindgut fermentation in herbivores. In Montgomery GC (ed): "Aboreal Folivares." Washington D.C.: Smithsonian Institute Press, pp 205-229.

Rackis JJ, Sasame HA, Mann RK, Anderson RL, Smith AK (1962): Soybean trysin inhibitors: Isolation, purification and physical properties. Arch Biochem Biophys 98:471-478.

Roe A (1977): "A Plague of Corn." New York: Harper.

Simoons FJ (1969a): Primary adult lactose intolerance and the milking habit: A problem in biological and cultural interrelationships. I. Review of the Medical Research. Am J Digest Dis 14:819-836.

Simoons FJ (1969b): Primary adult lactose intolerance and the milking habit: A problem in biological and cultural interrelationships. II. A culture history hypothesis. Am J Digest Dis 15:695-710.

Simoons FJ (1983): Geography and genetics as factors in the psychobiology of human food selection. In W Barker (ed): "Nutrition and Behavior." Hartford, Conn: Avi Press, pp 205-224.

SECTION II:
METHODOLOGICAL CONCERNS IN NUTRITIONAL ANTHROPOLOGY

Nutritional Anthropology, pages 67-84
© 1987 Alan R. Liss, Inc.

Methods for Determining Dietary Intake

Sara A. Quandt, PhD

Department of Anthropology, University of Kentucky,
Lexington, Kentucky 40506-0024

INTRODUCTION

Anthropologists use dietary intake data in a wide variety of research contexts. In general, cultural anthropologists employ it as a dependent variable in associations with economic and social factors, while biological anthropologists use dietary data as a complement to or approximation of nutritional status and as the independent variable in epidemiological investigations of health and disease. The purpose of this chapter is to examine currently available techniques for documenting dietary intake of humans in terms of their applicability to such issues in anthropological research. Those techniques which allow extrapolation from food to nutrient intake for individuals will be emphasized. After reviewing the strengths and weaknesses of various dietary assessment methods, recent developments in assessing and improving validity and reliability will be presented. Finally, the need for tailoring existing methods and research designs to the specific research needs and conditions of anthropologists will be discussed.

FACTORS GUIDING THE CHOICE OF DIETARY ASSESSMENT METHODS

There is no single *ideal* method for gathering dietary intake data. The ideal for any particular study will be dependent on the objectives of that study. Thus, research objectives must be clearly articulated before appropriate techniques for gathering, analyzing, and interpreting dietary data can be chosen

[Young and Trulson, 1960]. An overall consideration in all research is that the more detailed the desired data, the more expensive, time consuming, and subject to error the method required. The corollary of this is that "there is no merit in using a more elaborate or expensive method than is necessary to obtain the data needed to meet the defined objective of the study" [Young, 1981].

The major consideration dictating the choice of method is the specific kind of dietary knowledge needed. Is the research intended, for example, to document consumption of "foods" or intake of "nutrients"? If the former, the method must take into account these aspects of the specific foodway of the study population: 1) variability in food intake (day-to-day, seasonal, etc.); 2) differences in food consumption by sex, ethnicity, and age; and 3) differences between the informants and the interviewer in boundaries of the universe of "legitimate foods." If concern is with nutrients, the method must take account of all of the above, plus: 1) food preparation techniques (both the addition of condiments during preparation and the effect of the technique itself on nutrient composition); 2) sources of error in determination of amounts of foods consumed; 3) differences between nutrients in their distributions in various types of foods; and 4) the consumption of "nonfood" items (e.g., betel nut, coca leaves, laundry starch, and vitamin and mineral supplements) which may have a significant impact on nutrient intake levels. Limiting attention to single or few nutrients rather than many can help to streamline the method required.

Another significant consideration is whether data are required on the current diet—that is, foods or nutrients consumed during a restricted recent time period—or usual intake. It is possible to document "usual diet," but because it is a statistically defined abstraction, specific data collection strategies (discussed below) must be followed. Prior planning to incorporate them into the research design is important.

A further consideration in choosing a dietary assessment technique is the type of analysis to which data will be subjected. Methods such as correlation analysis, which attempt to relate dietary to other variables on an individual basis, require that data on individual informants be highly reliable. This requirement is less stringent, but still important, for classification analysis, where informants are assigned to groups (e.g., quantiles) based on dietary intake. Even lower reliability data from individuals can be tolerated when the analysis is designed to simply characterize the mean nutrient intake of the population. In this case, the greater the sample size, the less any imprecision in the data will distort the results.

Finally, the level at which data will be collected must also be chosen. Dietary intake can be measured and evaluated at a variety of levels, from populations to population subgroups, such as households, to individuals. Many of the same data collection techniques are used at each level, but their interpretations vary. After brief descriptions of the macrolevel techniques, this review will concentrate on those applicable to the individual.

Gathering Data on Groups

At the population level, data can come from food availability figures assessed by examining the food balance—the amount of food produced or imported by a population less that exported or converted for use as nonhuman food. Such data are necessarily crude indicators of diet, since they do not directly measure consumption itself. Another major approach to characterizing population diet has been large scale food consumption surveys, such as those conducted in the United States by the Department of Agriculture at 10-year intervals [Swan, 1983]. In these studies data from the food consumed by individuals or households are aggregated to obtain population intake estimates. In the past some of these surveys have suffered from inadequate assessment of validity and reliability [Young, 1981].

The most common population subgroup unit studied by anthropologists is the household. Indirect data on household intakes have been obtained in the past from food accounts, records of food brought into the household over a set period of time [Pekkarinen, 1970]. The use of computerized cash register tapes based on Universal Product Codes has been suggested as a possible technique for obtaining much of the same data in the future [Peal, 1981]. In nonwestern settings food consumption frequencies also have been used at the household level [Chassy et al., 1967; DeWalt and Pelto, 1976]. Extrapolation to individual intakes is not possible with all household level assessment, however, because of variations in intrahousehold distribution of foods [Cassidy, 1981; Ferro-Luzzi et al., 1981].

WIDELY USED METHODS OF DIETARY ASSESSMENT FOR INDIVIDUALS
Description of Methods

Commonly used techniques for assessing the dietary intake of individuals vary in terms of their timing relative to intake (record of current consumption vs recall of past consumption), duration (24 h to years), means of measuring food quantities (weights or estimates), and method of translating foods into nutrients consumed (direct chemical analysis or food composition tables). The most common techniques in two major types of assessment are discussed below.

Food record methods. The *weighed record* requires that all food items consumed be weighed before eating and plate waste be weighed after eating, to provide exact measures of foods consumed. Weighing is done either by the home food preparer or the researcher. The former requires training and compliance; the latter can be invasive in a home setting. Nutrient composition of the meals is calculated by direct laboratory analysis of an identical meal or sample of the food consumed or by using published food composition tables. (U.S. food composition tables are published and updated by the U.S. Department of Agriculture). An annotated bibliography of tables for over seventy countries has been published by F.A.O. [1975]. An international directory of food composition tables is maintained by the International Network of Food Data Systems (INFOODS), a United Nations University funded organization. A listing of approximately 150 entries from the directory plus information for obtaining INFOODS updates can be found in Quandt and Ritenbaugh [1986]. A recent review of computerized nutrient data bases can be found in the June, 1984 issue of the Journal of Nutrition Education.

While providing perhaps the most accurate data of any method on food actually consumed, any similarity of the diet to "usual consumption" is purely coincidental! Subjects are made highly conscious of food and food quantity choices and frequently simplify diets (e.g., by eliminating combination dishes) to streamline weighing procedures.

The weighed record technique has had two primary applications relevant to anthropology. The first is in short-term metabolic or body composition studies conducted in a laboratory setting [e.g., Viteri, 1971]. The second is in the study of infant diet. By providing parents with standard weight containers of formula, cow's milk or baby food and later collecting and weighing unused portions [e.g., Fomon et al., 1970, 1971], food weight data can be gathered with less disruption to the normal diet than is frequently the case with adults. In addition, pre- and post-feeding weighings of infants are frequently used to obtain amounts of breast milk consumed [e.g., Dewey and Lonnerdal, 1983]. These applications will be further discussed below.

The *estimated record* technique requires that subjects keep an ongoing record of foods consumed and their estimated weights or amounts. This may be done on a standard diary type form; recent work has included the use of small pocket notebooks and miniature cassette recorders [Todd et al., 1983]. While such a technique still assumes a cooperative, honest, and highly motivated subject, it has the advantage over the weighed record technique of not restricting food consumption to the home or laboratory. Further, long periods of data collection are both possible and practical. Estimated records are frequently kept for seven days. Estimated food weights can be converted into nutrients using food composition tables. As with weighed records, this technique is most appropriate when knowledge of actual rather than usual intake is required because keeping the record alters food habits.

Food recall methods. Recall techniques require that a subject give dietary intake information from memory. Several specific types of data collection fall within this category, including those designed to elicit usual consumption patterns over a relatively long time and those aimed at quantifying as precisely as possible actual intake for a finite time, usually one to three days. Collectively, these techniques differ from the weighed or estimated records in demanding less skill and long-term compliance of subjects and, by collecting data after the fact, in producing a record of freely chosen foods.

The *diet history* method was developed by Burke to obtain information reflecting "average dietary intake of the individual for the period under consideration, and/or the nutritional status of the individual just prior to the period considered" [Burke, 1947]. This dietary intake could then be compared with other indicators of nutritional status. The technique includes soliciting information regarding the subject's usual meal composition during a particular period of time. This is then "cross-checked" by obtaining quantity and frequency details for a list of specific food items. While Burke proposes that the food frequency data should "clarify and verify" that obtained in the more open-ended description of usual intake, there are no specific procedures for integrating the two bodies of data or for deciding which should be given priority. Quantification of intake data is not possible, and factors producing major fluctuations in intake (e.g., seasonal availability, feasting cycles) are not easily accommodated.

The *food frequency* method can be either used in an interview situation or as a self-administered questionnaire. Subjects report how frequently they consume specific foods on a list during a specified time limit (day, month, year, etc.). The list of foods used can encompass the general diet or be aimed at specific foods or nutrients of interest to the researcher. The data obtained in a food frequency are primarily qualitative. The National Cancer Institute has recently developed a food frequency method directed at the problem of quantification of nutrient intake. This lists a particular amount of a food for a medium serving (e.g., rice: 3/4 cup) and asks the respondents to rate their serving as relatively smaller or larger. Nutritional anthropologists at the University of Arizona are currently field testing a similar food frequency method in which the respondents specify their own usual serving size (Ritenbaugh, personal communication).

The *diet recall* is probably the most widely used technique in both clinical and research settings. This method requires that the subject recall all food, in as exact quantities as possible, for a specified period of time prior to the interview. Recalls of one to three days are most common. Skilled interviewing strategies are used to jog the memory of the respondent, and a variety of food and container models are frequently employed to improve recall of portion sizes. These models include natural looking food models [Moore et al., 1967] and graded shapes which can be used to represent surface area and volume [Sanjur, 1982].

Evaluation of Techniques. The evaluation of any data gathering technique involves two constructs, its reliability and its validity. Reliability is defined as the ability of the technique to produce identical results when repeated in similar situations. That is, how *representative* of the actual stream of human behavior is the portion which it samples? Validity, in contrast, is the degree to which the technique "reflects some underlying truth" [Rush and Kristal, 1982:1259]. That is, how accurate a measure is it of the actual behavior it records? In the case of dietary assessment, validity is usually operationalized to mean the extent to which data from one method agree with data from a control method, such as comparisons of recalls with weighed records. Data can be reliable without being valid, but the converse is not true: unreliable data cannot be valid [Keys, 1967].

The ideal dietary assessment technique would produce results both valid and reliable. However, methods (such as weighed records and direct chemical nutrient analysis) that are extremely accurate usually sacrifice reliability by disrupting normal dietary routine. Conversely, techniques which seek representative results, often through long-term data collection such as food frequency, do so at the expense of precision. The solution to this problem proposed most recently has been to choose a technique for which accuracy can be maximized with minimal disruption of eating behavior—the 24-h recall—and to incorporate it into a research design in such a way that the representativeness of the data produced is also maximized. The following discussion will concentrate on this particular approach in evaluating dietary methods. More complete reviews of other methods can be found in Burk and Pao [1976], Bazzarre and Myers [1980], and Pekkarinen [1970].

Validity. In general, validity studies indicate a moderate degree of agreement between 24-h recalls and measures of similar periods of time and much poorer agreement with longer term collection techniques such as diet histories and food frequencies. A review of the findings from a number of such studies suggests areas of potential problems with the 24-h recall.

Validity studies comparing *group intake averages* on the 24-h recall with those obtained by chemical analysis of duplicate portions, weighed records, or observed intake have demonstrated that the recall is indeed valid for getting at actual intake. Samuelson [1970], using chemical analysis of duplicate portions of school lunches of 8 and 13 year olds, found that the younger children on average significantly overestimated intake of energy, fat, and iron. Older children did not (although they tended to inflate protein intake), indicating increasing validity of the technique with subject age. In a similar study of first- to fourth-grade students, Emmons and Hayes [1973] found that recallability (i.e., the recalled percentage of items actually consumed) increased with age. However, older children had a tendency to show increasing normative behavior, reporting items usually available, such as bread and butter, even when they had not actually consumed them. Validity studies of the 24-h recall in adult populations have produced mixed results. In comparing weighed intakes and recalls for an elderly sample, Gersovitz et al. [1978] found that all nutrients were, on average, accurately reported with the exception of protein, which was overestimated. Using the technique of 24-h recall of a known menu with specific probing to elicit forgotten items, Campbell and Dodds [1967] found age and sex effects on validity. Among younger subjects (averaging about 40 years), substantially lower percentages of all macro- and micronutrients required probing for recall than among subjects in their seventies. Females recalled a greater percentage of all nutrients than did males among the younger group and of all nutrients except calcium and vitamin A among the older group.

Thus, for mean sample intakes, the validity of the 24-h recall technique seems to vary with the population. Younger children and the elderly seem more likely to forget food items and inaccurately estimate quantities consumed. Among adults, females are better able to report their intake, probably due to greater experience in food measurement and preparation. The level of validity for specific nutrients varies. Differences in research design make comparisons by nutrients between studies difficult.

Statistical analysis in validity studies which permit assessment of *individual* rather than group error further pinpoints problems to be expected using the 24-h recall. Using regression of actual intake (from weighed records) on recalled, a "flat slope syndrome" has been identified [Gersovitz et al., 1978; Linusson et al., 1974]. This is evident when regression of recall (Y) on actual intake (X) for individual nutrients or food quantities produces a regression line with an intercept greater than zero and a slope less than one (Fig. 1). This indicates that for intakes below the mean, respondents tend to overestimate quantities. In contrast, large intakes are underestimated. The result is an overall tendency for reported intakes to approximate the mean.

The flat slope syndrome appears to be a greater problem for some nutrients than others. Among an elderly population, Gersovitz et al. [1978] found

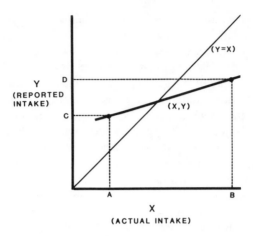

Fig. 1. Hypothetical illustration of over-reporting intake less than the mean and under-reporting intake greater than the mean (flat-slope syndrome) for group comparisons of dietary intake. (Reprinted with permission from Gersovitz et al. [1978]. ©The American Dietic Association.)

protein, cholesterol, and calcium most accurately recalled by individuals, with slope coefficients of .675 to .585 and vitamin A, energy, and iron least accurately recalled (slope coefficients .216 to .149).

Data gathered by Linusson et al., [1974] from a sample of lactating women suggest that accurate recall of some foods may be more problematic than of others, thus affecting accuracy of specific nutrients. Breakfast cereals (slope coefficient, .89), dairy products (.73), and combination main dishes (.60) were best recalled, while starches (.45), sweets (.45), and salads (.24) were least accurately recalled. These inaccuracies may reflect problems in estimating quantities (for example, salads composed of multiple, irregularly shaped items versus dairy products which are often served in standard sized portions). However, some recall inaccuracies may simply reflect adherence to cultural norms proscribing or prescribing consumption of particular foods. Most people can recite a "good" diet even if they don't consume it! Linusson et al.'s data [1974] support this, with a greater percentage of women *under*estimating sweets and desserts, and *over*estimating cereals and dairy products.

Reliability. In measuring the replicability of a technique, studies of reliability in human behavior are basically inquiries into whether the given technique measures "usual behavior" for individuals or for groups. In the case of diet, the reliability of the technique varies with the nature of the diet. It is common knowledge that the diet of every individual varies in composition or quantity every day. A number of factors cause this variation. First, foods may be consumed cyclically, in long-term cycles reflecting seasonal availability or feasting practices, or short-term cycles reflecting weeky activity patterns, pay periods, or the like. Further, the nature of the foods consumed influences day-to-day variation in nutrient intake. A number of interchangeable foods may be consumed or the diet may be fairly monotonous. In the former case, the pattern of distribution of nutrients among foods commonly interchanged becomes important. Those nutrients concentrated in only a few foods consumed sporadically may be more likely to go undetected in short-term dietary data collection or to appear more prevalent in the diet than is actually the case than nutrients which are more evenly distributed among foods.

In light of these factors causing day-to-day variation in reported nutrient intake, a series of recent studies has attempted to identify the magnitude and sources of variation in intake of different nutrients. Beaton et al. [1979; 1983] obtained six 24-h recalls for each of 30 males and 30 females in a study of urban Canadian adults. A Greco-Latin square design permitted isolation for both sexes of variation due to interviewer, "training effect" of sequential interviews and day of the week. Factorial analysis of variance found little or no interviewer or sequence effect. There was a strong day-of-the-week effect in females but none in males. Among females, day of the week contributed 9.4% to variance of energy and somewhat lower percentages to other nutrients, including iron (8.1%), thiamin (5.7%), fat (5.7%), protein (5.3%), and cholesterol (4.6%). Correction of nutrients for energy eliminated day-of-the week effects, indicating that the apparent day-to-day fluctuations in nutrient intake among females were simply due to their consuming more food on some days (especially Sunday) than others.

The greatest sources of variation in these studies were intraindividual, due to day-to-day differences in diet for each subject, and interindividual, due to real dietary differences between subjects. The variance ratio, the square of the ratio of intraindividual coefficient of variation to interindividual coefficient of variation, was found to differ widely among nutrients (Table I). However, for virtually all nutrients, intraindividual exceeded interindividual variation. This was most pronounced for vitamin A and cholesterol. Other studies of pregnant women [Rush and Kristal, 1982] and male graduate students [Todd et al., 1983] in which variance ratios have been computed have found values in the same range as those of Beaton et al. [1979; 1983].

The sources of variation in nutrient intake for infants seem to differ substantially from those for adults. Quandt used four random replicate 24-h recalls of infant diet to assess usual food intake within 1 month for 28 infants from four to six months of age [1985]. Participants were mothers of infants in the Special Supplemental Food Program for Women, Infants, and Children in Lexington,

TABLE I. Estimated Intraindividual and Interindividual Coefficients of Variability by Sex[a]

Nutrient	Mean	Coefficients of variation (%)			Variance ratio
		Total	Inter	Intra	
Males					
Energy (kcal/day)	2,639	35.8	24.9	25.7	1.0
Protein (g/day)	98.2	46.1	29.1	35.7	1.4
CHO (g/day)	264.4	37.7	23.4	29.5	1.7
Fat (g/day)	113.9	41.7	28.1	30.8	1.2
Cholesterol (mg/day)	521.1	59.4	28.2	52.3	3.6
Vitamin A (IU/day)	6,369	146.6	0	146.6	—
Vitamin C (mg/day)	111.5	76.0	35.9	67.0	3.6
Thiamin (mg/day)	1.75	51.2	27.3	43.4	2.6
Calcium (mg/day)	902.0	49.6	27.9	41.0	2.2
Iron (mg/day)	15.7	43.8	26.9	34.6	1.7
Females					
Energy (kcal/day)	1,793	40.9	26.4	31.3	1.4
Protein (g/day)	69.9	39.8	25.0	31.0	1.4
CHO (g/day)	180.6	47.4	30.8	36.0	1.4
Fat (g/day)	82.1	49.9	30.7	39.3	1.6
Cholesterol (mg/day)	396.3	60.7	26.3	54.7	4.4
Vitamin A (IU/day)	5,188	114.1	22.7	111.9	24.0
Vitamin C (mg/day)	105.9	79.9	46.2	65.2	2.0
Thiamin (mg/day)	1.29	58.1	25.0	52.4	4.4
Calcium (mg/day)	671.3	63.2	45.8	43.6	1.0
Iron (mg/day)	11.3	36.8	19.6	31.2	2.6

[a]From Beaton et al., [1979; 1983].

Kentucky. None was breast fed; most consumed formula plus a variety of baby and table foods. Interindividual variation exceeded intraindividual variation for all nutrients except vitamin C (Table II), producing variance ratios ranging from 0.3 to 1.3. The pattern was virtually the same when nutrients were expressed as percentage of the Recommended Dietary Allowance.

These studies of the variation documented by replicate recalls show that intake of certain nutrients is more variable and therefore subject to greater error than is intake of others. Vitamin A and cholesterol for adults and vitamin C for infants—nutrients whose concentrations vary sharply among foods—are particularly problematic. Subsets of populations, such as females, whose diets vary cyclically pose greater problems for getting at usual diet than do those with less variable diets. It also appears that intraindividual variability in nutrient intake increases with age. Among infants, each child generally consumes a relatively small number of items selected from the total universe of available foods. In contrast, adults each consume a wide range of foods. Thus greater

TABLE II. Estimated Variance Ratios and Coefficients of Variation for Total, Interindividual, and Intraindividual Variation for Lexington, Kentucky Infants[a]

Nutrient	Mean	Coefficients of variation %			Variance ratio
		Total	Inter	Intra	
Energy (kcal/day)	812.3	36	29	21	.5
Protein (g/day)	21.4	40	32	23	.5
Fat (g/day)	37.8	41	34	22	.4
Carbohydrate (g/day)	98.8	35	28	21	.6
Calcium (mg/day)	788.2	51	45	25	.3
Iron (mg/day)	22.3	52	41	32	.6
Vitamin A (IU/day)	273.7	78	67	40	.4
Vitamin C (mg/day)	88.8	40	26	30	1.3

[a]N = 112 recalls.

interindividual than intraindividual variation is found in infants and the opposite in adults.

These findings have been used to illustrate the ways and calculate the extent to which unreliable methods of dietary assessment are likely to bias research results. Low reliability presents the greatest problem in research designs which use either correlation or classification analyses. In both, accurate usual dietary intake for *individuals* is required. When this is not achieved, data analysis may produce distorted results. For example, the use of unreliable technique has been cited as a major cause of the failure of many epidemiological investigations to demonstrate the association between dietary lipids and serum cholesterol [Keys, 1967; Liu et al., 1978]. When intraindividual variation in a dietary factor is large, as it is for cholesterol, and each individual's mean intake is derived from a small number of measures, the error in the correlation coefficient will be high. Since intraindividual variation will be random in its distortion of estimated mean intakes, the correlation coefficient will be attenuated rather than skewed in a particular direction. When the other variable (in the case of Liu et al., serum cholesterol) also varies intraindividually, the likelihood of error in the correlation is exacerbated. Formulas for calculating the expected error in the correlation coefficient when variation is known [Liu et al., 1978], for estimating the "true" value of a correlation coefficient [Balogh et al., 1971], and for estimating the number of 24-h records needed to reduce attentuation to specific levels [Rush and Kristal, 1982] are available.

Classification, whether into quantiles or into risk groups defined by biologically significant cutoffs, is commonly used to analyze relationships between diet intake and outcome variables. When high intraindividual variation results in low reliability of dietary assessment, the chance of misclassifying substantial numbers of individuals increases [Garn et al., 1978]. Formulas are available to estimate the number of diet intake measures necessary for a specific level of classification accuracy [Liu et al., 1978]. Walker and Blettner [1985] demonstrate the extent to which imperfect measures of diet result in misclassification and suggest implications for research design.

Beaton [1982] illustrates the effect unreliable usual intake data will have on the assessment of the proportion of people with excessive or inadequate usual intakes of a nutrient (Fig. 2). Whether one uses either (A) a low reliability dietary data collection technique such as single 24-h recalls or (B) a highly reliable method of determining usual intake such as replicate records, the sample means should both equal the true mean of the individuals' usual intakes. However, the distributions will differ substantially. That employing single observations will have a weaker central tendency and the apparent prevalence of inadequate and excessive intakes will be inflated [Hegsted, 1972]. Moreover, the closer any individual's true mean intake is to the cutoff point, the greater the likelihood that she/he has been misclassified. This problem can be solved by increasing the number of measures per individual to make the dietary assessment technique more reliable but not by increasing the sample size.

Thus, the use of dietary assessment techniques which have a low level of reliability can distort research findings in a number of ways. If correlations are computed, the coefficients will be low, giving the impression of no relationship between diet and dependent variables when in fact significant relationships exist. When classification analysis is used, the number of false negatives and

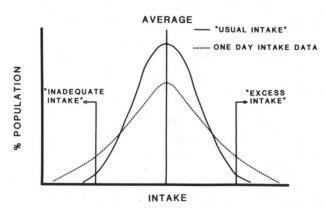

Fig. 2. Effect of duration of observation or number of replicate observations on apparent distribution of nutrient intakes. (Reprinted with permission from Beaton [1982].)

false positives will be high. Finally, the proportion of a population appearing to be at risk for low and high nutrient intake will be inflated.

PROBLEMS IN ANTHROPOLOGICAL APPLICATIONS

Most commonly used dietary assessment techniques were developed for use in Western adult populations. Anthropologists, however, frequently undertake research in populations where cultural and dietary differences and constraints on fieldwork exist which reduce the applicability of these techniques.

Food Consumption Cycles

Many data collection methods are based on time periods which are appropriate in Western culture—a day, a week, a month—but may not hold the same importance for food consumption cycles elsewhere. The difficulties posed by extremely uneven intake due to feasting and fasting cycles and seasonal food availability are quite apparent. More subtle temporal regulations of intake may be the scheduling of market days and their regulation of availability of particular foods [DeWalt and Pelto, 1976] or the ripening of wild plants which are still consumed by populations with otherwise agrarian diets [Messer, 1976]. Attention to available ethnography on relevant food cycles in the study population is crucial in designing the data collection procedures [Jerome and Pelto, 1981]. Proportionate inclusion of different parts of the food consumption cycle is necessary to document usual intakes, just as a balanced number of weekdays and weekend days is required in North American studies [Beaton, 1982].

Style of Food Consumption

One of the primary difficulties encountered is trying to obtain quantified intake data where food serving techniques differ from those in Western populations and where combination rather than single ingredient foods are the rule. In many cultures individuals in a household share a common bowl. While direct observation by the anthropologist will allow her/him to estimate quantities consumed, an additional problem exists if the shared food is a combination dish with a limited amount of food rich in particular nutrients (e.g., fat in meat) which is not shared equally. In using either direct observation or recall to obtain intake data, the anthropologist can increase the accuracy of such information by attending to household food preparation techniques. Valverde et al. [1980], for example, have demonstrated that significant between and within household variations exist in homemade tortilla sizes in Guatemala.

And Messer [1979] found significant variations in the customary sweetening of hot beverages consumed in different Mexican households.

Intake of Infants and Children

Obtaining the dietary intakes for children can be considerably harder than for adults. Volume and composition of milk consumed by breast fed infants presents a special case. Pre- and post-feeding infant weighings have been used to determine volume in a number of studies [Butte et al., 1983; Dewey and Lonnerdal, 1983; Picciano et al., 1981]. In validation with known quantities of milk consumed, 94.9 $\pm$ 13.2% of milk ingested was detected in weighings [Brown et al., 1982]. However, weighing is a labor intensive data collection technique for the mother or researcher. An alternative and less invasive technique which has been used in Africa in the Gambia is the measurement of changes in deuterium dilution in the infant's saliva over several days [Coward et al., 1979]. Evaluation of this method against test weighings for 24- or 48-h volumes indicates significant discrepancies which may limit the procedure's application to estimation of population milk volume rather than to that of individuals [Butte et al., 1983].

Because nutrient composition, particularly for fat, varies by time of day, phase of the feeding, and even from one breast to the other [Jelliffe and Jelliffe, 1979], representative milk composition data for individual infants are extremely difficult to obtain. Although the most representative milk sample is that obtained by a complete 24-h expression of milk [Lemons et al., 1980], many researchers (eg, Butte et al., 1983; Dewey and Lonnerdal, 1983] analyze a complete expression of milk from one breast at a standard time of day chosen to minimize fat variation. A more invasive method which is appropriate more for small scale research than for larger surveys is the nipple shield method [Lucas et al., 1980; Woolridge et al., 1982]. This allows for continuous sampling of milk as the infant sucks during the feeding through a specially constructed nipple shield. Given these problems in data collection, one might consider observing as indirect evidence breast feeding behaviors (eg, number of feedings per day and length of interval between feedings) which are known to be associated with volume and caloric density [De Carvalho et al., 1983; Quandt, 1984a].

A further challenge is obtaining dietary intake of children who consume much of their food away from home. Wilson [1974] recommends "child-following," in which the researcher directly observes and records the intake of a child. While this alleviates the problem of children's inability to report their consumption, it severely limits the number of children studied and the duration of data collection. Moreover, Bledsoe [1983] reports that among Mende foster children in Sierra Leone, who obtain much of their food by "tiefing" (stealing), child-following significantly inhibits this nutritionally important behavior. Despite difficulties in getting intake data on children's food consumed away from home, Baer and Ritenbaugh [1983] point out that with increasing consumption of processed and prepackaged snack foods, conversion of these data to nutrient values is often easier than for traditional foods consumed at home.

Data on such feeding transitions as weaning and introduction of solids are frequently obtained retrospectively from mothers of infants and children. Quandt [1986] and Persson and Carlgren [1984] have assessed the validity of such data and found high rates of recall error. Time since the feeding transition and salience of the event explain some but not all maternal errors.

Research Design

The preceding discussion of anthropological applications has concentrated on problems in obtaining valid nutrient data. For anthropologists conducting *long-term* fieldwork, the techniques suggested can be incorporated into research designs similar to those used by Rush and Kristal [1982], Beaton et al. [1979; 1983], and others to produce data on individuals which are also reliable. However, many researchers today find themselves operating under severe time and funding constraints or participating as a member of a research team which includes a nutritional anthropological component as only a small portion of the overall project. In such cases, it may be necessary to modify existing data collection techniques to suit research conditions. To obtain "usual" intake of nutrients for individuals, this could involve a prestudy of a subsample to document foods in which nutrients of greatest interest are most commonly consumed. If this is followed by construction of a food frequency index specific for those foods, assignment of informants to categories of intake should be relatively accurate due to the preliminary study which tailored the data collection instrument to the specific population's foodways. While information on precise intake of nutrients is lost, classification is frequently adequate for many purposes [Block, 1982].

Nutritionists have now taken dietary assessment methodology beyond the technical problems with individual data collection techniques to the critical analysis of the way these are incorporated into research design. Their emphasis is currently on understanding the nature of variation in human food consumption. Anthropologists, who recognize intracultural diversity as the norm [Pelto and Pelto, 1975] and identification of patterning as a primary goal [DeWalt, 1981], can make major contributions to these efforts through ethnographic research. They should be aware that specific methods developed by nutritionists are not intrinsically good or bad. Methods should be selected or rejected, or new ones developed, based on whether or not they can fit into a research design tailored to the constraints of the field situation. This will be most successful if the research design is formulated with a clear understanding of the questions to be answered.

REFERENCES

Baer RD, Ritenbaugh C (1983): The dietary effect of "eating out" in Sonora, Mexico. Paper presented at the annual meeting, American Anthropological Association, Chicago, Illinois.

Balogh M, Kahn HA, Medalie JH (1971): Random repeat 24-hour dietary recalls. Am J Clin Nutr 24:304-310.

Bazzarre TL, Myers MP (1980): The collection of food intake data in cancer epidemiology studies. Nutr Cancer 1(4):22-45.

Beaton GH (1982): What do we think we are estimating? In Beal VA, Laus MJ (eds): "Proceedings of the Symposium on Dietary Data Collection and Significance." Massachusetts Agricultural Experiment Station Research Bulletin 675, pp 36-48.

Beaton GH, Milner J, Corey P, McGuire V, Cousins G, Stewart D, de Ramos M, Hewitt D, Grambsch PV, Kassim N, Little JA (1979): Sources of variance in 24-hour dietary recall data: implications for nutritional study design and interpretation. Am J Clin Nutr 32:2549-2559.

Beaton GH, Milner J, McGuire V, Feather TE, Little JA (1983): Sources of variance in 24-hour dietary recall data: implications for nutritional study design and interpretation. Carbohydrate sources, vitamins, and minerals. Am J Clin Nutr 37:986-995.

Bledsoe CH (1983): Stealing food as a problem in demography and nutrition. Paper presented at the annual meeting, American Anthropological Association, Chicago, Illinois.

Block G (1982): A review of validations of dietary assessment methods. Am J Epidemiol 115:492-505.

Brown KH, Black RE, Robertson AD, Akhtar NA, Ahmed G, Becker S (1982): Clinical and field studies of human lactation: methodological considerations. Am J Clin Nutr 35:745-756.

Burk MC, Pao EM (1976): Methodology for large-scale surveys of household and individual diets. USDA: Home Economics Research Report No. 40.

Burke BS (1947): The dietary history as a tool in research. J Am Dietet Assoc 23:1041-1046.

Butte NF, Garza C, Smith EO, Nichols BC (1983): Evaluation of the deuterium dilution technique against the test-weighing procedure for the determination of breast milk intake. Am J Clin Nutr 37:996-1003.

Campbell VA, Dodds ML (1967): Collecting dietary information from groups of older people. J Am Dietet Assoc 51:29-33.

Cassidy CM (1981): Collecting data on American food consumption patterns: an anthropological perspective. In Committee on Food Consumption Patterns, Food and Nutrition Board, National Research Council (ed): "Assessing Changing Food Consumption Patterns." Washington, D.C.: National Academy Press, pp 135-154.

Chassy JP, van Veen AG, Young FW (1967): The application of social science research methods to the study of food habits and food consumption in an industrializing area. Am J Clin Nutr 20:56-64.

Coward WA, Sawyer MB, Whitehead RG, Prentice AM, Evans J (1979): New method for measuring milk intakes in breast-fed babies. Lancet ii:13-14.

De Carvalho M, Robertson S, Friedman A, Klaus M (1983): Effect of frequent breast-feeding on early milk production and infant weight gain. Pediatrics 72:307-311.

DeWalt KM (1981): Diet as adaptation: the search for nutritional strategies. Fed Proc 40: 2606-2610.

DeWalt KM, Pelto GH (1976): Food use and household ecology in a Mexican Community. In Fitzgerald TK (ed): "Nutrition and Anthropology in action." Assen: Van Gorcum, pp 79-93.

Dewey KG, Lonnerdal G (1983) Milk and nutrient intake of breast-fed infants from 1 to 6 months: relation to growth and fatness. J Pediatr Gastroent Nutr 2:497-506.

Emmons L, Hayes M (1973): Accuracy of 24-hr. recalls of young children. J Am Dietet Assoc 62:409-416.

Ferro-Luzzi A, Norgan NG, Paci C (1981): An evaluation of the distribution of protein and energy intakes in some New Guinean households. Nutr Rep Int 24:153-163.

Fomon SJ, Filer LJ, Thomas LN, Rogers RR (1970): Growth and serum chemical values of normal breastfed infants. Acta Paediatr Scand Supp 202.

Fomon SJ, Thomas LN, Filer LJ, Ziegler EE, Leonard MT (1971): Food consumption and growth of normal infants fed milk-based formulas. Acta Paediatr Scand Supp 223.

FAO (1975): Food Composition Tables. Updated Annotated Bibliography. Rome: Food and Agriculture Organization.

Garn SM, Larkin FA, Cole PE (1978): The real problem with 1-day diet records. Am J Clin Nutr 31:1114-1116.

Gersovitz M, Madden JP, Smiciklas-Wright H (1978): Validity of the 24-hr. dietary recall and seven-day record for group comparisons. J Am Dietet Assoc 73:48-55.

Hegsted DM (1972): Problems in the use and interpretation of the Recommended Dietary Allowances. Ecol Food Nutr 1:255-265.

Jelliffe DB, Jelliffe EFP (1979): Human Milk in the Modern World. Oxford: Oxford Unviersity Press.

Jerome NW, Pelto GH (1981): Integrating ethnographic research with nutrition studies. Fed Proc 40:2601-2605.

Journal of Nutrition Education (1984): Vol 16(2): Complete issue. Oakland, CA: Society for Nutrition Education.

Keys A (1967): Dietary epidemiology. Am J Clin Nutr 20:1151-1157.

Lemons JA, Schreiner RL, Gresham EL (1980): Simple method for determining the caloric and fat content of human milk. Pediatrics 66:626-628.

Linusson EEI, Sanjur D, Erickson EC (1974): Validating the 24-hour recall method as a dietary survey tool. Archivos Latinamer Nutr 24:277-294.

Liu K, Stamler J, Dyer A, McKeever J, McKeever P (1978): Statistical methods to assess and minimize the role of intraindividual variability in obscuring the relationship between dietary lipids and serum cholesterol. J Chron Dis 31:399-418.

Lucas A, Lucas PJ, Baum JD (1980): The nipple-shield sampling system: a device for measuring the dietary intake of breast-fed infants. Early Hum Dev 4:365-372.

Messer E (1976): The ecology of vegetarian diet in a modernizing Mexican community. In Fitzgerald TK (ed): "Nutrition and Anthropology in Action." Assen, The Netherlands: van Gorcum, pp 117-124.

Messer E (1979): Some like it sweet. Paper presented at the annual meeting, American Anthropological Association, Cincinnati, Ohio.

Moore MC, Judlin BC, Kennemur PMcA (1967): Using graduated food models in taking dietary histories. J Am Dietet Assoc 51:447-450.

Pearl, RB (1981): Possible alternative methods for data collection on food consumption and expenditures. In Committee on Food Consumption Patterns, Food and Nutrition Board, National Research Council (ed): "Assessing Changing Food Consumption Patterns." Washington, D.C.: National Academy Press, pp 198-203.

Pekkarinen M (1970): Methodology in the collection of food consumption data. World Rev Nutr Diet 12:145-171.

Pelto PJ, Pelto GH (1975): Intra-cultural diversity: some theoretical issues. American Ethnologist 2:1-19.

Persson LA, Carlgren G (1984): Measuring children's diets: evaluation of dietary assessment techniques in infancy and childhood. Int J Epidemiol 13:506-517.

Picciano MF, Calkins EJ, Garrick JR, Deering RH (1981): Milk and mineral intakes of breastfed infants. Acta Paediatr Scand 70:189-194.

Quandt SA (1984a): The effect of beikost on the diet of breast-fed infants. J Am Dietet Assoc 84:47-51.

Quandt SA (1984b): Nutritional thriftiness and human reproduction: beyond the critical body composition hypothesis. Soc Sci Med 19:177-182.

Quandt SA (1985): Strategies for collecting reliable infant dietary data. Paper presented at the annual meeting, American Anthropological Association, Washington, D.C.

Quandt SA (1986): Maternal recall accuracy for dates of infant feeding transitions. Human Organization, in press.

Quandt SA, Ritenbaugh C (eds) (1986): Training Manual in Nutritional Anthropology. Washington, D.C.: American Anthropological Association, Special Publication No. 20.

Rush D, Kristal AR (1982): Methodologic studies during pregnancy: the reliability of the 24-hour dietary recall. Am J Clin Nutr 35:1259-1268.

Samuelson G (1970): An epidemiological study of child health and nutrition in a northern Swedish county. Nutr Metabol 12:321-340.

Sanjur D (1982): Social and Cultural Perspectives in Nutrition. Englewood Cliffs, NJ: Prentice-Hall, Inc.

Swan PB (1983): Food consumption by individuals in the United States: Two major surveys. Ann Rev Nutr 3:413-432.

Todd KS, Hudes M, Calloway DH (1983): Food intake measurement: problems and approaches. Am J Clin Nutr 37:139-146.

Valverde V, Martorell R, Owens W, Klein RE (1980): Problems in the estimation of corn consumption in longitudinal studies in rural Guatemala. Archivos Latinamer Nutr 30:353-368.

Viteri FE (1971): Considerations on the effect of nutrition on the body composition and physical working capacity of young Guatemalan adults. In Scrimshaw NS, Altschul AM (eds): "Amino Acid Fortification of Protein Foods." Cambridge, MA: The M.I.T. Press, pp 350-375.

Walker AM, Blettner M (1985): Comparing imperfect measures of exposure. Am J Epidemiol 121:783-790.

Wilson C (1974): Child-following: a technic for learning food and nutrient intakes. J Trop Pediatr Environ Child Health 20:9-14.

Woolridge MW, How RV, Drewett RF, Rolfe P, Baum JD (1982): The continuous measurement of milk intake at a feed in breast-fed babies. Early Hum Dev 6:365-373.

Young CM (1981): Dietary methodology. In Committee on Food Consumption Patterns, Food and Nutrition Board, National Research Council (ed): "Assessing Changing Food Consumption Patterns." Washington, D.C.: National Academy Press, pp 89-118.

Young CM, Trulson MF (1960): Methodology for dietary studies in epidemiological surveys. II—Strengths and weaknesses of existing methods. Am J Publ Health 50:803-814.

Nutritional Anthropology, pages 85-99
© 1987 Alan R. Liss, Inc.

Purposeful Assessment of Nutritional Status

John H. Himes, PhD, MPH

Department of Health and Nutrition Sciences, Brooklyn College, City University of New York, Brooklyn, New York 11210

INTRODUCTION

Nutrition has become of great interest to workers in many basic and applied disciplines. The florescence of nutrition-related concerns probably has resulted as much from increased public awareness of health issues and growing involvement of academic disciplines not traditionally nutritionally oriented, e.g. economic and social sciences, as it has from technological and scientific advances per se. Accordingly, nutrition progressively has become more prominent in the anthropological literature, as have anthropological perspectives in the more traditional literatures of health and nutrition.

For some readers the logical extension of the title "Purposeful Assessment of Nutritional Status" may lead to the conclusion that there may be nutritional assessment without purpose or results. While this seems antithetical to the scientific method espoused by researchers, it is, nevertheless, common to see workers manifest their ethnographic training by including large collections of "nutrition-related" variables (for individuals and groups) without any guiding research questions, accompanying design, or predetermined analytical plans. Answering important nutrition questions from these data is usually serendipitous and always economically inefficient. In less extreme cases, less-than-purposeful nutritional assessment may result from: inappropriate matching of variables or analyses to stated study objectives, poorly chosen indicators, inadequately trained data collectors, confounding environmental factors, difficulties in the field, etc.

The intent of the present chapter is to consider selected practical factors that may contribute to more purposeful assessment of nutritional status of invididuals and groups. In this regard, the term purposeful relates to approaching assessment of nutritional status utilizing knowledge of basic characteristics of the concept of nutritional status and its indicators, of stated objectives guiding choices of indicators, and of considerations in field studies which may compromise results. The aim is to provide fundamentals which will aid in obtaining results that are meaningful and worthwhile (scientifically and economically). The selected aspects are not meant to be exhaustive, but they do provide perspectives and general principles that may be extended and applied to many situations.

NUTRITIONAL STATUS AND ITS ASSESSMENT

McLaren [1976] has defined *nutriture* as "the state resulting from the balance between supply of nutrition on the one hand and the expenditure of the organism on the other." Implicit in this definition is the notion that the body can use the nutritional supply provided.

Ideally, one would like to evaluate (preferably quantitatively) the physiological state of nutriture of individuals and groups for each nutrient and collectively across all nutrients. Because nutriture is a highly individualized and complex construct, it has been necessary to approach its assessment by selecting measurable variables that are manifestations of a single aspect of nutriture. Typically, these measures are body levels of the nutrients, their physiological compounds, their metabolities, or functional processes dependent upon them. If they are good measures, they have been validated over large ranges of nutriture and are well understood biologically and statistically. *Nutritional status,* then, is the expression of nutriture in a specific variable [Habicht et al., 1979]. By comparing these variables with known levels or patterns from appropriate reference data, *indicators of nutritional status* are derived.

By way of example, if one is interested in the iron nutriture of an individual, one may measure the hemoglobin concentration in a sample of whole blood. By comparing this value with appropriate reference data for those of a similar physiological state, age, sex, and perhaps race, one may obtain one indicator of iron status for this person. Other indicators of iron status are available, however, and one of these may provide a different answer, with different biological implications [INACG, 1981].

Conceptually, nutriture can be viewed globally, but practically, nutritional status cannot. Nutritional status is linked to a particular indicator or even a set of indicators which are limited in the nutrients they represent, as well as in the accuracy of representation. Indicators of nutritional status are only expressions of the physiological state of nutriture. Often, indicators of various nutrients are intercorrelated, they are indirect approximations, and they are imperfectly measured. Moreover, they are based on reference data collected with similar limitations. Thus, it is not surprising that certain nonnutritional information or nutritional information other than that intended may be included in indicators of nutritional status.

These imperfections in indicators are related to the epidemiologic concepts of sensitivity and specificity as they apply to assessment of nutritional status (Table I). *Sensitivity* is the porportion of those with *abnormal* nutriture that are identified as such using an indicator of nutritional status. Thus, a highly sensitive indicator is desirable so that those who require nutritional assistance can be correctly identified. When indicators are used as continuous variables to evaluate changes due to an intervention, a sensitive indicator changes with changes in nutriture in a predictable way and to an appreciable extent.

Specificity is related to sensitivity, but it refers to the proportion of individuals with *normal* nutriture who are identified as such using an indicator of nutritional status. High specificity is desirable so that normal individuals are not given unnecessary treatment; this may have adverse biological as well as economic implications. Further, high specificity facilitates unambiguous interpretation of existing nutritional problems.

For the hypothetical case in Table I, the indicator correctly identifies 93% of abnormal individuals (sensitivity), and , thus, one may have considerable confidence that almost all of those needing treatment or referral will be properly designated. In contrast, less than two-thirds of the normal individuals

TABLE I. Determination of Sensitivity and Specificity of a Hypothetical Indicator of Nutritional Status for a Population

Indicator of nutritional status	Actual nutriture	
	Abnormal	Normal
Positive (indicating abnormal nutriture)	A = 56	B = 176
Negative (indicating normal nutriture)	C = 4	D = 264
Totals	60	440

Sensitivity (%) $= \dfrac{A}{A + C} \times 100 = \dfrac{56}{60} \times 100 = 93.3\%.$

Specificity (%) $= \dfrac{D}{B + D} \times 100 = \dfrac{264}{440} \times 100 = 60\%.$

are considered so by the indicator (specificity). This means that only about one-fourth of all those considered abnormal by the indicator are, in fact, of abnormal nutriture $(100 \times A/A+ B)$. If treatment is the appropriate course of action for those considered abnormal, most of the money and time spent will be for those not requiring it, and most of those treated will be at risk if there are adverse consequences of unnecessary treatment. Sensitivity and specificity are important quantitative notions and an excellent discussion of these and related statistical issues as they relate to nutritional status has been presented by Habicht et al. [1979].

As a practical example of these concepts let us use children's stature relative to age and sex as an indicator. It is known that growth in stature is sensitive to caloric deficiency [Yarbrough et al., 1974]. In other words, caloric insufficiency is associated with relatively short stature and using short stature for age as an indicator will correctly identify a large proportion of those children with energy deficits. This growth–nutrition association primarily results because of the relatively low priority of somatic growth for available energy [Himes, 1982].

In addition to caloric deficiency, short stature may also reflect nonnutritional factors such as genetics or illness. Consequently, short stature is not specific to caloric adequacy per se, and attribution of all differences in stature to energy nutriture, or even primarily to energy nutriture may not be appropriate, especially if the general severity and prevalence of energy deficiencies are low. The sensitivity and specificity of a given indicator will vary according to the severity and prevalence of the nutritional abnormality. Hence, it is important to choose indicators of nutritional status that maximize the ability to detect differences in nutriture and which optimize interpretability and attribution of results in a particular situation.

A failure to recognize the importance of sensitivity and specificity has led to confusion in the literature between variables that are appropriate indicators of nutritional status and variables that are appropriate as outcomes related to nutritional factors. Head circumference, for example, is smaller in severely malnourished children than in normal controls [Engsner et al., 1974] and it is a reasonable measure of brain growth [Dobbing and Sands, 1978]. Thus, it is clear that the effects of severe undernutrition on growth in head circumference are probably very important for workers interested in neurological or behavioral impacts. Nevertheless, the circumference by itself is a poor indicator of nutritional status because of its low sensitivity to less extreme malnutrition [Yarbrough et al., 1974]. While variables may show some nutritional effect and be meaningful as outcomes, this does not ensure that they can be depended upon to be the basis for determining the nutriture of individuals or groups, i.e., indicators of nutritional status.

Recently, there has been an emphasis on developing functional indicators of nutritional status as opposed to static indicators. The traditional measures of nutrient levels in blood, urine, and other body tissues are examples of static indicators of nutritional status. Critics of static indicators argue that the cut-off points used to designate deficiency are arbitrary. Especially given the high degree of individual variability in physiological levels of adequacy, there seems to be little justification for accepting cut-off points as diagnostic criteria for the impairment of health status due to deficiency of a respective nutrient [Buzina, 1982]. This is especially true for individuals.

Solomons and Allen [1983] have reviewed functional indicators of nutritional status and define them as "…diagnostic tests to determine the sufficiency of host nutriture to permit cells, tissues, organs, anatomical systems, or the host him/herself to perform optimally the intended, nutrient-dependent biological function." The logic behind functional indicators of nutritional status is that the true significance of deficiency (or excess) is its impairment of physiological function rather than the levels of nutrients per se. Such functional variables include measures of structural integrity of cells and tissues, immune functions, nutrient transport and metabolism, hemostasis, nerve function, behavior, and work capacity [Solomons and Allen, 1983].

In general, most of the functional variables are probably not suitable for most field situations. Many are still in the research phase and require invasive procedures or elaborate and unconventional laboratory equipment. Moreover, for most of the functional variables the sensitivities and specificities are unknown. Consequently, at present, they cannot be considered well-developed indicators as defined in the present discussion. Nevertheless, this is a potentially fruitful area for further development and research. Exceptions to the above limitations of functional variables include some measures of somatic growth.

Finally, it should be noted that, historically, assessing nutritional status focused on the identification of individuals and groups with nutrient deficiency diseases [FAO/WHO, 1951]. More recently, it has become apparent that nutritional excess such as obesity and hypervitaminoses are important concerns in some areas, especially in developed countries [Young, 1979]. Thus, dependable indicators on nutritional status are required to evaluate these levels of nutriture also.

OBJECTIVES AND APPLICATIONS OF ASSESSMENT OF NUTRITIONAL STATUS

Purposeful assessment of nutritional status requires that specific study objectives be carefully formulated and that detailed research questions be defined in terms of specific variables. The level of specification here includes nutrients of interest, expected severity of problems, target groups, research design, confounding factors, etc. Appropriate indicators of nutritional status are then selected to answer the corresponding research questions.

In a single discussion, it is neither possible nor probably desirable to detail all possible objectives and research questions; nevertheless, a basic understanding of general objectives and their demands upon indicators of nutritional status is useful in selecting appropriate indicators. Moreover, understanding applications of indicators of nutritional status helps to define better their role in nutritional studies. Three general objectives for studies using indicators of nutritional status and referenced examples of their applications are presented in Table II. Clearly, these objectives are related and are not exclusive categories. Indeed, a single study may well include several components each with different objectives.

Descriptions of Populations or Groups

The most basic objective and application of indicators of nutritional status are to characterize or compare general levels of nutriture among groups or populations. This is usually based on statistics of central tendency (means or medians). Because it is the group statistics that are of main concern rather than those of individuals, less precision of measurement of indicators is required than for most individual-level applications.

TABLE II. General Objectives for Assessment of Nutritional Status and Examples of Application

Objectives	Examples of applications
Descriptions of populations or groups	Owen et al. [1974] Standal and Tiangha [1977] Martorell et al. [1984]
Identification of individuals and groups at risk	Lowenstein [1962] Bistrian et al. [1975] Yanochik-Owen and White [1977] CDC [1979] Chen et al. [1980] Salusky et al. [1983]
Evaluation of treatments and interventions	Rajalakshmi et al. [1973] Edozien et al. [1976] Gershoff et al. [1977] Edozien et al. [1979] Rush et al. [1980]

This reduced requirement for precision relates to the amount of *random* error resulting from observers, instruments, or procedures. Random error is always present in imperfect measurements. These errors are assumed to be independent of the true value of the measurement (although this is often untrue). They increase the observed variance terms of the measurements, i.e. standard deviation, but they do not affect the means or medians. Many data collectors, adverse field conditions, limited training, and inexperienced observers all tend to favor random error.

It is important that *systematic* error, or bias, be minimized among groups when describing their nutritional status. Systematic error results from consistent errors in one direction. For example, if some of the observers are systematically measuring high or low. These errors may not affect the variance of the indicator but they will shift the means or medians. Using the same data collectors for all groups to be compared will help in this regard, as will careful attention to standardization of data collection protocols. Of course, when results are compared to reference data, it is important to follow closely the measurement protocols specified.

The construction of reference data is an application that requires specialized attention to sampling, data collection, analysis, and presentation. Some of these concerns have been addressed in detail elsewhere and are beyond the scope of this discussion [Goldstein, 1979; Neumann, 1979). Similarly, the construction of reliable reference data, even for local purposes, should not be approached casually. Such an effort should include considerable consultation with statisticians experienced in these matters.

For meaningful interpretation of results, it is critical that indicators used to describe the nutritional status of groups or populations have demonstrated validity and that they are presented in conventional ways to facilitate comparisons. Validity in this context means that the indicators have been shown to really measure what they are intended to measure. Too often, "clever" or "innovative" approaches which allow little basis for comparison or for straightforward interpretation of nutritional status are used to describe groups. Such a conservative approach to describing nutritional status does not preclude true innovation *in addition* to a more conventional approach; rather, it allows a benchmark to aid in interpretation of less familiar indicators. Certainly, for most purely descriptive purposes, well-established indicators of nutritional status provide the surest bet for meaningful results.

Identification of Those at Risk

Accurately identifying individuals and groups at nutritional risk based on indicators of nutritional status is central to public health, and it is necessary to understand this basic application of indicators of nutritional status. The risk determination is based on cut-off points in the distribution of indicators of nutritional status relative to some acceptable standard of reference. These cut-off points mark the boundaries of acceptability of the nutriture reflected by the indicators and the probability of impaired function or adverse sequelae.

For example, Chen et al. [1980] have demonstrated rather marked thresholds in anthropometric indicators expressed as percentages of the Harvard standards as they relate to subsequent mortality of infants in Bengladesh. Below 70% of standard for weight for age, the mortality in the following year rose sharply. One might select 80% of standard as a cut-off point for weight for age in such a population. If the weight of an examined child falls below this level, the risk of imminent clinical malnutrition or death is considered unacceptable for that child and he or she is referred for appropriate treatment. Implicit in identifying individuals at nutritional risk is a suitable referral mechanism to allow these individuals to receive proper treatment and follow-up.

When the targets of assessment are groups rather than individuals, cut-off points may be combined with "trigger levels" to define criteria for intervention [WHO, 1976]. Here, trigger levels refer to the proportion of the examined population that fall beyond some established cut-off point. In the case of weight for age, we may specify 10% of the population below 80% of the standard as our trigger level. If greater than 10% of the examined target population then fall below 80% of the standard, a predetermined intervention is initiated (or triggered) in response.

In assessing groups, it is important that the sample included is representative, in a statistical sense, of the larger population. Using a single source for the sample, like a clinic population, will likely lead to an unrepresentative sample. Careful attention should be given to establishing the appropriate sampling frame.

Clearly, the reference data, cut-off points, and trigger levels need to be chosen with great care because the effectiveness of the risk assessments depend on these determinations. Special care must be taken in the measurement of indicators used to assess individuals, as slight errors one way or another can determine whether or not the individual receives needed treatment. On the one hand, liberal cut-off points will increase sensitivity of indicators and reduce the number of individuals who are false negatives, i.e., really malnourished but not determined as such by the indicators. On the other hand, a too-liberal cut-off point leads to reduced specificity, unnecessary expense, and an inefficient program.

Nutritional surveillance includes risk identification, but extends to much broader goals as well [WHO, 1976]. Here, surveillance refers to a continuous effort to collect and report information regarding nutritional status, usually on a large scale. This information is then used to select preventive or ameliorative measures, to set priorities for planning purposes, and to assist in the formulation of policy.

There is a growing interest in developing indicators of nutritional status for chronically ill or hospitalized patients [Salusky et al., 1983; Bistrian et al., 1975]. These individuals may have unique needs due to their specific disease or to hypermetabolism not seen in most ambulatory patients and otherwise unanticipated based on reduced activity levels.

Another special application of risk identification is the use of indicators of nutritional status as the basis of triage in managing emergencies with nutritional implications in large populations [de Ville de Goyet et al., 1978]. This approach has been successfully applied, e.g. in Africa [Lowenstein, 1962; Aall, 1970], and some countries have now incorporated such schemes in their emergency planning.

Evaluation of Treatments or Intervention Programs

The demands upon indicators used in evaluating impacts on individuals and groups are more rigorous than in the applications described above. These requirements of indicators arise from technical issues in the general design of evaluations and from the need for unambiguous interpretations of results.

Customarily, evaluations of individuals and groups compare change in indicators between those receiving treatments or group interventions and those not receiving them. Differences then, between treatment and control groups are attributable to the intervention. This is, of course, a greatly simplified description and there are many complex designs and important technical issues regarding evaluations [Klein et al., 1979; Campbell and Stanley, 1963], most of which are beyond the scope of the present discussion.

Detecting changes in indicators generally requires that indicators be measured relatively more precisely than when the same indicators are used in a one-time survey. In the simplest case, change in an indicator may be described as an increment or difference score: postintervention level less preintervention level. Whereas a single measurement of the indicator is accompanied by a single measurement error term, the increment is accompanied by two error terms, one on each measurement occasion. The relative difficulty in detecting change is twofold: 1) Increments are usually smaller than attained values, but their standard deviations are relatively larger; and 2) The error variance of increments is a relatively larger proportion of the total variance of increments than is the error variance of the attained values relative to their total variance.

An example of differences between attained values and increments in the same variable is given in Table III. These are data for attained values and

TABLE III. Measurement Error for Attained Values and Increments of Periosteal Diameter (mm) of Second Metacarpal of Malnourished Children[a]

Components	Attained values	Annual increments
Mean	4.62	0.34
SD	0.40	0.15
Error variance[b]	0.0036	0.0072
Error SD[c]	0.0600	0.0849
% Error[d]	1.30	24.97
Coefficient of variation[e]	11.55	2.27
R[f]	0.15	0.57

[a]From Himes et al [1975].

[b]$\dfrac{\Sigma d^2}{2n}$, where d, difference between replicate measurements; n, number of pairs (25).

[c] $\sqrt{\dfrac{\Sigma d^2}{2n}}$

[d](Error SD/mean) 100.
[e]Mean/SD.
[f]R, Error SD/SD.

annual increments in periosteal diameters of the left second metacarpal, based on measurements from radiographs of malnourished Guatemalan children [Himes et al., 1975]. In absolute terms the error variance for the increments is twice that for the attained values. The observed mean and standard deviation of the increments are smaller than those for the attained values but this difference is relatively greater for the means.

Virtually all parametric tests of means use a function of the standard deviation as a denominator (usually standardized for sample size). Thus, as the standard deviation increases relative to its mean, it is progressively more difficult to detect significant differences between means. For the example in Table III, it is clear that the mean attained value (4.62) is much larger relative to its standard deviation (0.4) than is the mean increment (0.34) relative to its standard deviation (0.15). These relationships are demonstrated by comparing the coefficients of variation in Table III (11.55 vs 2.27). The contribution of the measurement error per se to this disparity between attained values and increments is shown by the % errors: the measurement error standard deviation is almost 25% of the mean increment while it is little more than 1% of the mean attained value.

For statistics focusing on shared variance, e.g. analysis of variance, correlation, regression, a more important concern is that the measurement error standard deviation is a rather large proportion of the observed standard deviation in increments (R 0.57) compared to the corresponding ratio for attained values (R 0.15). The fact that a large proportion of the observed variance is error makes it difficult to detect true variation because of extraneous noise or error.

A practical implication of the foregoing is that some satisfactory indicators for assessing static nutritional status may not be adequate for evaluating change in nutritional status. In some cases, this problem can be overcome by increasing sample sizes or by reducing probable sources of error, although one may have practical limitations to modifying these aspects. This issue has been addressed for selected indicators by Yarbrough et al. [1974].

It is difficult to extrapolate from changes in indicators of nutritional status in individuals in response to interventions to those of group responses [Habicht and Butz, 1979]. Group responses depend upon the distribution of individuals who will actually respond to the intervention and upon the distribution of the intervention treatment. In nutritional supplementation studies, for example, not all individuals ingest the same amount of supplement [Rush et al., 1980], nor is the supplement necessarily consumed in proportion to needs.

If only a small percentage of an intervention group responds to nutritional supplementation, these improvements in nutritional status may not be reflected in appreciable changes in the group means of indicators of nutritional status. For example, of those women classified as anemic, probably less than 10% would benefit from iron therapy [Meyers et al., 1979]. It is this variability in the proportion of those identified who respond to intervention that contributes to the differences between the sensitivity of an indicator on an individual level and the sensitivity of the indicator on a population or group level.

Evaluations of impact on nutritional status may be restricted to a very small number of individuals and focus on a single nutrient treatment effect. Alternatively, evaluations may be extended to very large population studies in which a variety of social, economic and medical interventions are taking place. In the latter case, the direct nutritional treatment may be only a small portion of the overall intervention. Clearly, as the program to be evaluated grows in size and complexity, the demands on design, specificity of indicators, and sophistication of analysis increase also.

FIELD CONSIDERATIONS

Often conditions in the field interfere with purposeful assessment of nutritional status. Recognizing and dealing with some of these situations favor meaningful results.

The problems of choosing the most appropriate measurements and protocols are often magnified in field situations for logistical reasons. Delicate or bulky equipment is difficult to transport satisfactorily. Specific needs for some procedures that are accomodated easily in a clinical or city setting may pose enormous problems in the field. Particularly, biochemical indicators of nutritional status customarily require at least a power source and refrigeration for preparing samples to be sent to laboratories. Some procedures require specialized equipment and experienced personnel that are usually not found in most commercial or hospital laboratories. In some cases, portable equipment is available, i.e., generators, centrifuges, etc, but consideration of such limitations in the planning stages will aid in selecting the most appropriate indicators and may obviate subsequent problems.

Much of the usefulness of indicators of nutritional status depends upon the care with which measurements are taken. In some large field surveys, many individuals with little or no previous experience may need training to collect the necessary data. One must assess beforehand the degree of sophistication of measurements that will best accommodate the project objectives and the level of expertise of the data collectors, and then choose the appropriate measurement protocols. As a rule, one must plan on greater observer variability in field studies compared to that expected in more controlled situations. This, of course, increases the sample sizes necessary to achieve a degree of statistical precision and sensitivity similar to that attained in more controlled studies. Systematic training and standardization of data collectors can help reduce these problems and useful guidelines have been described [Habicht, 1974].

For a field study of nutritional status to be successful, one must obtain the support of the communities involved. This includes cooperation from governing and administrative officials, as well as acceptance and support from the populace [Townsend et al., 1979]. To stress a need for careful consideration of local cultural and linguistic factors to anthropologists seems redundant. Nevertheless, it is clear that many local practices can confound and vitiate the results, e.g. personal hygiene, weaning, child rearing, sanitation, food and other taboos, etc. Similarly, a knowledge of local environmental factors is necessary for meaningful interpretation of results, e.g. quality and availability of water, crops cultivated, pattern of rainfall, season of this year, etc.

Many indicators of nutritional status are linked to categories of chronological age, especially those taken during the childhood years. In many developing countries, one is faced with the problem of accurate determination of chronological age of children because of no formal birth or age registration. In these areas, approximations of a child's age should be obtained whenever possible. Inquiries should be made of parents or other relatives regarding important events or other calendar-related associations that may be linked with the child's birth. An approximate age is better than no age at all.

Accurate assessment of age is especially important during the periods of rapid growth (infancy and adolescence). Most indirect methods, such as counting of deciduous teeth in young children may be appropriate for groups but are unsatisfactory for individuals because of the wide individual variation in the timing of deciduous eruption [Meredith, 1946; Delgado et al., 1975]. In reporting all studies, care should be taken to explain how age was determined.

CONCLUSIONS

Clearly, many factors contribute to purposeful assessment of nutritional status and to successful nutritional studies. The aim of the foregoing has been to address some factors frequently overlooked in studies incorporating assessment of nutritional status. There are certainly many factors contributive to purposeful assessment of nutritional status that have not been included.

Recommending specific indicators of nutritional status has been avoided intentionally. There are many good references dealing with various indicators of nutritional status and these should be referred to by the interested reader [Jelliffe, 1966; WHO, 1976; Beaton and McHenry, 1966; Himes, 1980; Johnston, 1981; Pi-Sunyer and Woo, 1984].

Although it seems trite to recommend intensive and detailed preparation before nutritional studies, it is, nonetheless, clear that most of the difficulties, especially in interpretation of results, could be avoided with competent planning beforehand. Too often, statistical and analytical issues are not anticipated with the same degree of concern as are logistical issues. Assessment of nutritional status is an important tool with wide applications in nutrition-related studies. Its potential contribution is enhanced if it is sharp and purposeful.

REFERENCES

Aall C (1970): Relief, nutrition and health problems in the Nigerian/Biafran war. J Trop Pediat 16:70-90.

Beaton GH, McHenry EW (eds) (1966): "Nutrition. A Comprehensive Treatise. Vol III. Nutritional Status: Assessment and Application." New York: Academic Press.

Bistrian BR, Blackburn GL, Sherman M, Scrimshaw NS (1975): Therapeutic index of nutritional depletion in hospitalized patients. Sur Gynecol Obstet 141:512-516.

Buzina R (1982): Nutrition in health and disease and international development. In Harper AE, Davis GK (eds): "XII International Congress of Nutrition." New York: Alan R Liss, pp 285-303.

Campbell DT, Stanley JC (1963): "Experimental and Quasi-Experimental Designs for Research." Boston: Houghton Mifflin Co.

CDC (1979): Centers for Disease Control Nutritional Surveillance. Annual Summary 1979. Washington, D.C.: U.S. Gov't Printing Office.

Chen LC, Chowdhury AKM, Huffman SL (1980): Anthropometric assessment of energy-protein malnutrition and subsequent risk of mortality among preschool-aged children. Am J Clin Nutr 33:1836-1845.

Delgado H, Habicht J-P, Yarbrough C, Lechtig A, Mortorell R, Malina RM, Klein RE (1975): Nutritional status and the timing of deciduous tooth eruption. Am J Clin Nutr 28:216-224.

Dobbing J, Sands J (1978): Head circumference, biparietal diameter and brain growth in fetal and postnatal life. Early Hum Develop 2:81-87.

Edozien JC, Khan MAR, Waslien CI (1976): Human protein deficiency: results of a Nigerian village study. J Nutr 106:312-328.

Edozien JC, Switzer BR, Bryan RB (1979): Medical evaluation of the special supplemental food program for women, infants and children. Am J Clin Nutr 32:677-692.

Engsner G, Relete S, Sjogren I, Vahlquist B (1974): Brain growth in children with marasmus. Uppsala J Med Sci 79:116-128.

FAO/WHO (1951): "Food and Agriculture Organization and World Health Organization Joint Expert Committee on Nutrition Report." WHO Tech Rpt Ser 44, Geneva: World Health Organization.

Gershoff SN, McGandy RB, Sullapreysri D, Promkutkao C, Nondasuta A, Pisolyabutra U, Tantiwongse P, Viraviadhaya V (1977): Nutrition studies in Thailand. II. Effects of fortification of rice with lysine, thrionine, thiamin, riboflavin, vitamin A, and iron on preschool children. Am J Clin Nutr 30:1185-1195.

Goldstein H (1979): "The Design and Analysis of Longitudinal Studies." New York: Academic Press.

Habicht J-P (1974): Estandarización de métodos epidemiológicos cuantitativos sobre el terreno. Bol of San Pan 76:375-384.

Habicht J-P, Butz WP (1979): Measurement of health and nutrition effects of large-scale nutrition intervention projects. In Klein RE, Read MS, Riecken HW, Brown JA, Pradilla A, Daza C (eds): "Evaluating the Impact of Nutrition and Health Programs." New York: Plenum Press, pp 133-170.

Habicht J-P, Yarbrough C, Martorell R (1979): Anthropometric field methods: Criteria for selection. In Jelliffe DB, Jelliffe EFP (eds): "Nutrition and Growth." New York: Plenum Press, pp 365-387.

Himes JH (1980): Subcutaneous fat thickness as an indicator of nutritional status. In Green LS, Johnston FE (eds): "Social and Biological Predictors of Nutritional Status, Physical Growth, and Neurological Development." New York: Academic Press, pp 9-32.

Himes JH (1982): Energy as a factor limiting growth of children. "Food in Contemporary Society: Energy, the Critical Factor." Proceedings of Stokley-Van Camp Annual Symposium. Knoxville Tenn: University of Tennessee, pp 40-55.

Himes JH, Martorell R, Habicht J-P, Yarbrough C, Malina RM, Klein RE (1975): Patterns of cortical bone growth in moderately malnourished preschool children. Hum Biol 47:337-350.

INACG (1981): "Iron Deficiency in Women." The International Nutritional Anemia Consultive Group. New York: The Nutrition Foundation.

Jelliffe DB (1966): "The Assessment of the Nutritional Status of the Community." Geneva: World Health Organization.

Johnston FE (1981): Anthropometry and nutritional status. In: "Assessing Changing Food Consumption Patterns." Washington DC: National Academy Press, pp 252-264.

Klein RE, Read MS, Riecken HW, Brown JA, Pradilla A, Daza C (1979): "Evaluating the Impact of Nutrition and Health Programs." New York: Plenum Press.

Lowenstein FW (1962): An epidemic of kwashiorkor in the South Kasai, Congo. Bull Wld Hlth Org 27:751-758.

Martorell R, Leslie J, Moock PR (1984): Characteristics and determinants of child nutritional status in Nepal. Am J Clin Nutr 39:74-86.

McLaren DS (1976): "Nutrition in the Community." New York: Wiley.

Meredith HV (1946): Order and age of eruption for the deciduous dentition. J Dent Res 25:43-58.

Meyers L, Habicht J-P, Johnson CL (1979): Components of the difference in hemoglobin concentration in blood between black and white women in the US. Am J Epidemiol 109:539-549.

Neumann C (1979): Reference data. In Jelliffe DB, Jelliffe EFP (eds): "Human Nutrition: A Comprehensive Treatise, Vol 2. Nutrition and Growth." New York: Plenum Press, pp 299-328.

Owen GM, Kram KM, Garry PJ, Lowe JE, Lubin AH (1974): A study of nutritional status of preschool children in the United States, 1968-1970. Pediat (Suppl) 53:597-645.

Pi-Sunyer FX, Woo R (1984): Laboratory assessment of nutritional status. In Simko MD, Lowell C, Gilbride JA (eds): "Nutrition Assessment. A Comprehensive Guide for Planning Intervention." Rockville MD: Aspen System Corp, pp 139-174.

Rajalakshmi R, Sail SS, Shar DG, Ambody SK (1973): The effects of supplements varying in carotene and calcium content on physical, biochemical and skeletal status of preschool children. Brit J Nutri 30:77-86.

Rush D, Stein Z, Susser M (1980): "Diet in Pregnancy: A Randomized Controlled Trial of Nutritional Supplements." BD: OAS, Vol XVI, No. 3, New York: Alan R. Liss.

Salusky IB, Fine RN, Nelson P, Blumenkrantz MJ, Kopple JD (1983): Nutritional status of children undergoing continuous ambulatory peritoneal dialysis. Am J Clin Nutr 38:599-611.

Solomons NW, Allen LH (1983): The functional assessment of nutritional status: Principles, practice and potential. Nutr Rev 41:33-50.

Standal BR, Tiangha MF (1977): Assessing the anthropometric status of Hawaii's preschoolers participating in feeding programs in day care centers. Am J Clin Nutr 30:2101-2107.

Townsend JW, Farrell WT, Klein RE (1979): Special issues for the measurement of program impact in developing countries. In Klein RE, Read MS, Riecken HW, Brown JA, Pradilla A, Daza C (eds): "Evaluating the Impact of Nutrition and Health Programs." New York: Plenum Press, pp 99-123.

de Ville de Goyet C, Seaman J, Geijer U (1978): "The Management of Nutritional Emergencies in Large Populations." Geneva: World Health Organization.

WHO (1976): "Methodology of Nutritional Surveillance." Report of a joint FAO/UNICEF/WHO Expert Committee. WHO Tech Rept Ser 593. Geneva: World Health Organization.

Yanochik-Owen A, White M (1977): Nutrition surveillance in Arizona: Selected anthropometric and laboratory observations among Mexican-American children. Am J Pub Health 67:151-154.

Yarbrough C, Habicht J-P, Martorell R, Klein RE (1974): Anthropometry as an index of nutritional status. In Roche AF, Falkner R (eds): "Nutrition and Malnutrition: Identification and Measurement." New York: Plenum Press, pp 15-26.

Young CM (1979): Overnutrition. In Rechcigel M (ed): "Nutrition and the World Food Problem." Basel: S Karger, pp 195-217.

Nutritional Anthropology, pages 101-116
© 1987 Alan R. Liss, Inc.

Assessment of Energy Expenditure and Physical Activity Pattern in Population Studies

Angelo Tremblay, PhD and Claude Bouchard, PhD

Physical Activity Sciences Laboratory and Center for Research on Nutrition,
Laval University, Quebec, Canada G1K 7P4

Energy expenditure of the human organism is a complex phenotype that includes the contribution of several components. Among these, it is generally recognized that basal energy expenditure, energy expenditure associated with adjustment to cold or heat, energy expenditure related to food consumption, and energy expenditure of work and leisure activities are the most important to consider. This review will focus on the assessment of energy expenditure associated with work or occupational and leisure activities in large groups or for the purpose of population studies.

The assessment of energy expenditure in humans as well as in animals is basically undertaken under the assumption that the oxidation of substrates is necessary to replenish high energy phosphate bonds in nucleotides, particularly in ATP. Energy expenditure is generally determined in the laboratory by measuring heat production and respiratory gases, that is, by direct and indirect calorimetry, respectively. These procedures are accurate to assess work and leisure caloric expenditure but their applicability is very limited for testing in population studies. In these cases, investigators have developed more practical methods such as heart rate measurement, the use of portable recording instruments, diaries, and questionnaires.

The estimation of energy expenditure is often performed to characterize the physical activity pattern of individuals and to determine the association with health indicators, socioeconomic factors, cultural differences, and other biosocial correlates. In such situations, the quantification of energy expenditure can tolerate a reasonable level of error, one which is generally higher than in metabolic experiments conducted in a small number of subjects under well controlled laboratory conditions. The question that may be raised is to what extent can these more practical methods satisfy the requirements of population studies. It is the purpose of this chapter to briefly describe these methods and to discuss their characteristics in terms of applicability, validity, and reproducibility.

DIRECT CALORIMETRY

Lavoisier was probably the first to try to measure animal heat production and he used an ice chamber [Lusk, 1931]. During the second half of the last century, Pettenkofer and Voit initiated the construction of a calorimeter for the determination of heat dissipated by the human body. The thermally insulated chamber designed by these investigators was small to assure adequate sensitivity of measurements. This principle still remains valid today. From a practical point of view, the calorimeter is thus reserved for the assessment of energy expenditure in the resting state or during stationary activities, like exercising on a cycle ergometer. Direct calorimetry remains an important procedure and it can also be used to validate field techniques like the heart rate method [Dauncey and James, 1979].

The use of direct calorimetry is also restricted due to the cost of the device, which probably explains in part the fact that few calorimeters are operating today. An alternative to the conventional calorimeter has been proposed by Webb et al [1972]. Their calorimeter is a clothing assembly consisting of a water cooled undergarment and overlying insulating garments. Water flows through tubes in contact with the skin, and from the flow rate of water and its temperature change, heat loss can be computed. This system is less expensive than the conventional calorimeter and is convenient for energy balance studies in man [Webb et al., 1980].

INDIRECT CALORIMETRY

The indirect measurement of energy expenditure from respiratory gases can be performed in the laboratory as well as in the field. This technique has often been used to assess the caloric cost of various actvities, thus allowing the preparation of tables which are currently employed to estimate energy expenditure from physical activity records [Passmore and Durnin, 1955; Consolazio et al, 1963; Durnin and Passmore, 1967]. Many investigators have also applied indirect calorimetry to evaluate the resting components of energy expenditure, particularly resting metabolic rate (RMR) and dietary-induced thermogenesis (DIT). In addition to the well-established role of age and body weight on RMR and/or DIT, several studies have indicated that they can be influenced by the state of nutrition [Miller and Mumford, 1967; Apfelbaum et al., 1971], composition of diet [Nair et al., 1983], exercise training [Tremblay et al., 1983; Leblanc et al., 1984], body composition [Hoffmans et al., 1979; Ravussin et al., 1982], and by conditions like obesity [Kaplan and Léveillé, 1976; Shetty et al., 1981] and diabetes mellitus [Golay et al., 1982]. From these research efforts, it should be obvious that one has to take into account several factors when interpreting energy expenditure data obtained by one method or another.

HEART RATE METHOD

Heart rate and oxygen consumption are linearly associated, particularly above the resting level and below maximal work power. On the basis of this relationship, heart rate has been widely used to predict energy expenditure in various activities. The procedure requires that a regression line of heart rate versus energy expenditure be derived for each activity or family of activities. Indirect calorimetry, and occasionally direct calorimetry have been used to measure energy expenditure. Thereafter, heart rate is recorded during normal daily life activities, and heart rate values are referred to the appropriate regression lines to determine their energy equivalents.

Several experiments have been performed to estimate the accuracy of this procedure and the conditions under which its application is most appropriate. Bradfield et al [1969] showed that during 4 h of controlled steady-state activities, the accumulated pulse measurement and a respirometer diary provided results that were within 10% of each other. Similar results were obtained by Astrand [1971] who observed that in activities requiring approximately 0.8 $1 O_2 \cdot min^{-1}$, a regression of heart rate on $\dot{V}O_2$ overestimated by about 0.1 1 $O_2 \cdot min^{-1}$ the energy cost determined by air collection. Using energy intake and body composition changes as reference measurements, Acheson et al. [1980] also found that the heart rate method overestimated energy expenditure. With seven different regression lines, the overestimation ranged between 150 and 930 kcal, or about 5 to 30% of error.

In the field, one has the possibility to perform individual or group regression lines. Between these two procedures, substantial variations can be observed. Goldsmith et al [1966] showed that the regression derived from data obtained in one individual differed from that of another subject. Bradfield et al. [1970] demonstrated that the use of individual regression improved the predictability of heart rate as an indirect measure of energy expenditure when compared to a group regression. The selection of techniques then becomes a choice between the speed and convenience of group regression versus the accuracy of individual regression lines.

The body position and the type of work tasks involved must be taken into account when applying the heart rate method. Thus, heart rate is influenced when changing from the supine to the standing position [Payne et al., 1971]. Moreover, Andrews [1967] showed that, for a given heart rate, energy expenditure is different when legs are active compared to when they are passive, a difference which could be attributed to homeostatically related factors. These observations tend to support the notion that there are numerous regressions depending upon position and work tasks involved. The specificity of the heart rate—$\dot{V}O_2$ relationship probably accounts for some of the variation found by Acheson et al. [1980] between seven regression lines calculated using different activities.

Maxfield [1971] pointed out that heart rate is a valid predictor of energy expenditure when it is associated with a change in work load. Standard heart rate-energy expenditure regression lines traditionally ignored or used only few points of calibration in the vicinity of resting energy expenditure. Under these conditions, the prediction of energy expenditure tends to be unreliable. Thus, Dauncey and James [1979] found that in sedentary individuals, with 24-h mean heart rate typically close to the resting level or at the lower end of the calibration curve, considerable overestimates and underestimates were observed. However, the use of linear regression fitted to points obtained at the lower end of the energy expenditure improved the prediction of the 24-h heat production. In another experiment [Booyens and Hervey, 1960], it has been demonstrated that the relationship between heart rate and heat production during quiet activities such as lying and sitting showed more variation than during exercise.

The above observations emphasize the need to obtain several reference points in the resting state and, perhaps, even to calculate specific regression for sedentary and vigorous activities [Malhotra, 1963]. In this case, however, a diary would have to be completed concomitantly with heart rate measurements to calculate the time spent in each category of activities. Intensity and percent time spent in each activity category could also be registered with a special heart rate counter. An example of this type of device has been developed by the World Health Organization [Masironi and Mansourian, 1974]. Briefly, this apparatus subdivides into eight categories of intensity the heart rates recorded over a period of time. The use of such a system would provide more detailed information than that obtained by using only heartbeat totalizers.

In their review of literature concerning the assessment of energy requirements, Buskirk and Mendez [1980] qualified the heart rate method as moderate and weak in terms of applicability and accuracy, respectively. Durnin [1982] recently indicated that when accurate measurements of energy expenditure are needed, one would be naive using the heart rate method. Therefore, the application of this method appears to be appropriate only when some error can be tolerated in the quantification of energy expenditure. The method was used in studies attempting to discriminate between the expenditure of obese and nonobese subjects [Bradfield et al., 1971]. The procedure has also been applied by Griffiths and Payne [1976] to evaluate the relationship between obese and normal-weight parents and the activity level of their children.

MOVEMENT RECORDING DEVICES

A substantial fraction of the daily energy expenditure is related to movement of trunk or limbs. Based on this observation, several instruments have been designed to assess movement in an effort to quantify energy expenditure or pattern of participation in activities.

Pedometer

One of these recording devices is the pedometer, an instrument the size of a pocket watch which is inexpensive and easy to use. Movement is recorded by a balance arm which is displaced in the vertical plane. The apparatus is generally worn suspended from the waist, other sites such as the ankle being likely less appropriate [Saris and Binkhorst, 1977a]. During walking or running, each step transmits an impulse to the balance arm.

Even after appropriate calibration, some practical problems are observed using the pedometer. Thus, movements other than walking can influence pedometer counting. This complicates the interpretation of what is actually measured by the instrument. For instance, results ranging between 0.3 and 1.3 units per stride were reported when walking at different speeds [Saris and Binkhorst, 1977a]. In that case, the instrument underestimated the actual step rate by 0.2 to 0.7 counts per step during slow walking, but an overestimation of 0.1 to 0.3 counts per step was noted during fast walking. Finally, these investigators showed that the relationship between estimations of energy expenditure and pedometer counts varied considerably depending on the activity performed.

From these observations, it is clear that the pedometer should not be used when accuracy is needed, even for the measurment of distance walked. However, the instrument remains convenient to estimate physical activity pattern since pedometer counts are generally well correlated with habitual physical activities as appraised by observation [Saris and Binkhorst, 1977b]. In field studies, several investigators have used the pedometer to compare physical activity habits of obese and nonobese subjects. In general, obese individuals tended to be less active compared to their controls [Dorris and Stunkard, 1957; Chirico and Stunkard, 1960; Wilkinson et al., 1977], although other investigators failed to reproduce this finding [Maxfield and Konishi, 1966].

Actometer

The impulses generated by movements like walking and running can also be converted in energy units using an actometer. As for the pedometer, this instrument resembles a watch and is sensitive to acceleration and deceleration. When fixed at the ankle, it responds in proportion to walking and running speeds and with their respective energy costs [Saris and Binkhorst, 1977a]. This sensitivity is not observed when it is placed on the wrist. Thus, the actometer fixed at the ankle appears better than the pedometer to reflect locomotion. Moreover, high correlations were reported between ankle actometer measurements and those of usual physical activities [Saris and Binkhorst, 1977b]. For the wrist actometer, the correlations were also significant but lower than when the instrument was fixed on the ankle. In population studies, the applicability of the actometer is comparable to that of the pedometer to assess physical activity pattern. For instance, Massey et al. [1971] developed an inexpensive actometer for the assessment of activity participation in mentally deficient persons. Since the actometer can reflect changes in intensity during activities of locomotion, it should preferably be used over the pedometer.

Accelerometer

Recently, Montoye et al. [1983] described an accelerometer designed to assess energy expenditure. These investigators observed that the instrument was not sensitive to changes in slope during walking and running and that the energy cost of static exercise and of body support was not appraised by the accelerometer. These limitations probably also characterize other procedures using acceleration and deceleration to assess energy expenditure.

Large Scale Integrated Activity Monitor (LSI)

Body movement has also been measured using an instrument called LSI. This apparatus, described by Laporte et al. [1979] resembles a wrist watch in which a ball of mercury has been placed. A 3° inclination or declination from the horizontal produces closure of the mercury switch, which is registered by an internal counter. The LSI can be placed on various sites of the body. Laporte et al. [1979] reported that trunk movements are more correlated with energy expenditure estimated from logging activities than ankle movements. In another study, Laporte et al. [1983] compared LSI values to those provided by the diary described by Paffenberger et al. [1978]. Even though the two methods were found to be very stable, their results were not well correlated. Their weak association was explained by the fact that each procedure is measuring different aspects of physical activity. Indeed, while the LSI monitors movement, the Paffenbarger method evaluates the intensity of activities. Thus, as for the other instruments discussed above, the LSI ignored the energy expenditure that is not associated with movement.

DIARIES

Records of physical activities can be obtained following one of several standardized procedures. Current methods include the recording by the subject or by an observer [Bradfield et al., 1971], the classification by occupation [Mayer et al., 1956], and the analysis from a filmed record of activities [Bullen et al., 1964]. Among these methods the following are believed to be the most appropriate for this review.

Diary - Calorimetry

Theoretically, the most accurate procedure in this category should be a combination of the diary and the calorimetric measurements. Briefly, this method requires that the cost of activities recorded be individually determined by respiratory movements. It is an elaborate procedure since new measurements are needed for each activity introduced in the diary. To be accurate, the laboratory determinations of oxygen uptake must match closely the activity recorded at the time of the diary, which may cause some problems [Andrews, 1971]. Satisfactory results were, however, reported by Acheson et al. [1980] who found that the method overestimated, by only 3%, reference values obtained from dietary records and body composition changes over a period of 6 to 12 months. The method was also used to estimate energy expenditure in a small group of obese housewives over a 4-week period [Curtis and Bradfield, 1971]. However, the method is not suited for application in large groups of subjects but, once the laboratory measurements have been obtained, it would seem advantageous to use them in conjunction with diary records over a long period of time.

Diary - RMR

A practical modification of the above method has been to use a diary concomitantly with the assessment of RMR. RMR can be easily and accurately determined during a short laboratory session using indirect calorimetry. Tables describing the cost of activities as multiples of RMR are utilized to derive caloric expenditure [Blackburn and Calloway, 1976]. This technique assumes that the intensity of activities, as quantified in multiples of RMR, is similar in the subjects of the study compared to that of the reference population from which the tables were derived. Even though data are lacking concerning this assumption, the estimates of energy costs are probably close to the more direct laboratory measurements of the diary-calorimetry method. If proven true, a gain in practicability would be achieved without a marked loss of accuracy. This would be of great importance, since the method is suitable for application to groups of moderate size. Gorsky and Calloway [1983] have apparently obtained satisfactory evaluation of energy expenditure changes in ten men submitted to 30 days of restricted diet using this approach.

Diary-Tables

Energy expenditure can also be calculated strictly from a diary and tables of caloric cost of activities [Passmore and Durnin, 1955; Consolazio et al., 1963; Durnin and Passmore, 1967]. This method is widely used as no laboratory measurements are needed to estimate energy expenditure. In this case, however, it is assumed that values obtained in the reference population, i.e., data of tables, would not be different from those of subjects on which the estimation is applied to. As no interindividual differences are controlled by this procedure, the accuracy of the method is probably lower than that of the diary-calorimetry or the diary-RMR techniques. However, Acheson et al. [1980] found only a small difference between estimates provided by a diary in conjunction with data of the literature and a diary-calorimetry procedure. Surprisingly, they found that the diary-table method provided a better prediction of mean daily expenditure as determined from dietary records and body composition changes over a period of 6 to 12 months than the diary-calorimetry method.

When the diary-table technique is applied to subjects performing regularly walking and/or running at different intensities, it is advantageous to assess the energy cost of these activities with more refined formulas instead of simple tables. Such formulas [Silverman and Anderson, 1972; Falls and Humphrey, 1976; Pandolf et al., 1977] take into account the intensity of the activity, which is undoubtedly better than using the fixed values of some tables. Moreover, as a close relationship exists between body weight and energy expenditure while walking and running, a suggestion is to apply a formula that controls for this variable.

From a practical point of view, a diary is acceptable to determine the physical activity pattern of an individual. When this approach is taken to quantify energy expenditure, errors are expected, but the mean estimate of daily energy output should be close to the values provided by more accurate techniques [Acheson et al., 1980]. However, if the purpose of a study is to obtain a summary of the overall activity level, a diary is sufficient [Hueneman et al., 1967] and, perhaps, even unnecessary. Indeed, in such cases, a questionnaire, which is easier to apply, could then be sufficient to meet the objective [Bishop et al., 1975].

Categorial Scoring

A semiquantitative diary which simplifies the recording of activities is sometimes used in large population studies. This is generally achieved by using a simple coding system which facilitates the analysis of data. An example of this approach is the system recently described by Bouchard et al. [1983]. This system requires recording on a 1 to 9 scale, the energy cost of the dominant activity performed during each 15 min period over 3 days. Each categorical value of the scale refers to a class of activities grouped together because of their comparable energy cost. The approximate median energy cost associated with each of the nine categorical scores is utilized to compute the daily energy expenditure of an individual. This method was shown to be highly reproducible. Moreover, energy expenditure estimates derived with this system were moderately but significantly correlated with physical working capacity. More recently, it was suggested that the sum of the categorical scores could be used to rank order individuals according to levels of energy expenditure [Bouchard, 1983]. This method presents some similarities with the recall technique described by Yasin [1967] and can be considered as intermediate between a complete diary and the questionnaire method.

However, when a categorical score is used to represent the energy cost of activities in a given category, estimates of energy expenditure may differ somewhat from quantitative diary assessments. Thus, it was recently observed that the method tended to overestimate energy expenditure in male and female adults [Tremblay et al., 1983b]. This can probably be explained by the fact that subjects frequently performed activities whose energy cost was lower than the median energy value for the category. Thus, it was concluded that the procedure is likely not appropriate to quantify exact energy expenditure. On the positive side, the method can be applied to rank order subjects and assess intraindividual changes over a given period of time. In addition, the numerical system used in this method provides a simple approach for the study of patterns of usual physical activities.

QUESTIONNAIRES AND INTERVIEWS

Categorical scoring procedures, questionnaires, and interviews all share in that they are convenient for epidemiological investigation. Questionnaire and interview will generally classify activities into various categories to characterize past and present activity habits.

Questionnaire

Several developments have taken place with this method as participation in physical activities had to be evaluated in several epidemiological studies. Thus, Yasin [1967] applied a recall technique with British Civil servants to assess their activity pattern during the past 2 days. Even though this procedure is generally considered as a questionnaire [Taylor et al., 1978], it bears some resemblance to the Bouchard et al. [1983] categorical scoring system, as noted above. In the Health Insurance Plan (HIP) study of New York, two questionnaires were developed for the assessment of physical activity at work and leisure, respectively [Shapiro et al., 1965]. Data about habitual physical activity were associated with those in maximal oxygen uptake [Taylor et al., 1978].

For the purpose of establishing the relationship between physical activity habits and the risk of a heart attack, a self administered questionnaire was developped by Paffenbarger et al. [1978]. The questionnaire, which was mailed to Harvard male alumni, investigated three categories of activities: climbing stairs, walking blocks, and sports. The energy cost of these activities was derived from standard tables, and a physical activity index was computed using multiples of 2,000 kcal/week expenditure on activities as the unit of measure. Using this index, a higher risk of heart attack was observed in less active persons.

Questionnaire and Interview

A different approach combining both a questionnaire and an interview was used in the Tecumseh community study. As described by Montoye [1971] and Reiff et al. [1967], the procedure included the following steps: first, the interviewer delivered a self-administered questionnaire inquiring about occupations, hours worked, transportation to and from work, and participation in major home repairs and maintainance. Leisure-time sports, gardening, and other physical activities were also checked on a list. Second, a trained interviewer spent from 30 to 60 min with each subject inquiring about leisure activities and occupation. The two procedures together inquired about the activities performed during the preceding year. The scoring system used tables of work to basal metabolic rate ratio. The reliability of the method, as appraised by three judges who analysed data of two groups of 20 subjects, was shown to be satisfactory. Moreover, indirect validity reflected by correlations with cholesterol, blood pressure, and fatness looked promising. The Tecumseh study procedure has been compared to the HIP questionnaire by Buskirk et al. [1971]. They found that correlations between the two methods did not exceed 0.5, indicating that the two techniques were probably not measuring the same dimensions of energy expenditure.

Taylor et al. [1978] adapted the Tecumseh procedure to assess leisure time physical activity. From the questionnaire data, an activity metabolic index taking into account intensity and duration of exercise was developed to discriminate between light, moderate, and heavy activities. It was demonstrated that the procedure was valid to study the relationship of physical activity with disease and in weight control clinics when administered by trained interviewers. Moreover, Laporte et al. [1979] showed that data obtained by this questionnaire were significnatly correlated with body movement measurements estimated by the LSI technique.

In a recent study, Baecke et al. [1982] developed a short questionnaire to evaluate habitual physical activities subdivided into three major components: 1) physical activity at work, 2) sport during leisure time, and 3) physical activity during leisure time excluding sport. The reliability of these three indices was found to be adequate. Moreover, physical fitness indices were differently associated with the indices, which would tend to support the relevance of such a subdivision of activities.

In summary, questionnaires and/or interviews are useful to classify individuals on the basis of usual activity habits, even though data represent only a summary of activities instead of an accurate measurement of energy costs. These techniques are generally reliable and associated with physical fitness indices and health risk factors such as the predisposition to develop heart attack. Finally, it is interesting to note that the supplementary energy intake associated with exercise training can also be well predicted by a questionnaire [Taylor et al., 1978].

DIETARY RECORD

Even though dietary record is generally used to assess energy input instead of caloric expenditure, it has sometimes been used to predict energy expenditure and participation in physical activities. Buskirk et al. [1971] compared data obtained from a 7-day dietary record with those derived from the HIP questionnaire and the Tecumseh study procedure. No significant correlations were, however, observed between the activity questionnaire estimates and the 7-day energy intake measurements. Similarly, Laporte et al [1983] found no significant correlation between 3-day energy intake data and activity indices provided by the Paffenbarger method and the LSI measurement.

However, it has been suggested that when used in conjunction with regular assessments of body composition over a long period of time, the dietary record provides a more accurate picture of energy expenditure. In their studies performed in the Antarctic, Acheson et al. [1975, 1980] used energy intake and skinfold thickness changes over 6 to 12 months as a reference measurement to validate other techniques. The same procedure was employed by Malhotra et al. [1976] to determine energy requirements of soldiers.

SUMMARY

The methods discussed in the present review have been used to assess the pattern of habitual physical activities. Except for the pedometer, the reliability of the procedures has generally been described as satisfactory. In contrast, large variations were noted between techniques for their applicability and validity in measuring work and leisure-related energy expenditure. In an attempt to illustrate these variations, we have qualified these procedures for validity and applicability in population studies on a scale from 1 to 5 (Table I). Such an approach had been taken earlier by Buskirk and Mendez [1980]. Even though this evaluation represents only the views of the authors, it will probably be useful in indicating the strong and weak features of the methods

TABLE I. Validity and Applicability of Methods to Assess Work and Leisure Energy Expenditure in Population Studies[a]

Methods	Validity	Applicability
1 Direct calorimetry	5	1
2 Indirect calorimetry	5	2
3 Heart rate	3	3
4 Movement recording devices		
-Pedometer	1	4
-Actometer	2	4
-Accelerometer	2	4
-LSI	2	4
5 Diaries		
-Diary-calorimetry	4	2
-Diary-RMR	3	3
-Diary-tables	2	4
-Categorical scoring	2	5
6 Questionnaires and interviews		
-Questionnaire	1	5
-Questionnaire and interview	1	4
5 Dietary record	1	3

[a]The methods are qualified on a scale from 1 to 5 (1, low; 5, high). This represents a modification of the procedure previously used by Buskirk and Mendez [1980].

currently available to assess work and leisure energy expenditures in population studies. As a rule, accuracy decreases when applicability improves.

ACKNOWLEDGMENTS

Thanks are expressed to Dr. H.J. Montoye and the late Dr. H.L. Taylor for having provided us with a preprint copy of their manuscript [Montoye and Taylor, 1984] published in *Human Biology*. A. Tremblay and C. Bouchard are supported by grants from FCAC-Québec (EQ-1330), NSERC of Canada (A-0139, G-0850, A-8150).

REFERENCES

Acheson KJ, Campbell IT, Edholm OG, Miller DS, Stock MJ (1980): The measurement of daily energy expenditure—an evaluation of some techniques. Am J Clin Nutr 33:1155-1164.

Acheson AJ, Miller DS, Stock MJ (1975): Energy balance studies over a period of one year. In Jequier E (ed): "Régulation du bilan d'énergie chez l'homme." Genève: Editions Médecine et Hygiène, pp 209-211.

Andrews RB (1967): Estimation of values of energy expenditure rate from observed values of heart rate. Hum Factors 9:581-586.

Andrews RB (1971): Net heart rate as a substrate for respiratory calorimetry. Am J Clin Nutr 24:1139-1147.

Apfelbaum M, Bostsarron J, Lacatis D (1971): Effect of caloric restriction and excessive caloric intake on energy expenditure. Am J Clin Nutr 24:1405-1409.

Astrand I (1971): Estimating the energy expenditure of housekeeping activities. Am J Clin Nutr 24:1471-1475.

Baecke JAH, Burema J, Frijters JER (1982): A short questionnaire for the measurement of habitual physical activity in epidemiological studies. Am J Clin Nutr 36:936-942.

Bishop C, Jeanrenaud C, Lawson K (1975): A comparison of a time diary and a recall questionnaire for surveying leisure activities. J Leisure Res 7.

Blackburn NW, Calloway DH (1976): Energy expenditure and consumption of mature, pregnant and lactating women. J Am Diet Assoc 69:29-37.

Booyens J, Hervey GR (1960): The pulse rate as a mean of measuring metabolic rate in man. Can J Biochem Physiol 38:1301-1309.

Bouchard C (1983): Letter to the editor. Am J Clin Nutr 38:815.

Bouchard C, Tremblay A, Leblanc C, Lortie G, Savard R, Thériault G (1983): A method to assess energy expenditure in children and adults. Am J Clin Nutr 37:461-467.

Bradfield RB, Huntzicker PB, Fruehan GJ (1969): Simultaneous comparison of respirometer and heart-rate telemetry techniques as measures of human energy expenditure. Am J Clin Nutr 22:696-700.

Bradfield RB, Huntzicker PB, Fruehan GJ III (1970): Errors of group regressions for prediction of individual energy expenditure. Am J Clin Nutr 23:1015-1016.

Bradfield RB, Paulos J, Grossman L (1971): Energy expenditure and heart rate of obese high school girls. Am J Clin Nutr 24:1482-1488.

Bullen BA, Reed RB, Mayer J (1964): Physical activity of obese and non-obese adolescent girls appraised by motion picture sampling. Am J Clin Nutr 14:211-223.

Buskirk ER, Harris D, Mendez J, Skinner J (1971): Comparison of two assessments of physical activity and a survey method for caloric intake. Am J Clin Nutr 24:1119-1125.

Buskirk ER, Mendez J (1980): Caloric requirements. In Alfin-Slater RB, Kritchevsky D (eds): "Human nutrition, a comprehensive treatise." New York: Plenum Press, pp 49-95.

Chirico AM, Stunkard AJ (1960): Physical activity and human obesity. New Engl J Med 263:935.

Consolazio CF, Johnson RE, Pecora LJ (1963): "Physiological measurements of metabolic functions in man." New York: McGraw-Hill, pp 29-32.

Curtis DE, Bradfield RB (1971): Long-term energy intake and expenditure of obese housewives. Am J Clin Nutr 24:1410-1417.

Dauncey MJ, James WT (1979): Assessment of the heart-rate method for determining energy expenditure in man, using a whole-body calorimeter. Br J Nutr 42:1-13.

Dorris RJ, Stunkard AJ (1957): Physical activity: Performance and attitudes of a group of obese women. Am J Med Sci 233:622.

Durnin JVGA (1982): Energy consumption and its measurement in physical activity. Ann Clin Res 14:6-11.

Durnin JVGA, Passmore R (1967): "Energy, work and leisure." London: Heinemann Educational Books, pp 25-103.

Falls HB, Humphrey LD (1976): Energy cost of running and walking in young women. Med Sci Sport 8:9-13.

Golay A, Schutz Y, Meyer HU, Thiébaud D, Curchod B, Maeder E, Felber JP, Jéquier E (1982): Glucose-induced thermogenesis in nondiabetic and diabetic obese subjects. Diabetes 31:1023-1028.

Goldsmith R, Miller DS, Mumford P, Stock MJ (1966): The use of long-term measurements of heart rate to assess energy expenditure. Proc Physiol Soc December: 35P-36P.

Gorsky RD, Calloway DH (1983): Activity pattern changes with decreases in food energy intake. Hum Biol 55:577-586.

Griffiths M, Payne PR (1976): Energy expenditure in small children of obese and non-obese parents. Nature 260:698-699.

Hoffmans M, Pfeifer WA, Gundlack BL, Jijkrake HGM, Oude Ophius AJM, Hautvast SGAJ (1979): Resting metabolic rate in obese and normal weight women. Int J Obes 3:111-118.

Hueneman RF, Shapiro LR, Hampton MC, Mitchell BW (1967): Teen-agers' activities and attitudes toward activity. J Am Diet Assoc 51:433-440.

Kaplan ML, Levéillé GA (1976): Calorigenic response in obese and nonobese women. Am J Clin Nutr 29:1108-1113.

Laporte RE, Black-Sandler R, Cauley JA, Link M, Bayles C, Marks B (1983): The assessment of physical activitiy in older women: Analysis of the interrelationship and reliability of activity monitoring, activity surveys, and caloric intake. J Gerontol 38:394-397.

Laporte RE, Kuller LH, Kupfer DJ, McPartland RJ, Matthews G, Caspersen C (1979): An objective measure of physical activity for epidemiologic research. Am J Epidemiol 109:158-168.

Leblanc J, Mercier P, Samson P (1984): Diet-induced thermogenesis with relation to training state in female subjects. Can J Physiol Pharmacol 62:334-337.

Lusk G (1931): "The elements of the science of nutrition." Philadelphia: W.B. Saunders, pp 14-74.

Malhorta MS (1963): Pulse count as a measure of energy expenditure. J Appl Physiol 18:994-996.

Malhorta MS, Chandra U, Rai RM, Venkataswamy Y, Sridhavan K (1976): Food intake and energy expenditure of Indian troops in training. Br J Nutr 35:229-244.

Masironi R, Mansourian P (1974): Determination of habitual physical activity by means of a portable r-r interval distribution recorder. Bull World Health Organ 51:291-298.

Massey PS, Lieberman A, Batarseh G (1971): Measure of activity level in mentally retarded children and adolescents. Am J Mental Def 76:259-261.

Maxfield ME (1971): The direct measurement of energy expenditure in industrial situations. Am J Clin Nutr 24:1126-1138.

Maxfield E, Konishi F (1966): Patterns of food intake and physical activity in obesity. J Am Diet Assoc 49:406-408.

Mayer J, Roy R, Prasad Mitra K (1956): Relation between caloric intake, body weight, and physical work: Studies in an industrial male population in West Bengal. Am J Clin Nutr 4:169-175.

Miller DS, Mumford P (1967): Gluttony 1. An experimental study of overeating low- or high-protein diets. Am J Clin Nutr 20:1212-1222.

Montoye HJ (1971): Estimation of habitual physical activity by questionnaire and interview. Am J Clin Nutr 24:1113-1118.

Montoye HJ, Taylor HL (1984): Measurement of physical activity in population studies: A review. Hum Biol 56:195-216.

Montoye HJ, Washburn R, Servais S, Ertl A, Webster JG, Nagle FJ (1983): Estimation of energy expenditure by a portable accelerometer. Med Sc Sport Ex 15:403-407.

Nair KS, Halliday D, Garrow JS (1983): Thermic response to isoenergetic protein, carbohydrate or fat meals in lean and obese subjects. Clin Sci 65:307-312.

Paffenbarger RS, Wing AL, Hyde RT (1978): Physical activity as an index of heart attack risk in college alumni. Am J Epidemiol 108:161-175.

Pandolf KB, Givoni B, Goldman RF (1977): Predicting energy expenditure with loads while standing or walking very slowly. J Appl Physiol 43:577-581.

Passmore R, Durnin JVGA (1955): Human energy expenditure. Physiol Rev 35:801-840.

Payne PR, Wheeler EF, Salvosa CB (1971): Prediction of daily energy expenditure from average pulse rate. Am J Clin Nutr 24:1164-1170.

Ravussin E, Burnand B, Schutz Y, Jéquier E (1982): Twenty-four-hour energy expenditure and resting metabolic rate in obese, moderately obese, and control subjects. Am J Clin Nutr 35:566-573.

Reiff GG, Montoye HJ, Remington RD, Napier JA, Metzner HL, Epstein FH (1967): Assessment of physical activity by questionnaire and interview. In Karvonen MJ, Barry AJ (eds): "Physical activity and the heart." Finland: Charles C. Thomas, pp 336-371.

Saris WHM, Binkhorst RA (1977a): The use of pedometer and actometer in studying daily physical activity in man. Part I: Reliability of pedometer and actometer. Eur J Appl Physiol 37:218-219.

Saris WHM, Binkhorst RA (1977b): The use of pedometer and actometer in studying daily physical activity in man. Part II: Validity of pedometer and actometer measuring the daily physical activity. Eur J Appl Physiol 37:229-235.

Shapiro S, Weinblatt E, Frank CW (1965): The H.I.P. study of the incidence of myocardial infarction and angina. J Chron Dis 18:527.

Shetty PS, Jung RT, James WPT, Barrand MA, Callingham BA (1981): Postprandial thermogenesis in obesity. Clin Sci 60:519-525.

Silverman M, Anderson SD (1972): Metabolic cost of treadmill exercise in children. J Appl Physiol 33:696-698.

Taylor HL, Jacobs Dr, Shucker B, Knudsen J, Leon AS, Debacker G (1978): A questionnaire for the assessment of leisure time physical activities. J Chron Dis 31:741-755.

Tremblay A, Côté, J, Leblanc J (1983a): Diminished dietary thermogenesis in exercise-trained human subjects. Eur J Appl Physiol 52:1-4.

Tremblay A, Leblanc C, Sévigny J, Savoie JP, Bouchard C (1983b): The relationship between energy intake and expenditure: A sex difference. In Landry F (ed): "Health risk estimation, risk reduction and health promotion." Ottawa: Canadian Public Health Association, pp 115-119.

Webb P, Annis JF, Troutman SJ (1972): Human calorimetry with a water cooled garment. J Appl Physiol 32:413.

Webb P, Annis JF, Troutman SJ (1980): Energy balance in man measured by direct and indirect calorimetry. Am J Clin Nutr 33:1287-1298.

Wilkinson PW, Parkin JM, Pearlson G, Strong H, Sykes P (1977): Energy intake and physical activity in obese children. Br Med J March: 756.

Yasin S (1967): Measuring habitual leisure-time physical activity by recall questionnaire. In Karvonen NJ, Barry AJ (eds): "Physical activity and the heart." Finland: Charles C. Thomas, pp 372-373.

SECTION III: NUTRITION AND THE LIFE CYCLE

Nutritional Anthropology, pages 119-154
© 1987 Alan R. Liss, Inc.

Nutrition in the Reproductive Years

Linda S. Adair, PhD

Department of Anthropology, Rice University, Houston, Texas 77251

Nutritional status is one of many interacting variables that influence reproductive success of individuals and populations. Not only does nutrition play an important role in fertility, it also affects the health, growth, and development of offspring. This chapter examines nutrition in the reproductive years. Data are drawn from the medical, nutritional, and anthropological literature to provide a biocultural view of the ways in which malnutrition—both over- and undernutrition—affects reproductive outcomes. The major focus is on maternal nutrition during pregnancy and lactation. Topics include biological and cultural determinants of maternal nutritional status, assessment of nutritional risk, and consequences of maternal malnutrition for both mother and child. A secondary focus in on the relationship between nutrition and fertility in both males and females.

INTRODUCTION

One view of pregnancy states that the pregnant woman is basically a normal adult who "happens to be pregnant" [Munro, 1981]. Thus, her nutrient needs include those usual for the adult plus an added component to support the pregnancy. The way in which recommended dietary intakes for pregnancy are presented (Table I) supports this approach. According to this view, it is appropriate to refer to standard "normal" (nonpregnant) values for laboratory and clinical assessments of nutritional status during pregnancy. Using such criteria, many women appear to be manifesting pathological states which may, in fact, reflect the normal physiology and biochemistry of pregnancy. For example, even in well-nourished women, serum iron and hemoglobin levels fall in the 14th to 28th weeks of pregnancy. Maternal folate,

TABLE I. Recommended Dietary Allowances: U.S. RDA and FAO/WHO

Age (years)	Weight (kg)	Height (cm)	Protein (g)	Vitamin A (RE)	Vitamin D (µg)	Vitamin E (mg)	Vitamin C (mg)	Thiamin (mg)	Riboflavin (mg)	Niacin (mg equiv)	Vitamin B_6 (mg)	Folacin (µg)	Vitamin B_{12} (µg)	Calcium (mg)	Phosphorus (mg)	Magnesium (mg)	Iron (mg)	Zinc (mg)	Iodine (µg)
Males																			
11-14	45	157	45	1,000	10	8	50	1.4	1.6	18	1.8	400	3.0	1,200	1,200	350	18	15	150
15-18	66	176	56	1,000	10	10	60	1.4	1.7	18	2.0	400	3.0	1,200	1,200	400	18	15	150
19-22	70	177	56	1,000	7.5	10	60	1.5	1.7	19	2.2	400	3.0	800	800	350	10	15	150
23-50	70	178	56	1,000	5	10	60	1.4	1.6	18	2.2	400	3.0	800	800	350	10	15	150
51+	70	178	56	1,000	5	10	60	1.2	1.4	16	2.2	400	3.0	800	800	350	10	15	150
Females																			
11-14	46	157	46	800	10	8	50	1.1	1.3	15	1.8	400	3.0	1,200	1,200	300	18	15	150
15-18	55	163	46	800	10	8	60	1.1	1.3	14	2.0	400	3.0	1,200	1,200	300	18	15	150
19-22	55	163	44	800	7.5	8	60	1.1	1.3	14	2.0	400	3.0	800	800	300	18	15	150
23-50	55	163	44	800	5	8	60	1.0	1.2	13	2.0	400	3.0	800	800	300	18	15	150
51+	55	163	44	800	5	8	60	1.0	1.2	13	2.0	400	3.0	800	800	300	10	15	150
Pregnant			+30	+200	+5	+2	+20	+0.4	+0.3	+2	+0.6	+400	+1.0	+400	+400	+150		+5	+25
Lactating			+20	+400	+5	+3	+40	+0.5	+0.5	+5	+0.5	+100	+1.0	+400	+400	+150		+10	+50
FAO/WHO																	(Range)		
Males																			
10-12	36.9		30		2.5		30	1.0	1.6	17.2		100	2.0	650			5-10		
13-15	51.3		37		2.5		30	1.2	1.7	19.1		200	2.0	650			9-18		
16-19	62.9		38		2.5		30	1.2	1.8	20.8		200	2.0	550			5-9		
Adult	65.0		37		2.5		30	1.2	1.8	19.8		200	2.0	450			5-9		
Females																			
10-12	38.0		29		2.5		30	0.9	1.4	15.5		100	2.0	650			5-10		
13-15	49.9		31		2.5		30	1.0	1.5	16.4		200	2.0	650			12-24		
16-19	54.4		30		2.5		30	0.9	1.4	16.2		200	2.0	550			14-28		
Adult	55.0		29		2.5		30	0.9	1.3	14.5		200	2.0	450			14-28		
Pregnant (later half)			38		10		30	+.1	+.2	+2.3		400	3.0	1,100			14-28[a]		
Lactating (first 6 months)			46		10		30	+.2	+.4	+3.7		300	2.5	1,100			14-28[b]		

[a]If iron stores are adequate prior to pregnancy.

[b]Iron supplement recommended.

calcium, and albumin concentrations may also appear abnormally low during pregnancy without resulting in any adverse effects on the fetus.

An alternative view is that pregnancy needs to be afforded a more special status; one that sees the mother and fetus as interlocking systems and recognizes that there may be maternal physiological adjustments during pregnancy which are fundamentally different from those of the nonpregnant state. Such adjustments may involve increases in the efficiency of absorption or utilization of particular nutrients. In addition, the developing fetus can maintain adequate levels of some nutrients at the expense of the mother. For example, cord blood folate levels in the neonate may be normal despite signs of deficiency in the mother [Lind, 1981]. Observations such as these emphasize the need for pregnancy-specific norms for nutrient levels.

In either view, maternal nutrient needs during pregnancy reflect growth of both maternal and fetal tissues and associated increased costs of metabolism. The following sections describe specific needs and how they have been determined.

Energy

Estimates of the net energy equivalents of tissue increments and maintenance costs are presented in Figure 1. The total energy cost of pregnancy in the well-nourished woman has been estimated to be about 80,000 kcal [Hytten and Leitch, 1971]. Recommended energy intakes for pregnancy are based on this value divided by the average duration of pregnancy (280 days), suggesting a requirement for 300 kcal per day over nonpregnant intake. In fact, energy needs are not uniform throughout the pregnancy but vary with

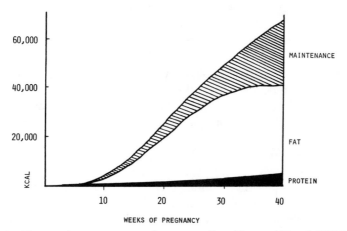

Fig. 1. The cumulative energy cost of pregnancy (from Hytten and Leitch [1971]).

the types and amounts of maternal and fetal tissues being formed. Components of the average pregnancy weight gain of women on unrestricted diets are presented in Table II. The "weight not accounted for" category is thought to represent maternal fat stores. Significant increases in skinfold thicknesses occur between weeks 10 and 30 [Taggart et al., 1967]. Coupled with maximal increments in the placenta, breasts, and blood volume and with a large gain in fetal weight during the third 10 weeks, the average cost during this period is about 390 kcal per day. As maternal tissue growth falls off in the final 10 weeks, daily needs drop to about 250–300 kcal per day.

Using indirect calorimetry, Emerson et al. [1972] have also calculated the energy cost of normal pregnancy. Their estimate of $27,120 \pm 2,175$ kcal corresponds well with the Hytten and Leitch [1971] oxygen consumption (i.e., metabolic cost) estimate, but does not account for the energy equivalents of maternal and fetal tissues. Emerson's recommended supplemental energy intakes are for 10, 85, and 220 kcal/day in the first, second, and third trimesters, respectively.

It is possible for the well-nourished pregnant woman to meet the increased needs of the final trimester of pregnancy without significantly increasing her energy intake. First, she enters the final months with a significant store of energy (about 30,000 kcal) in the form of subcutaneous fat. Second, she can decrease physical activity. The energy requirement of 220 of 300 kcal per day represents about 25% of daily activity costs estimated by the WHO, and 40% of the energy costs measured by Emerson et al. [1972]. These strategies may not be possible for women in developing countries. If undernourished, they may not build substantial energy reserves early in pregnancy. Moreover, the demands of agricultural economies may not allow a significant decrease in physical activity in the last trimester of pregnancy. Nonetheless, there is accumulating evidence that in populations with chronic low energy intakes, women develop a set of adaptations—probably involving increased metabolic efficiency—that allow them to achieve a considerable degree of reproductive success despite their low intakes [Prentice, 1984; Prentice et al, 1983, 1984; Adair 1984]. The results of these studies raise questions about the global validity of established estimates of nutrient needs.

Protein

Contrary to earlier views, Hytten and Chamberlain [1980] argue that unlike energy, protein is not stored during pregnancy beyond that which is found in maternal reproductive and fetal tissues. Nitrogen retention studies in metabolic wards give estimates of mean daily nitrogen retention that are in close accord with estimates based on tissue increments [Zuspan and Goodrich, 1968;

Johnstone et al., 1972]. Protein needs vary through pregnancy according to the demands of tissue synthesis. In the final 10 weeks of pregnancy, Hytten and Leitch [1971] estimate that the average British woman needs an additional 8.5 g per day to account for the protein increments in maternal and fetal tissues (Table II). This value is based on actual increments of 6.1 g/day in fully assimilated tissue protein. Dietary protein in Britain has a NPU (net protein utilization) value of 70%. With lower NPU value diets, such as those based primarily on nonlegume vegetable product staples (eg, cassava), dietary protein needs will be significantly higher. On the other hand if, as suggested by studies in animals, there is an increased efficiency of protein utilization during pregnancy [Naismith, 1977], needs may be substantially less. This may help to explain the reproductive success of many populations judged to be nutritionally at risk based on their low intakes of protein.

Other Nutrients

Needs for other nutrients may be associated with increased energy and protein intakes or with a direct role in tissue formation. For example, niacin, thiamin, and riboflavin are related to energy intake, folic acid plays a role in DNA synthesis, and vitamin B_6 is important in amino acid metabolism and protein synthesis (see recommended intakes of these nutrients in Table I).

Calcium and phosphorus are needed primarily for the calcification of the fetal skeleton. Widdowson [1968] has estimated that the fetus draws about 250 to 300 mg of calcium per day from the maternal circulation in the last

TABLE II. Components of Weight Gain During Pregnancy

Tissues and fluids accounted for	Weight increase at (weeks)							
	10		20		30		40	
	g	%	g	%	g	%	g	%
Fetus	5	0.1	300	9	1,500	44	3,400	100
Placenta	20	4	170	26	430	66	650	100
Amniotic fluid	140	4	350	44	750	94	800	100
Uterus	140	14	320	33	600	62	970	100
Mammary glands	45	11	180	44	360	89	405	100
Blood	100	8	600	48	1,300	104	1,250	100
Extracellular fluid[a]	0	0	30	2	80	5	1,680	100
Total	340	4	1,950	21	5,020	55	9,155	100
Total weight gain	650	5	4,000	32	8,500	68	12,500	100
Weight not accounted for	310	9	2,050	61	3,480	104	3,345	100

[a]With no edema or leg edema only.
Modified from Hytten and Leitch [1971].

trimester of pregnancy. In the presence of adequate vitamin D, maternal absorption of dietary calcium increases to meet the demands of the fetus and protect the maternal skeleton from mineral losses. Iron is needed for expanded maternal blood volume and to meet needs of the developing fetus and placenta. Even in the well-nourished mother, serum iron and hemoglobin levels drop during the second trimester of pregnancy due to the effects of hemodilution as maternal blood volume expands. In the latter half of pregnancy, the efficiency of iron absorption is significantly increased among women not taking iron supplements [Svanberg, 1975]. The greatest accumulation of iron in the fetus occurs during the last trimester of pregnancy (see Table III for a quantitative breakdown of iron needs). The fetus tends to be an efficient parasite with respect to iron, maintaining adequate iron status even if the mother is slightly anemic. There is at present no convincing evidence that supplemental iron benefits the mother with adequate iron status, however, iron supplementation is needed in cases of maternal anemia to prevent fatigue and cardiac stress.

CONSEQUENCES OF MALNUTRITION

This section deals with the consequences for the mother and fetus of imbalances between nutrient needs and nutrient intakes resulting from dietary inadequacies or excesses during pregnancy. The assessment of nutritional status of the mother during pregnancy is a necessary first step in understanding the effects of malnutrition.

Determining the Nutritional Risk Status of Populations

Dietary intake relative to standards is often used as a first approximation of the nutritional risk status of a population. Hytten and Leitch [1971] and Prentice [1984] have summarized data on energy intakes of pregnant women

TABLE III. Iron Requirements During Pregnancy

Expansion of maternal red cell mass	570 mg
Losses in skin, feces, urine	270 mg
Transfer to the fetus	200–370 mg
Placental and umbilical cord content	35–100 mg
Maternal blood loss at delivery	100–180 mg
Total	1,175–2,490 mg
Savings from amenorrhea	240–480 mg
Estimated requirements: 4 mg/day for the first two trimesters, 6.6 mg/day in the last trimester	

From Hytten and Chamberlain [1980].

living in a wide range of environments. There are many populations throughout the world in which mean daily intake of individuals falls considerably below 1974 FAO/WHO (2,250 kcal) or 1980 U.S. (2,200 kcal) recommendations. For example, mean daily energy intakes during the wet season in the Gambia are only about 1,300 kcal [Prentice et al. 1980]. Intakes in the range of 1,500 to 1,600 kcal per day have been reported for women in India [Venkatachalam, 1962; Devadas et al., 1978], New Guinea [Norgan et al., 1974], Guatemala [Lechtig et al., 1972], Ethiopia [Gebre-Mehdin and Gobezie, 1975] and Colombia [Mora et al., 1978]. In contrast, women from more privileged populations often exceed recommendations, e.g., 2,633 kcal in wives of white collar workers in Aberdeen [Thomson 1958, 1959], and 2,770 kcal in rural Dutch women (den Hartog et al., 1953 in Hytten and Leitch [1971]). Using these data to make inferences about nutritional status is problematic. First, recommended intakes are estimates of average energy requirements based on a reference person who may differ significantly in body composition and activity levels from women in developing countries. Second, we do not fully understand the ways in which populations adapt to low nutrient intakes (cf. Adair [1984] and Prentice [1984]). Third, there is a need for more information on how nutrient requirements are influenced by variables such as climate, nutritional history, disease, and physical activity. Finally, estimates of dietary intake may be unreliable, particularly if based on dietary recall methods.

Because of these difficulties, more direct measures of nutritional status are needed. A second commonly used assessment strategy is measurement of maternal anthropometric status, particularly weight for height relative to standards. This method has its own set of problems. Choice of relevant standards for comparison is important since populations differ significantly in size and body composition due to genetic factors. It is vital to discern whether mothers are small due to their own nutritional histories and adaptation to low nutrient intakes or due to genetic factors. The degree to which maternal body size is predictive of fetal outcomes may reflect the underlying causes of small body size.

The best strategy for assessment of nutritional risk may involve assessment of functional indicators of nutritional status. Weight gain during pregnancy correlates well with birthweight in infants in cases of both low and high weight gain. Moreover, long-term weight changes provide an index of energy balance over time. In some populations of women living under conditions of chronic deprivation, there tends to be a slow decline in maternal body weight with increasing parity [Venkatachalam et al., 1960]. Birth outcomes including size, body composition, developmental maturity, and health of the offspring are further important retrospective functional indicators of maternal nutritional status during pregnancy.

Maternal Malnutrition and Pregnancy Outcome

There has been a long-standing controversy concerning the relationship between maternal and fetal nutritional status. For a time, the fetus was viewed as the perfect parasite with respect to all nutrients and was thought to be relatively immune to the nutritional status of the mother.

Evidence to the contrary comes from several different sources: animal studies in which maternal dietary restriction during pregnancy resulted in impaired fetal growth and development [McCance and Widdowson, 1962], physician-prescribed diets to restrict intrauterine growth, retrospective studies of human populations subjected to severe food shortages during World War II, epidemiological studies of pregnancy outcomes in poorly nourished communities, and studies of the effects of nutrition supplementation on pregnant women.

Beginning in the latter part of the 19th century, a German physician named Prochownick advocated a diet that would restrict intrauterine growth and thereby promote easier births. This was desirable in women who had contracted pelves as a result of ricketts during childhood. The "Prochownick diet" [Hytten and Leitch, 1971] was high in protein (130–160 g per day), low in calories (1,800–2,000) and fluids. It was designed to restrict maternal weight gain during pregnancy and prevent the transfer of "fat and fluids" to the fetus during the last trimester. The diet was indeed successful in lowering birth weight, but Hytten and Leitch [1971] have suggested this was due to the severe fluid restriction rather than to limited calories. The diet does, however, indicate an early awareness of a relationship between maternal diet and size of the offspring at birth.

During World War II, a military blockade lasting from October 1944 to May 1945 caused severe restrictions in food availability throughout most of Holland. As a result, there was a marked decline in fertility compared to pre-war levels: only one third of expected births occurred. About 50% of women of reproductive age experienced amenorrhea, and only about 30% had normal menstrual cycles. Those who did conceive or gestate during the famine were probably among the better nourished members of the population. Birth outcomes were markedly influenced by the adverse nutritional conditions. Compared to before the war, there was a significant drop in mean birthweight of 240 g and an increase in miscarriage, stillbirths, and neonatal deaths. The phase of pregnancy during which food restriction occurred was an important factor. Famine conditions during the first trimester increased the incidence of prematurity, stillbirths, and congenital abnormalities, while deprivations in the later trimesters resulted in a higher incidence of low birthweight (LBW, < 2500 g) [Stein et al., 1975].

Similar conditions prevailed during the siege of Leningrad from 1941 to 1943. Fertility declined, amenorrhea was common, and rates of prematurity and infant mortality increased. Birthweights declined from pre-war levels by an average of 410 g in females and 500 g in males [Antonov, 1947].

Maternal Nutrition Supplementation During Pregnancy

Numerous populations around the world live under less severe but chronic conditions of poor nutrition. The incidence of LBW and perinatal mortality is significantly higher in those populations compared to well nourished populations. The precise role played by nutrition is difficult to separate from other environmental conditions. Poorly nourished communities tend to have a high incidence of infectious disease due to poor sanitary conditions and limited access to health care.

Nutrition intervention studies attempt to isolate the effects of poor nutrition from other environmental variables that influence reproductive success. Results from several supplementary feeding programs targeted to pregnant and lactating women are presented below. Reviews of maternal and supplementation studies have been published by Brozek et al. [1977], Lechtig [1982], Stein et al. [1978], and Osofsky [1975].

Guatemala: The INCAP Four Villages Study [Lechtig et al., 1972, 1975, 1978]. Women from four rural Ladino villages were given energy supplements in the form of a sweetened beverage (fresco) or energy plus protein supplements consumed as a gruel (atole). Presupplementation energy intakes among pregnant women were about 1,400 kcal/day. Supplement intake was ad libitum and took place by voluntary attendance at a distribution center. Total supplement intake for pregnancy varied widely between individuals, ranging from 0 to over 40,000 kcal. (These values do not represent net intake since substitution of the supplement for usual dietary items was not measured). Calories alone were found to be as effective as protein plus calories in increasing mean birthweights (28 g/ 10,000 supplemental kcal) and in decreasing the incidence of LBW and infant mortality. Supplementation was also positively correlated with maternal weight gain during pregnancy, leading investigators to conclude that supplemental calories during pregnancy improve both maternal nutritional status and pregnancy outcomes.

Bogota, Colombia [Mora et al., 1978, 1979, 1981, Mora, 1983]. In Bogota, families were provided with weekly supplies of food, including powdered skim milk, enriched bread, and vegetable oil. The supplemental foods raised energy intakes in pregnant women by about 9%, from 1,623 to 1,773 kcal/day. Mean birthweights of male offspring of supplemented women were 63 g heavier than those of unsupplemented controls.

The Gambia [Prentice et al., 1983a]. Supplement in the forms of a groundnut-based biscuit and vitamin-fortified tea drink resulted in a mean net daily increase of 431 kcal among pregnant women. This represented a 30% increase over presupplement intakes of 1,467 kcal/day. Increased intake was associated with a 120 g improvement in mean birthweights, year round. In the wet season when nutritional stress is more severe, the improvement in birthweight, which occurred in both males and females, was 225 g.

Taiwan: The Bacon Chow Study [Adair and Pollitt 1983, 1985; McDonald et al., 1981; Mueller and Pollitt, 1983, Adair et al., 1983, 1984]. Marginally nourished women living in rural, agricultural villages of Taiwan were given either a nutrient rich (800 kcal, 40 g protein per day) supplement (A) or a low-calorie, protein-free placebo (B) beginning 3 weeks after birth of one infant and continuing through the lactation period following birth of a second infant. Thus, it is possible to make intergroup (A–B) comparisons and to compare the results of unsupplemented and supplemented pregnancies in the same woman. Supplementation in the A group significantly improved birthweights of male infants, and reduced the degree to which siblings resembled one another at birth due to modification of the intrauterine nutritional environment during the supplemented pregnancy. Furthermore, as in the Gambia, supplementation buffered the effects of season, lessening maternal weight losses and dysmorphic prenatal growth in the offspring associated with the stressful summer months.

Mexico [Chavez and Martinez, 1973]. Pregnant women living in rural villages were given daily supplements of skim milk which provided an average of 210 kcal and 15 g of protein per day. Mean presupplement intakes were 1,950 kcal/day. Compared to the offspring of matched controls, infants of supplemented mothers weighed an average of 180 g more at birth. Supplementation decreased the incidence of LBW and improved maternal weight gain during pregnancy by 6.4 kg.

Montreal [Rush, 1983]. The Montreal intervention study provided free foods on a prescription basis and nutrition education to pregnant, low income urban women attending a public prenatal clinic. The average increment in birthweight was small (40 g) but statistically significant due to the large sample size (> 1,000). Supplementation had no significant effect on pregnancy weight gain in the mothers.

New York [Stein et al., 1978; Rush et al. 1980]. In a randomized controlled trial, urban black women at risk for giving birth to LBW infants were given liquid supplement (470 kcal, 40 g protein per day) or complement (322 kcal, 6 g protein per day). The women were not nutritionally at risk judging from their mean presupplement dietary intake of 2,200 kcal, 80 g protein per day. Thus it is not surprising that the intervention produced no significant increases in birthweight or maternal weight gain during pregnancy. It did, however, prevent the usual decrease in birthweight that occurs in infants of mothers who smoked heavily during pregnancy. An unexpected effect was the increase in prematurity and neonatal deaths among supplement group mothers who previously had a LBW infant.

Interpretation of these studies as a group is complicated by differences in research design, methods of delivering supplements, nature of the supplements, nutritional history and genetic makeup of the population, presupplement energy intakes, health, and nutritional status of the subjects. In most cases, the net increase in dietary intake attributable to supplementation was not measured accurately. Despite these factors, the variability in outcome is less that one might expect. With the exception of wet season births in the Gambia, supplementation effects on mean birthweight did not exceed 200 g.

These results raise several important questions about the relationship between maternal nutritional status and birth outcomes. Populations targeted for nutrition intervention are often selected on the basis of low nutrient intake relative to standards. As previously noted, standards may overestimate needs, particularly in cases in which there may be behavioral and physiological adjustments to long-term low energy intakes. If populations are indeed well adapted to their low intakes, supplementation may have limited effects on mean outcome variables. Within populations, individuals or subgroups may vary in adaptability and nutritional risk status. For example, several of the studies cited above have shown a greater response to supplementation in male fetuses compared to females [Mora et al., 1981; McDonald et al., 1981; Mueller and Pollitt, 1983] and in infants born to relatively tall mothers [Mora, 1983; Adair and Pollitt, 1985].

Episodic or periodic stresses imposed by disease or seasonal fluctuations in food availability and physical activity associated with agricultural cycles may further challenge adaptive mechanisms and represent significant risk. Thus nutrition may vary in importance relative to other environmental factors through time. Data from the Gambia and Taiwan show differential effects of nutritional supplementation by season.

Timing and severity of nutritional stress relative to the stage of gestation also play a significant role in pregnancy outcome. While severe nutritional deprivation early in pregnancy increases risk of miscarriage and prematurity, deprivation later in pregnancy affects tissues undergoing critical periods of growth. Growth in length of the fetus is most affected by poor nutrition in the second trimester, while growth in weight is limited (primarily due to decreased deposition of subcutaneous fat) if malnutrition occurs in the third trimester [Villar et al., 1983, Adair and Pollitt, 1985]. Finally, the biological significance of 100 to 200 g increments in mean birthweight are unknown. Such increments may be attributable to a decrease in the number of preterm and LBW infants and may have particular health or survival consequences for infants in these categories.

The relationship between maternal nutritional status and pregnancy outcome is not a simple one. While certain nutritional conditions have a direct effect on outcome, others are involved in a complex web of interactions and adaptations that ultimately determine the reproductive success of a population.

MATERNAL MALNUTRITION AND FETAL BRAIN DEVELOPMENT

Because of methodological and ethical issues associated with deprivation studies in human subjects, much of what is known about the relationship between malnutrition and the growth and development of the brain derives from animal studies. Experiments in laboratory rats have shown that maternal dietary restriction during pregnancy and restriction of intake in the offspring during the suckling period impairs brain growth and neuromotor development [Dobbing, 1972; Winick, 1976; Winick and Noble, 1965; McCance and Widdowson, 1962, Zamenhof et al., 1971]. The brain is most susceptible to the effects of malnutrition during its period of most rapid growth [Dobbing, 1972]. Permanent deficits in the number of brain cells occur when dietary restriction is imposed during hyperplastic growth. When malnutrition occurs during hypertrophic growth, cells are small, but recovery is possible if adequate nutrition is restored [Winick, 1976]. Functional consequences of biochemical and structural alterations in the brains of the offspring include decreased exploratory behavior and problem solving abilities and heightened irritability [Levitsky and Barnes, 1972].

There are difficulties in extrapolating from these studies to humans. First, rats and humans differ in timing of the brain growth spurt relative to birth. In the rat, the critical period occurs during the suckling period, while in the human, it spans a period fron the second trimester of pregnancy when there is a spurt in neuronal growth through the second year of postnatal life when glial cell development, synaptic formation, and myelination take place [Dobbing, 1972]. Thus the effects of maternal dietary restriction during pregnancy may vary widely between the two species.

Secondly, the degree of dietary restriction necessary for permanent neurological impairment in the rat occurs infrequently in human populations. In the rat, diets were sufficiently restricted to produce a 40 to 50% deficit in body weight. In human populations this would occur only in cases of severe intrauterine growth retardation resulting in birthweights of less than 2 kg or in cases of marasumus or failure to thrive in the postnatal period. The effects of less severe deprivation are poorly understood.

Thirdly, the effects of nutrition cannot be understood in isolation from other environmental variables. For example, Barnes [1976] has shown that recovery from early nutritional deprivation is possible when animals are handled and stimulated.

Direct evidence of the effects of poor prenatal nutrition on brain growth and development in humans is scanty. Most studies have focused on the effects of malnutrition in the postnatal period. For example, Winick's [1976] data on the size and biochemical composition of brains of infants who died from marasmus shows deficits in total weight and lower concentrations of RNA, DNA, and protein compared to well-nourished infants who died from other causes. The relative contribution of prenatal versus postnatal malnutrition cannot be isolated using these data.

Supplementation studies are useful in providing additional data, but they suffer from problems similar to those mentioned in the data above since, in most designs, a supplement is provided during both pregnancy and lactation. Nonetheless, the available data indicate an association between maternal nutrition supplementation during pregnancy and improved infant performance in visual attention tests, higher visual–habituation traits associated with later intellectual development [Vuori et al., 1979], and increased head circumference in the offspring [Lechtig et al., 1975]. Although the relationship between head circumference and brain development is not straightforward, Winick and Rosso [1969] have shown that the diminution in brain cell number in malnourished infants is directly proportional to reduction in head circumference.

Effects of Specific Nutrient Deficiencies and Excesses

The focus so far has been on the effects of protein–calorie malnutrition. Specific nutrients, including vitamins, minerals, and trace elements also play an important role in reproductive success. Deficiencies or excesses of certain nutrients may have physiologic or metabolic consequences for the fetus, while imbalances in others may have structural or teratogenic effects. Much of the available evidence on the role of specific nutrients in reproduction comes from studies of laboratory animals [Hurley, 1980]. Nutrients known to influence human prenatal growth and development are treated briefly below.

Fat-soluble vitamins. Vitamin A deficiency is common in India and parts of Africa where diets are low in carotene-containing foods. The resulting incidence of night blindness and corneal damage is high. Mothers with deficiency-induced blindness may produce offspring with abnormalities of the eye as severe as anopthalmia. Excess vitamin A may also be teratogenic, causing abnormalities of the urogenital [Bernhardt and Dorsey, 1974] and central nervous systems [Strange et al., 1978].

Vitamin D is essential for absorption of dietary calcium and mineralization of developing bone. A maternal deficiency of this vitamin can result in abnormal development of the fetal skeleton, ricketts [Ford et al., 1973], and tooth enamel hypoplasia [Purvis, 1973]. Evidence of the effects of excess vitamin D during pregnancy in animals have not been confirmed in humans.

Interest in vitamin E as an agent to prevent miscarriage in humans has been generated by the knowledge that vitamin E deficiency in animals is known to cause spontaneous abortion. Vitamin E deficiency rarely occurs in humans, and no therapeutic role has yet been demonstrated. When vitamin E deficiency does occur in infancy, it can cause a hemolytic anemia that becomes apparent at about 6 weeks of age. Attempts at prevention through maternal supplementation with vitamin E during pregnancy have not been successful since maternal levels must be significantly elevated before cord blood levels in the neonate are affected [Malone, 1975].

Deficiency of vitamin K can result in hemorrhagic disease of the newborn. Newborn infants are particularly susceptible to vitamin K deficiency because they lack the intestinal bacteria which normally synthesize this vitamin. Mothers are sometimes given supplements of natural vitamin K in the last week of pregnancy to prevent deficiency in the newborn.

Water-soluble vitamins. Water soluble vitamins must be provided on a regular basis since they are not stored in the body. Consequences of excess intake of these vitamins are potentially less serious, due to urinary excretion. Relatively little is known about the effects of deficiencies of the water soluble vitamins during pregnancy.

Riboflavin deficiency has been associated with an increase in vomiting during pregnancy, prematurity, and stillbirths, while thiamin deficiency, prevalent in Southeast Asia, can cause congenital beriberi in the neonate [Van Gelder and Darby, 1944; Thanagkul and Amatayakul, 1975].

Folic acid, a nutrient found primarily in leafy green vegetables, is involved in all aspects of DNA and RNA synthesis. Needs are increased during pregnancy to support erythropoesis and growth of the fetus and placenta. Low serum folate levels are common during pregnancy, but relatively few women develop megaloblastic anemia, the major abnormality caused by deficiency. There is controversy concerning the effects of low folate levels on pregnancy outcome. Although cord blood levels in the neonate may be normal despite low maternal levels, more severe deficiency in the mother may be associated with abruptio placenta, spontaneous abortion, and an increased incidence of small for dates infants and neural tube defects [Gross et al., 1974; Hibbard, 1975, Hibbard and Smithells, 1965, Smithells et al., 1976] Other studies have failed to show an association between these disorders and low maternal folate levels [Scott et al., 1970; Giles, 1966].

Vitamin B_{12} is found only in animal products. Strict vegans are therefore at risk for deficiencies. Studies in South India have shown an association of B_{12} deficiency with infertility, miscarriage, and possibly with chronic tropical sprue. Megaloblastic anemia and its sequlae are usually the consequence of combined folate and B_{12} deficiencies in communities with very poor diets [Chanarin, 1969]

Therapeutic use of vitamin B_6 has been advoacted by some researchers to treat morning sickness in the early months of pregnancy [Wheatley, 1977]. Its effectiveness is, however, controversial. In a study of infants born to mothers who differed in vitamin B_6 levels during pregnancy and at parturition, a higher incidence of low Apgar scores was associated with low maternal dietary intake and serum levels of B_6 [Roepke and Kirksey, 1979].

Finally, there is evidence that excess intake of vitamin C during pregnancy can alter metabolism of this vitamin and cause a conditioned scurvy in the infant after birth [Cochrane, 1965].

Minerals and trace elements

Calcium. Dietary deficiency is not common. Furthermore, since maternal efficiency of absorption and utilization of calcium increases during pregnancy, the fetus is likely to get sufficient calcium to meet its needs. When calcium deficiencies occur, they are most often due to malabsorption or vitamin D deficiency. In some areas of Asia and among Asian immigrants to Britain, dietary intakes of calcium are extremely low, resulting in osteomalacia in high parity mothers and in hypocalcemia and ricketts in their infants [Krisnamachari and Iyengar, 1975; Ford et al., 1973].

Iron. Anemia due to iron deficiency is one of the most common nutritional problems of pregnancy. Anemia, defined by hematocrit values less than 32% and hemoglobin less than 11 g/dl, occurs in one-half to one-third of all pregnant women not taking iron supplements [Worthington-Roberts et al., 1981]. For mothers, anemia increases the risk of infection and cardiac stress and decreases ability to tolerate hemorrhage at delivery. Studies in India have shown moderate to severe anemia to be associated with an increase in the incidence of spontaneous abortion, prematurity, LBW, and perinatal mortality [Rosario, 1971; Achari and Rani, 1971], while another study in Africa indicated a direct relationship between anemia and weight and skinfold thicknesses of the infant at birth [Reinhardt, 1978]. Since the fetus tends to be an efficient parasite where iron is concerned, fetal consequences are mild unless maternal iron stores are heavily depleted.

Iodine. Iodine deficiency during pregnancy can result in neurological impairment or cretinism in the offspring depending on its severity [Pharoah et al., 1971; Greene, 1980]. The incidence of endemic cretinism in highest in several mountainous areas of the world (Ecuador, Peru, New Guinea, and Switzerland) where soils and, thus, the plants grown in them are iodine deficient. Since similar maternal dietary intakes of iodine produce effects of varying severity in the offspring, it is assumed that other environmental and genetic factors play a role in manifestation of deficiency disease. Excess iodides taken during pregnancy can cause congenital goiter, hypothyroidism, and increased neonatal mortality [Carswell et al., 1970].

Sodium. In the past, physicians called for restriction of sodium intake during pregnancy to prevent edema and pre-eclampsia [Pitkin et al., 1972]. Moderate edema in the extremities is now recognized as normal during the latter part of pregnancy and dietary sodium intake is not directly related to pre-eclampsia. Moreover, sodium restriction may be detrimental, causing stress to the maternal renal system and low blood sodium levels in infants [Lelong-Tissier, 1977]. Thus, routine recommendations of low sodium intake during pregnancy are no longer made.

Zinc. Although zinc deficiency is highly teratogenic in rats, its precise role in human prenatal development is unclear. In the Middle East where zinc deficiency is common, there is an increase in the frequency of central nervous system abnormalities at birth [Sever and Emanuel, 1973]. A study in Sweden also showed an association between low maternal serum zinc levels and postterm deliveries and malformations in the infants [Hurley, 1977].

Interpretation of the results of population studies on the role played by specific nutrients in reproductive outcomes is complicated by the fact that the overall diet may be poor. It is therefore difficult to rule out effects of nutrient interactions and multiple deficiencies in the etiology of disorders observed. Nonetheless, the available evidence leaves little doubt that maternal nutrition during pregnancy plays a significant role in pregnancy outcome. While the effects of severe deficiencies of energy and specific nutrients are clear, there is much to be learned about the consequences of moderate to mild malnutrition and the role of adaptation to low nutrient intakes in human populations. Furthermore, nutrition is but one of many variables that influence reproductive success.

Maternal Malnutrition and Immunity in the Infant

Infants suffering from intrauterine growth retardation due to poor maternal nutrition during pregnancy have impaired immune systems and show increased susceptibility to infection. These effects parallel those found in older children suffering from malnutrition. Specific defects include low IgG levels, depression of cell-mediated immunity due to a reduction in T lymphocytes [Chandra, 1975; Chandra et al., 1977], and a decrease in rosette-forming lymphocytes [Ferguson et al., 1974].

Nutrition and Maternal Health

Pre-eclampsia. Pre-eclampsia is a disorder of pregnancy characterized by hypertension, proteinuria, and generalized edema, usually beginning after the 20th week of pregnancy. If untreated, it can result in maternal and fetal death. It tends to occur most frequently in women living in poor socioeconomic conditions, in which suboptimal nutrition, inadequate prenatal care, and overall poor health occur in combination. The exact role played by nutrition is poorly understood. Pre-eclampsia has been associated with poor nutrition and low pregnancy weight gain [Tomplins et al., 1955; Eastman, 1970], and with overnutrition and excessive weight gain [Thomson and Billewicz, 1957]. The current view is that risk is represented not by the overall amount of weight gain but by its pattern and components. Other studies have suggested a role for vitamin B_6. Placentas from toxemic patients contain only about one third of the normal content of vitamin B_6 and also lack the enzyme necessary to convert this vitamin to its active form.

NUTRITION AND LACTATION

Lactation success, judged by the adequacy of child growth and development depends on a variety of nutritional and nonnutritional aspects of the maternal environment. The quantity and quality of milk produced reflect maternal nutritional status prior to and during lactation as well as maternal health, demands of physical activity, and environmental and psychosocial stress [Jelliffe and Jelliffe, 1978]. Lactation places considerable demands on the mother. With the exception of energy and some specific nutrients that can be drawn from maternal stores, the lactating woman must consume a diet adequate to meet her own needs plus provide all of the raw materials necessary for production of milk that will meet all of the nutritional needs of her infant. Recommended dietary intakes to meet those needs are presented in Table I.

The total energy cost of lactation includes both synthesis and energy content of the milk itself. Older FAO/WHO recommendations for energy intake during lactation are based on the assumption that the energy efficiency of milk production is only about 60%. Thus, a mother would need about 1,000 additional calories per day to produce 850 ml of milk containing 75 kcal/100ml. More recent recommendations of the FAO/WHO [1974] for 550 kcal and of the U.S. National Research Council (1980) for 500 additional kcal per day reflect revised estimates of efficiency (90%): Thomson et al. [1970], a lower estimate of daily milk output (600-700 ml/day): Thomson and Black [1975], and assume that lactation costs can be subsidized by about 200 to 300 kcal per day during the first 3 months of lactation from maternal fat stores deposited during pregnancy [Hytten and Leitch, 1971].

The protein content of human milk, determined by amino acid analysis, is now thought to be about 0.9 g/100 ml [Hambraeus et al., 1978]. Higher estimates of 1.0 to 1.6 g are based on techniques that measure total nitrogen and tend to ignore the fact that nearly 25% of milk nitrogen is nonprotein nitrogen. Recommended protein intakes for lactation are variable, with FAO/WHO [1974] values (46 g/day) significantly lower than U.S. RDA'S (66 g/day). Either estimate should be adequate to cover needs for milk protein synthesis if dietary protein is of good quality.

Needs for vitamins, minerals and trace elements are elevated due to their role in biosynthesis and presence in the milk.

Effects of Maternal Nutritional Status on Lactation Performance

Milk volume. The volume of milk produced by well-nourished women during the first postpartum year is about 600 to 700 ml/day [Thomson and Black, 1975] but varies widely between individuals. Reliable determinations of milk output are difficult due to problems of methodology. Until the recent development of methods using double-labelled water, there have been no measurement techniques that do not in some way disrupt the mother-child interaction which strongly influences the course of a feeding. Relying primarily on test weighing methods, numerous studies (summarized in Jelliffe and Jelliffe [1978]), have shown that milk output tends to be lower in women from malnourished communities, during famine conditions, and during seasonal food shortages [Vis, 1976, Prentice et al., 1983]. Several studies have shown a positive effect of maternal protein supplementation on milk volume [Gopalan, 1958; Bassir, 1975; Edozien et al., 1976; Sosa et al., 1976], while a recent study in the Gambia showed no change in milk output with supplementation even during wet season when milk production is generally lower [Prentice et al, 1983b].

Milk composition. Comparative studies of the effects of maternal nutritional status on milk composition are hindered by the fact that milk composition varies within a single feeding, over the course of a day, seasonally, and by stage of lactation. The milk nutrients most influenced by maternal diet are the water soluble vitamins. Protein, fat, and calcium are affected only to a minor degree, while lactose is most invariable [Jelliffe and Jelliffe, 1978].

Milk protein content has been the focus of special concern because of its importance to postnatal child growth. When comparable methods are used to determine the concentration of protein in human milk, little variability is observed. For example, Lindblad and Rahimtoola [1974] found a milk protein content of 0.8 g/100 ml in poorly nourished women from Karachi, Pakistan, a value comparable to estimates of 0.8 to 0.9 g/100 ml from Sweden, Belgium, and Japan. In general, it is assumed that amino acid deficits will be subsidized by maternal tissue, but the Pakastani women mentioned above produced milk with lower levels of lysine and methionine compared to well-nourished women.

Maternal protein supplementation during lactation has produced inconsistent results. In India, Goplan [1958] found a decrease in milk concentration coupled with an increase in volume such that overall protein content in 24 h remained the same. Edozien et al., [1976] found no effect of a 50 g/day dietary protein supplement on protein concentration, while Prentice et al., [1983b] observed a 6.6% increase in protein concentration when undernourished Gambian women were given a protein–calorie supplement. Additional data from India indicate that dietary protein supplementation produced a drop in milk creatinine levels along with a nonsignificant increase in total protein nitrogen [Belavady and Gopalan, 1960; Belavady, 1979].

Although the amount of fat in milk is relatively resistant to dietary manipulation, the fatty acid composition can vary widely [Insull et al., 1959; Potter and Nestel, 1976; Sanders and Naismith, 1976; Sanders et al., 1978]. Vegetarian diets and diets which substitute corn oil for animal fats result in milk with elevated linoleic acid content. Furthermore, comparative data from Africa have shown that when a high percentage of dietary energy is derived from carbohydrate rather than fat, milk is high in lauric and myristic acids [Read et al., 1965]. When maternal fat and energy intakes are restricted, the fatty acid composition of milk tends to resemble maternal depot fat [Insull et al., 1959]. The long-term consequences of fatty acid composition for the infant are not well known. Crawford et al., [1977] have suggested that the diminished levels of polyenoic fatty acids in the milk of malnourished women may have consequences for brain growth in the offspring. Furthermore, while maternal dietary manipulation does not alter milk cholesterol levels, milk high in linoleic acid lowers blood cholesterol levels in the infants consuming it [Picciano, 1978].

The milk content of most water-soluble vitamins directly reflects maternal dietary intake. Deficiency symptoms in breastfed infants tend to mirror those in the adult with respect to thiamin, which is associated with infantile beriberi in South Asia [Simpson and Chow, 1956], and vitamin B_{12} deficiency, which is related to the "syndrome of tremors" [Jadhav et al., 1962]. Milk content of folic acid, vitamin B_6, and riboflavin also tracks maternal dietary intake of these nutrients.

Milk levels of vitamin C vary seasonally with the available of fresh fruits and vegetables [Squires, 1952]. There is, however, evidence of adaptation to low maternal intake of vitamin C [Rajalakshmi, 1974]. The ascorbate content of breast milk tends to be higher than maternal plasma levels, suggesting that the breast has the ability to synthesize vitamin C [Jelliffe and Jelliffe, 1978].

Supplementation studies have shown significant improvements in milk levels of water soluble vitamins when they are provided in quantities sufficient to correct maternal deficits [Belavady, 1979; Prentice et al., 1983b].

The fat soluble vitamins pass less readily into the milk, but can be influenced by maternal stores and dietary intake. Vitamin A content varies seasonally with the availability of fresh fruits and vegetables. Dietary excess of plants containing carotenoids can significantly raise vitamin A levels in milk [Honda et al., 1975]. Milk levels of vitamin D tend to be low and are little affected by maternal intake of this nutrient. Ricketts in totally breastfed infants has been reported, but it is most common when infants are not regularly exposed to sunlight.

Milk calcium content varies minimally with maternal dietary calcium intake. Deficiencies are made up by resorption of maternal bone. Over time, osteoporosis and osteomalacia may develop in high parity women with low intakes of calcium and vitamin D. This problem is particular apparent in Asian women [Jelliffe and Jelliffe, 1978; Atkinson and West, 1970].

Long-Term Consequences of Malnutrition

Effects of maternal supplemental programs have most often been evaluated in terms of their effects on the offspring. One important but overlooked consequence of supplementation may be its positive contribution to long-term maternal health; i.e., it may prevent deterioration of maternal health and nutritional status with repeated reproductive cycles [Prentice et al., 1983b]. In some poorly nourished populations that fail to develop adequate adaptations to chronic low nutrient intakes, the energy and nutrient costs of pregnancy and lactation can create energy deficits manifested by weight loss with increasing parity [Venkatachalam et al., 1960, Bailey, 1962]. Specific nutrient deficiencies may also be exacerbated by repeated reproductive cycles and short birth intervals. Osteomalacia and osteoporosis are common in high parity women whose diets are chronically low in calcium and/or vitamin D [Krishnamachari and Iyengar, 1975; Ford et al, 1973]. Goiter and nutritional edema are worsened by repeated pregnancies [Jellife and Maddocks, 1964]. It may be difficult for poorly nourished women to replenish iron lost to the fetus, in blood during parturition, and to milk during lactation. The resulting chronic anemia may adversely affect maternal health status by increasing susceptibility to infection. Prentice et al., [1983c] found that supplementation of lactating women decreased the incidence of gastrointestinal complaints and upper respiratory infections and increased the mothers' overall sense of well being. In the long term, maternal nutrition may also have an important impact on fertility in human populations (see section on nutrition and fertility below).

Overnutrition during pregnancy may also have long-term consequences. Excess fat deposited during pregnancy may not be lost, particularly in women who do not breastfeed their infants. The onset of obesity in adult females may typically be dated to the reproductive years. Furthermore, diabetes mellitus increases with both obesity and increasing parity.

NUTRITION AND FERTILITY

A relationship between nutrition and fertility has been inferred from a wide range of observations made on humans in laboratory and field studies. Nutritional status appears to play a role in the onset and maintenance of menstrual cycles and pregnancy outcome in females and in sexual development and performance in males.

Although the evolutionary logic of a nutrition-fertility relationship is appealing, the exact mechanism by which nutrition may influence fertility is unclear. Reproduction is costly in terms of energy and nutrients. If a woman's health and work capcity are already compromised by poor nutrition, she is more likely to experience a poor reproductive outcome. It makes sense, therefore, that she not reproduce unless her energy reserves are adequate to subsidize a pregnancy and lactation period. This type of logic forms the basis of the appeal of Frisch's critical weight hypothesis which states that the initiation and maintenance of ovulatory cycles is dependent on the attainment of a critical level of body fat [Frisch and Revelle, 1970; Frisch and McArthur, 1974]. According to this hypothesis, nutrition is related to fertility by its influence on the body's energy reserves. Numerous critiques of the Frisch hypothesis (cf. Scott and Johnston [1982], Johnston et al. [1975], and, Huffman et al. [1978]) have raised doubts about a causal relationship between fatness and the onset or maintenance of menstrual cycles, but they do not question the existence of a basic relationship between nutritional status and fertility. To date, no completely satisfactory hypotheses have been offered to explain the mechanisms involved in this relationship. Moreover, it is well known that nutrition is but one of many interacting variables that influence fertility in human populations. The following section summarizes the evidence for a nutrition-fertility relationship.

Total fertility is related to the span of reproductive years. Delayed menarche or early menopause can thus significantly influence fertility. Over the past century, the age at menarche has declined by about 3 to 4 months per decade. This trend toward earlier menarche associated with accelerated physical growth and maturation has been attributed to improved nutrition from infancy through the childhood years [Tanner, 1973]. Furthermore, studies of adolescents in developing countries show that malnourished girls experience menarche later than those who are well nourished [Frisch, 1972; Malcolm, 1970]. Within populations, menarche occurs earlier in girls who are heavier and fatter [Frisch, 1972]. In all of these cases, the relationship between nutrition and menarche is inferred from body size and/or composition, which is assumed to reflect nutritional history and nutritional status at the time of menarche.

A somewhat more direct relationship is seen in data on secondary nutritional or lactation amenorrhea. As previously mentioned, the incidence of amenorrhea and irregular menstrual cycles increased dramatically in those populations subjected to severe food shortages in Holland, Germany, and Leningrad during World War II [Antonov, 1947; Stein et al., 1975]. Secondary amenorrhea also occurs with anorexia nervosa and severe weight loss [Frisch, 1972; Lev-Ran, 1974].

It has been hypothesized that in poorly nourished communities, maternal nutritional status interacts with lactation to prolong postpartum amenorrhea and thereby increase birth intervals and reduce overall fecundity [Delgado et al., 1978]. Lactation suppresses ovulation through hormonal mechanisms involving prolactin and the hypothalamic-pituitary-gonadal axis. Since the frequency of suckling and feeding of supplemental foods to nursing infants influences the duration of lactation amenorrhea, any study which attempts to isolate the role of maternal nutrition in the duration of amenorrhea must account for these variables. Unfortunately, few studies have done so, thus inconsistent results are not surprising. Based on their study of noncontracepting women in Bangladesh, Huffman et al., [1978] concluded that maternal nutrition played only a minor role in the duration of postpartum amenorrhea. Maternal age, supplemental feeding of the infant, and socioeconomic status were more strongly related. In contrast, Prema et al., [1981], in their study of the effects of maternal nutritional status on postpartum amenorrhea in a population of low income, noncontracepting Indian womens, found that when duration of lactation was held constant, there was a decline in the duration of postpartum amenorrhea with increasing body weight of the mother. This effect was not observed in nonlactating women.

Several maternal nutrition supplementation trials have also evaluated effects of nutrition on the duration of postpartum amenorrhea. Chavez and Martinez [1973] found that caloric supplements amounting to about 300 kcal/day significantly reduced the mean duration of postpartum amenorrhea from 14 to 7.5 months. Data from Guatemala also show a similar effect of maternal supplementation, but the magnitude of the effect was much less: postpartum amenorrhea had an average duration of 12.4 months with supplementation, 13.9 months without [Delgado et al., 1978]. Differences may also reflect variability in infant food and supplement consumption. In their study of lactating women in the Gambia, Lunn et al. [1980, 1981] and Prentice et al. [1983c] found a decline in serum prolactin, cortisol, insulin, and thyroid hormone levels with maternal supplementation, and a 6-month decrease in the duration of postpartum amenorrhea. Since feeding frequency was not significantly altered by supplementation, Lunn and colleagues have suggested that undernutrition may have a direct effect on prolactin levles. High prolactin levels in undernourished lactating women may selectively channel nutrients to the breast for milk production. With supplementation, milk output may be maintained with less metabolic stress on the mother compared to the unsupplemented, undernourished state [Prentice et al., 1983c].

In addition to these studies which focus specifically on the duration of postpartum amenorrhea, there are data which relate malnutrition to fertility in general. For example, based on historical data from England and Scotland, Frisch [1978] has argued that the lower than expected fertility of the mid 19th century is a result of undernutrition and "hard living." Fertility was lowest in the lower classes, where diets tended to be especially poor, and where women are less likely to consume quality foods than men. Eaton and Mayer [1953] have shown a significant increase in fertility in Hutterite populations as their standard of living increased from 1880 to 1950. Similarly, Chen at al. [1974] in Bangladesh and Gopalan and Naidu [1972] in India have related changing patterns of fertility to variations in the food supply and nutritional status of the populations.

A variety of effects of poor nutrition on the reproductive capacity of males have been reported. These include loss of libido, decreased production of prostate fluid, decreased sperm counts, loss of sperm motility, and cessation of sperm production, depending on the severity of nutritional stress [Bishop, 1970; Keys et al., 1950]. In addition, delayed onset of sexual maturity and a decline in fecundity with age—possibly a more rapid decline than that observed in females—are associated with poor nutrition [Frisch, 1978]. Specific nutrient deficiencies have also been related to reproductive ability in males. In the Middle East, for example, a relatively high frequency of hypogonadal dwarfism and delayed sexual maturation has been attributed to zinc deficiency [Prasad et al., 1963; Sandstead et al., 1967; Halsted et al., 1972, Ronaghy, 1974].

CULTURAL DETERMINANTS OF DIETARY INTAKE DURING PREGNANCY AND LACTATION

Pregnancy and lactation are generally recognized as times of heightened vulnerability and needs for both the mother and her offspring. One rarely finds a human group that does not alter usual dietary habits in some way during pregnancy and lactation. A plethora of culturally based prescriptions and food taboos are found around the world. Although not intended as a comprehensive review, what follows is an overview of the general categories of beliefs found cross-culturally, with culture-specific examples.

Dietary Beliefs and Practices During Pregnancy

Dietary practices during pregnancy are culturally shaped to fulfill one or more of the following goals: 1) To meet perceived "nutrient" needs of the mother or developing fetus; 2) To protect the fetus from malformation; 3) To promote easy delivery; and 4) To prevent ill health in the mother.

The conventional medical wisdom and nutritional counselling offered to pregnant women by western biomedical health practitioners falls into the first category. Women are taught that they must increase their dietary intake of fresh fruits and vegetables, dairy products, meats and grains, plus take a vitamin mineral supplement in order to meet the nutrient needs of the developing fetus and ensure a favorable pregnancy outcome. A variety of folk beliefs fit this category as well. For example, increased consumption of calcium-rich foods is thought to prevent the loss of "one tooth per pregnancy," and pregnant women are thought to be "eating for two."

The pregnant woman is popularly thought to experience a variety of food cravings, [Dickens and Trethowan, 1971]. Hook [1978, 1980] studied dietary cravings and aversions in a group of pregnant women in Albany, New York. Cravings were most often for milk, ice cream, sweets (especially chocolate), fruits, and fish. In an earlier study of Black women in Tuskeegee, Alabama, the most commonly reported cravings were for clay, fish, chicken, corn starch, and apples [Edwards et al., 1959]. Taggart [1961] found cravings for fruit to be most common, with sweets mentioned only occasionally by the Scottish women in her study.

A great deal of interest has been generated by the fairly common practice of geophagy or clay eating during pregnancy [O'Rourke et al., 1967; Ferguson and Keaton, 1950; Edwards et al., 1959; Posner et al., 1957; Halstead, 1968; Crosby, 1971]. Picas for substances such as clay have been associated with poor nutrition. For example, 94% of the clay-eating women in Mississippi surveyed by Ferguson and Keaton were judged to have inadequate diets. Hunter [1973] has offered a " cultural-nutrition" hypothesis for geophagy. It has been suggested that dietary cravings are manifestations of specific physiological needs. Hunter contends that such needs form the basis for the establishment (but not necessarily the maintenance) of cultural practices. Geophagy is thus seen as a form of mineral and trace element supplementation of the diet (as well as a form of therapy for gastrointestinal disorders). Certain clays are high in calcium, iron, magnesium, zinc, or copper. After accounting for poor absorption due to a high presence of chelating compounds, Hunter found that the average clay consumption of African women (30 g/day) could fulfill up to 33% of daily copper needs and up to 65% of iron needs. The mineral and trace element content of clays and their contribution to the diet varies extensively. Some reports have suggested that due to the presence of chelating agents, some clays cause rather than alleviate mineral deficiencies [Crosby, 1971]. Moreover, corn or laundry starch, which contains no usable nutrients, has been substituted for clay in parts of the U.S. [Edwards et al., 1959]. Thus, although some food cravings may be explained by physiologic need, the basis for others remains a mystery. Other explanations offered by the consumers of clay or starch are that they relieve indigestion [Vermeer, 1971] or soothe the gatrointestinal tract; fill the stomach, eliminating hunger [Hunter, 1973]; taste good, relieve nervous tension, or prevent birth marks [O'Rourke et al., 1967].

Numerous food proscriptions during pregnancy are based on the belief that certain foods will harm the developing fetus. Some of these beliefs are well founded and based on knowledge of the teratogenic effects of certain substances. For example, current recommendations of the medical establishment include restriction or avoidance of caffein and alcohol to prevent birth defects and fetal alcohol syndrome. Hook [1978, 1980] has argued that natural aversions exist for foods with possible embryotoxic effects. This is how he explains the decline in consumption of coffee and alcoholic beverages during pregnancy in the absence of specific medical recommendations.

Other beliefs represent folk wisdom passed from generation to generation. Many of the 200 pregnant women attending prenatal clinics in Charleston,

South Carolina surveyed by Bartholomew and Poston [1970] avoided particular foods to protect the fetus: Milk was believed to cause cancer, eggs cause
sores on the baby's head that could lead to brain damage, collards "mark" the
baby, and diet colas can poison the fetus. Similar beliefs are common cross-
culturally and may have their basis in sympathetic magic. For example,
consuming the flesh of a particular animal may result in a child who takes on
the characteristics of that particular animal: bony-headed fishes, antelope with
twisted horns, and snakes are forbidden to Mbum women of Africa [O'Laughlin, 1974]. In a number of cases, particularly in Africa, chicken and goat are
prohibited because they are thought to cause pain or death in childbirth or
abnormal children [O'Laughlin, 1974; Douglas, 1966].

A third set of dietary practices is believed to promote easy delivery. One
strategy is to limit the size of the fetus by restricting maternal food intake. This
was the goal of the Prochownick diet discussed earlier. Mace and Mace [1959]
cite the example of the mother-in-law in India who starved her sons's wife to
promote an easier birth. Similar practices of food restriction to limit fetal size
are described by May [1961] and Mead [1955] for Cambodia, Burma, and
Vietnam. Other beliefs center around preventing the fetus from "sticking" to
the womb. For example, cheese was avoided by about 7% of the women
surveyed by Bartholomew and Poston [1970] because it was thought to make
the baby's head stick to the womb and cause a "dry birth." Rice cake was also
thought to cause a difficult labor because of its stickiness.

A fourth set of beliefs focus on the prevention of ill health in the mother.
Recommendations made by obstetricians concerning optimal weight gain fall
into this category. Several decades ago, it was common to restrict pregnancy
weight gain to about 7 kg to prevent pre-eclampsia (by those who associated
pre-eclampsia with excessive weight gain [Hytten and Leitch, 1971]). Recommendations changed with the accumulation of data on the relationship
between low pregnancy weight gain and LBW in infants and work detailing
the components of pregnancy weight gain in the well-nourished woman
[Hytten and Leitch, 1971]. Current recommendations are for a gain of about
12.5 kg. Gains in excess of that are thought to contribute to obesity in the
mother.

Dietary practices associated with humoral theories are also concerned with
maternal well-being. According to humoral theories, pregnancy, birth, and
lactation can disrupt humoral balance. A proper diet must be consumed to
restore balance and preserve maternal health. In most humoral systems (Asian
and Latin American), pregnancy is seen as a hot state which must be balanced
by consumption of cold foods [Manderson, 1981; Laderman, 1981]. For
example, Malay dietary practices involve the avoidance of hot foods in the

first trimester to prevent miscarriage and in the third trimester to promote easy delivery [Manderson, 1981].

The psychological well-being of the mother may also be served by dietary practices during pregnancy. Ayres [1967] contends that the frustration and anxiety of pregnancy create an increased demand for nurturance that is manifested in the form of food cravings which must be met by the husband and other relatives. She goes on to suggest that indulging those cravings may result in overconsumption of food, increasing the threat of toxemia, which then necessitates social sanctions in the form of food taboos to safeguard the mother and child. Although there may be some truth to the first part of her argument, that is, indulgence of food cravings may serve a nurturant function and perhaps acknowledge the special status of the pregnant woman, the second part is fallacious given what we know about the dangers of toxemia. Furthermore, the societies that form the basis for her hypothesis tend to have more problems with poor nutrition than with overnutrition. One final suggestion about the role of food taboos for the pregnant woman is that they reinforce male-female separateness [O'Laughlin, 1974].

Dietary Beliefs and Practices During Lactation

Dietary beliefs and practices during lactation tend to be somewhat less common than those for pregnancy [Ford, 1945]. In general, they seek to protect the mother during what is viewed as a particularly vulnerable period, to promote a good milk supply, or to protect infants from foods that may harm them through the milk.

A postpartum period of confinement with restricted activity, social contacts, and a special diet is common cross-culturally. According to humoral theories, parturition involves loss of heat, which must be restored by a proper diet rich in hot foods and avoidance of cold foods [Manderson, 1981]. Thus in many parts of Asia, heavily spiced teas (e.g., ginger roots) are drunk, and most fruit and vegetables, which are categorized as cold, are avoided. The diet may be higher than usual in animal proteins, since these foods are considered hot. Osgood [1963] noted that in China, foods considered of high quality (pork, eggs, chicken, and brown sugar) were given to women in the early postpartum period.

A number of foods and beverages are thought to promote good milk production. In the U.S. and British Isles, beer—particularly dark beer—is thought to be good for lactating women, in part because of its B vitamin content and ability to promote relaxation. Another common belief in the U.S. is that mothers need to drink milk to make milk.

Finally, some foods are avoided because they are believed to cause distress in the infant. Common advice to lactating women in the U.S. is to avoid "gassy vegetables" (cabbage, broccoli, etc.) to prevent gastrointestinal distress, caffein to prevent wakefulness in the infant, and citrus fruits to prevent skin rashes.

Cultural - Ecological Factors

In populations with limited food availability or where quality foods are sold as cash crops, there may be a systematic diversion of quality foods, particularly animal protein, to adult males [Rosenberg, 1980]. Pregnancy and lactation are not always perceived as states requiring increased food intakes. The pattern of intrafamilial food distribution observed by Mora et al. [1983] in Bogota may illustrate this point. Although 850 kcal/day was targeted to them, pregnant women supplemented their diets with only about 150 of the calories provided to the family unit.

Consequences of Dietary Beliefs and Practices

It is difficult to ascertain the degree to which dietary prescriptions and taboos during pregnancy and lactation influence maternal nutritional status and reproductive outcomes. Most of the studies that describe dietary beliefs fail to measure actual dietary practices, nutritional status, or biological outcomes [Rosenberg, 1980]. Furthermore, although there are data on the presence and nature of beliefs in many groups, there is relatively little information on the adherence to those practices. One might expect that, due to evolution and adaptation, a majority of beliefs serve to ensure positive outcomes, that is, they protect the fetus and promote maternal health. In fact, there are cases where this is not true. Bartholomew and Poston [1970] estimated that the diets of 10% of the prenatal clinic patients they surveyed had substandard diets due to "folklore." In particular, avoidance of dairy products prevented adequate intake of calcium. The aforementioned avoidance of fruits and vegetables by women in the postpartum period and of animal protein during pregnancy may serve to compromise maternal nutritional status when needs for the nutrients that could be provided by those foods are particularly high. Additional practices with possible detrimental effects include overzealous restriction of sodium intake and diets that excessively limit maternal weight gain during pregnancy.

Although it may be argued that women in some populations have adapted to poor-quality diets and maintain a high level of reproductive success, it is important to recognize that the adaptations may have long-term costs. For example, if activity is significantly reduced, work output and ultimately food production or purchasing power may be compromised. Under these circumstances, dietary practices that would be advantageous would divert quality foods *to* rather than *away from* pregnant women.

CONCLUSIONS

Nutrition during the reproductive years plays an important role in the reproductive success of human populations. Numerous cultural, biological, and ecological factors interact to create situations of nutrition risk. Although individuals and populations are capable of adapting to a wide range of nutritional circumstances, both over- and undernutrition—particularly when extreme—can curtail reproductive success. The nutritional status of both males and females influences overall fertility of populations either by preventing conception or by increasing fetal and neonatal losses. Interacting with other environmental variables, maternal nutrition during pregnancy and lactation can have a profound effect on both long- and short-term maternal health, pregnancy outcomes, and the subsequent health, growth, and development of offspring.

REFERENCES

Achari K, Rani U (1971): Maternal anemia and the fetus. J Obstet Gynecol India 21:305.

Adair LS (1984): Adaption to low energy intakes during pregnancy and lactation: The case of rural Taiwan. In Pollitt E, Amante P (eds): "Energy Intake and Activity." New York: Alan R. Liss, pp 33-55.

Adair LS, Pollitt E (1983): Seasonal variation in maternal body measurements and infant birth weight. Am J Phys Anthr 62:325-331.

Adair LS, Pollitt E (1985): Outcome of maternal nutrition supplementation: A comprehensive review of the Bacon Chow study. Am J Clin Nutr 41:948-978.

Adair LS, Pollitt E, Mueller WH (1983): Maternal anthropometric changes during pregnancy and lactation in rural Taiwanese population. Hum Biol 55:771-787.

Adair LS, Pollitt E, Mueller WH (1984): The Bacon Chow study: Effect of maternal nutritional supplementation on maternal weight and skinfold changes during pregnancy and lactation. Brit J Nutr 51:357-369.

Antonov A (1947): Children born during the siege of Leningrad in 1942. J Pediatr 30:250-259.

Atkinson PJ, West RR (1970): Loss of skeletal calcium in lactating women. J Ob Gyn Brit Cwlth 77:555-560.

Ayres B (1967): Pregnancy magic: A study of food taboos and sex avoidances. In Ford CS (ed): "Cross Cultural Approaches." New Haven: HRAF Press, pp 111-125.

Bailey KV (1962): Rural nutrition surveys in Indonesia (6) Field studies of lactating women. Trop Geog Med 14:11-19.

Barnes RH (1976): Dual role of environmental deprivation and malnutrition in retarding intellectual development. Am J Clin Nutr 29:912-917.

Bartholomew MJ, Poston FE (1970): Effect of food taboos on prenatal nutrition. J Nutr Educ 2:15-17.

Bassir O (1975): Nutritional studies on breast milk of Nigerian women. Determination of the output of breast milk. W Afr J Biol Chem 1:15.

Belavady B (1979): Dietary supplementation and improvements in the lactation performance of Indian women. In Aebi H, Whithead RG (eds): "Maternal Nutrition During Pregnancy and Lactation." Bern: Hans Huber Publishers. pp 274-284.

Bernhardt IB, Dorsey DJ (1974): Hypervitaminosis A and congenital renal anomalies in a human infant. Obstet Gynecol 43:750-755.

Bishop MWH (1970): Aging and reproduction in the male. J Repro Fertil (suppl) 12:65-87.

Brozek J, Coursin DB, Read MS (1977): Longitudinal effects of malnutrition, nutrition supplementation and behavioral stimulation. PAHO Bull 11:237-249.

Carswell F, Kerr MM, Hutchinson JH (1970): Congenital goiter and hypothyroidism produced by maternal ingestion of iodides. Lancet 1:1241-1243.

Chanarin I (1969): "The Megaloblastic Anemias." Oxford: Blackwell Scientific.

Chandra RK (1975): Fetal malnutrition and postnatal immunocompetence.. Am J Dis Child 129:450-454.

Chandra RK, Ali SK, Kutty KM (1977): Thymus dependent lymphocytes and delayed hypersensitivity in low birthweight infants. Biol Neonate 31:15-18.

Chavez A, Martinez C (1973): Nutrition and development of infants from poor rural areas III. Maternal nutrition and its consequence on fertility. Nutr Rep Int 7:1-8.

Chen LC, Ahmed S, Gesche M, Mosley WH (1974): A prospective study of birth interval dynamics in rural Bangladesh. Pop Studies 28:277-297.

Cochrane WA (1965): Overnutrition in prenatal and neonatal life. Can Med Assoc J 93:893-899.

Crawford MA, Hassam AG, Hall BM (1977): The metabolism of essential fatty acids in the human foetus and neonate. Nutr Metab 21 (suppl one):187-188.

Crosby WH (1971): Food pica and iron deficiency. Arch Int Med 127:960-961.

Delgado H, Lechtig A, Martorell R, Brineman E, Klein RE (1978): Nutrition, lactation and postpartum amenorrhea. Am J Clin Nutr 31:322-327.

Devadas RP, Vijayalakshmi P, Vanitha R (1978): Impact of nutrition on pregnancy, lactation and growth performance of the exterogestate foetus. Ind J Nutr Dietet 15:31-37.

Dickens G, Trethowan WH (1971): Cravings and aversions during pregnancy. J Psychosomat Res 15:259-268.

Dobbing J (1972): Vulnerable periods of brain development. In Von Muralt A (ed): "Lipids, Malnutrition and the Developing Brain." Amsterdam: Associated Scientific.

Douglas M (1966): "Purity and Danger." Baltimore: Pelican Press.

Eastman NJ (1970): In Committee on Maternal Nutrition, National Research Council, National Academy of Sciences: "Maternal Nutrition and the Course of Pregnancy." Washington, D.C.: U.S. Government Printing Office.

Eaton JW, Mayer AJ (1953): The social biology of very high fertility among the Hutterites: The demography of a unique population. Hum Biol 25:206-264.

Edozien JC, Khan MAR, Waslien CI (1976): Human protein deficiency: Results of a Nigerian village study. J Nutr 106:312-328.

Edwards CH, McDonald S, Mitchell JR, Jones L, Mason L, Kemp AM, Laing D, Trigg L. (1959): Clay and cornstarch eating women. J Am Diet Assoc 35:810-815.

Emerson K, Saxena BN, Poindexter EL (1972): Caloric cost of normal pregnancy. Obstet Gynecol 40:786-794.

FAO/WHO (1974): Handbook on human nutritional requirements. Monograph series No. 61. Geneva:WHO.

Ferguson AL, Lawlor GJ, Neumann CG, Oh W, Stiehm ER (1974): Decreased rosette forming lymphocytes in malnutrition and intrauterine growth retardation. J Pediatr 85:717-723.

Ferguson JH, Keaton A (1950): Studies of diets of pregnant women in Mississippi. Ingestion of clay and laundry starch. New Orleans Med Surg J 103:81-87.

Ford CS (1945): "A comparative Study of Human Reproduction." New Haven: Yale University Publications in Anthropology 32. HRAF Press.

Ford JA, Davidson DC, McIntosh WB, Fyfe WB, Dunnigan MG (1973): Neonatal ricketts in an Asian immigrant population. Brit Med J 3:211-212.

Frisch RE, Revelle R (1970): Height and weight at menarche and a hypothesis of critical body weights and adolescent events. Science 169:397-398.

Frisch RE, McArthur J (1974): Menstrual cycles: fatness as a determinant of minimum weight for height necessary for their maintenance or onset. Science 185:949-951.

Frisch RE (1972): Weight at menarche: Similarity for well nourished and undernourished girls as evidence for historical constancy. J Pediatr 50:445-450.

Frisch RE (1978): Population, food intake and fertility. Science 199:22-30.

Gebre-Mehdin M, Gobezie A (1975): Dietary intake in the third trimester of pregnancy and birthweight of offspring among non-privileged and privileged women. Am J Clin Nutr 28:1322-1329.

Giles C (1966): An account of 335 cases of megaloblastic anemia of pregnancy and the puerperium. J Clin Pathol 19:1-11.

Gopalan C (1958): Studies on lactation in poor Indian communities. J Trop Ped 4:87-97.

Copalan C, Naidu AN (1972): Nutrition and fertility. Lancet 2:1077-1079.

Greene LS (1980): Social and biological predictors of physical growth and neurological development in an area where iodine and protein-energy malnutrition are endemic. In Greene LS, Johnston FE (eds): "Social and Biological Predictors of Physical Growth and Neurological Development." New York: Academic Press, pp 223-256.

Gross RL, Newberne PM, Reid JVO (1974): Adverse effects on infant development associated with maternal folic acid deficiency. Nutr Rep Int 10:241-248.

Halsted JA (1968): Geophagia in man: Its nature and nutritional effects. Am J Clin Nutr 21:1384-1393.

Halsted JA, Ronaghy HA, Abadi P, Haghshenass M, Amirhakemi GH, Barakat RM, Reinhold JG (1972): Zinc deficiency in man. The Shiraz experiment. Am J Med 53:277-284.

Hambraeus L, Lonnerdal B, Forsum E, Gebre-Mehdin M (1978): Nitrogen and protein components of human milk. Acta Ped Scand 61:561-565.

Hibbard BM (1975): Folates and the fetus. S Afr Med J 49:1223-1226.

Hibbard ED, Smithells RW (1965): Folic acid metabolism and human embryopathy. Lancet 1:1254.

Honda T, Kawakami T, Kohno T, Morishima N, Osumi K (1975): A study of aurantiasis in Japanese children. Proc Xth Int Cong Nutr 706.

Hook EB (1978): Dietary cravings and aversions during pregnancy. Am J Clin Nutr 31:1355-1362.

Hook EB (1980): Influence of pregnancy on dietary selection. Int J Obesity 4:338-340.

Huffman SL, Chowdhury AKM, Mosley WH (1978): Postpartum amenorrhea: How is it affected by maternal nutritional status? Science 200:1155-1157.

Hunter JM (1973): Geophagy in Africa and in the United States: A Cultural-nutrition hypothesis. Geog Rev 63:170-195.

Hurley LS (1977): Zinc deficiency in prenatal and neonatal development. In Brewer GJ, Prasad AS (eds): "Zinc Metabolism: Current Aspects in Health and Disease." New York: Alan R. Liss, pp 47-58.

Hurley LS (1980): "Developmental Nutrition." Englewood NJ: Prentice Hall.

Hytten FE, Leitch I (1971): "The Physiology of Human Pregnancy." 2nd Ed. Philadelphia: F.A. Davis.

Hytten FE, Chamberlain G (1980): "Clinical Physiology in Obstetrics." Oxford: Blackwell.

Insull W, Hirsch J, James T, Ahrens EH (1959): The fatty acids of human milk II. Alteration produced by manipulation of caloric balance and exchange of dietary fats. J Clin Invest 38:443-450.

Jadhav M, Webb JKG, Vaishnava S, Baker SJ (1962): Vitamin B_{12} deficiency in Indian infants. A new syndrome. Lancet II 903-907.

Jelliffe DB, Jelliffe EFP (1978): "Human Milk in the Modern World." London: Oxford University Press.

Jelliffe DB, Maddocks I (1964): Ecologic malnutrition in the New Guinea Highlands. Clin Pediatr 3:432-438.

Johnston FE, Roche A, Schell LM, Wettenhall Ne (1975): Critical weight at menarche: Critique of a hypothesis. Am J Dis Child 129:19-23.

Johnstone FD, MacGillivray I, Dennis KJ (1972): Nitrogen retention in pregnancy. J Obstet Gynecol Brit Cwlth 79:777-784.

Keys A, Brozek J, Henschel A, Mickelson O, Taylor HL (1950): "The Biology of Human Starvation, Vol 1.," Minneapolis: University of Minnesota Press.

Krishnamachari KAVR, Iyengar L (1975): Effect of maternal malnutrition on the bone density of the neonates. Am J Clin Nutr 28:482-486.

Laderman C (1981): Symbolic and empirical reality: A new approach to the study of food avoidances. Am Ethnol 30:468-493.

Lechtig A (1982): Studies of nutrition intervention in pregnancy. Birth 9:115-119.

Lechtig A, Habicht J-P, Yarbrough C, Delgado H, Guzman G, Klein RE (1972): Influence of food supplementation during pregnancy on birthweight in rural populations of Guatemala. Proc 9th Int Congr Nutr 2:44-52.

Lechtig A, Habicht J-P, Delgado H, Klein RE, Yarbrough C, Martorell R (1975): Effect of food supplementation during pregnancy on birthweight. Pediatr 56:508-520.

Lechtig A, Martorell R, Delgado H, Yarbrough C, Klein RE (1978): Food supplementation during pregnancy, maternal anthropometry and birthweight in Guatemala rural population. J Trop Ped 24:217-222.

Lelong-Tissier M (1977): Hyponatremie maternofoetal carientielle par regime desode. Arch Fr Pediatr 34:64.

Levitsky DA, Barnes RH (1972): Nutritional and environmental interactions in the behavioral development of the rat: Long term effects. Science 176:68-71.

Lev-Ran A (1974): Secondary amenorrhea resulting from uncontrolled weight reducing diets. Fertil Steril 25:459-469.

Lind T (1981): Nutrient requirements during pregnancy I. Am J Clin Nutr 34:669-678.

Lindblad BS, Rahimtoola RJ (1974): A pilot study of the quality of human milk in a lower socioeconomic group in Karachi, Pakistan. Acta Ped Scand 63:125-128.

Lunn PG, Prentice AM, Austin S, Whitehead RG (1980): Influence of maternal diet on prolactin levels during lactation. Lancet I:623-625.

Lunn PG, Watkinson M, Prentice AM, Morrell P, Austin S, Whitehead RG (1981): Maternal nutrition and lactational amenorrhea. Lancet I:1428-1429.

Mace D, Mace V (1959): "Marriage East and West." New York: Doubleday Dolphin Press.

Malcolm LA (1970): Growth and development in the Bundi child of the New Guinea Highlands. Hum Biol 42:293-328.

Malone JI (1975): Vitamin passage across the placenta. Clin Perinat 2:295-307.

Manderson L (1981): Roasting, smoking and dieting in response to birth: Malay confinement in cross-cultural perspective. Soc Sci Med 15B:509-520.

May J (1961): "The Ecology of Malnutrition in the Far and Near East." New York: Hafner Press.

McCance RA, Widdowson EM (1962): Nutrition and growth. Proc Soc Biol 156:326-337.

McDonald EC, Pollitt E, Mueller WH, Sherwyn R (1981): The Bacon Chow study: Maternal nutritional supplementation and birth weight of offspring. Am J Clin Nutr 34:513-517.

Mead M (1955): "Cultural Patterns and Technical Change." New York: Mentor Books.

Mora JO, de Navarro L, Clement J, Wagner M, de Paredes B, Herrera MG (1978): The effect of food supplementation on the calorie and protein intake of pregnant women. Nutr Rep Int 17:217-228.

Mora JO, deParades B, Wagner M, deNavarro L, Vuori J, Susecum J, Christiansen N, Herrera MG (1979): Nutrition supplementation and the outcome of pregnancy. I. Birthweight. Am J Clin Nutr 32:455-462.

Mora JO, Sanchez R, de Paredes B, Herrera MG (1981): Sex related effects of nutritional supplementation during pregnancy on fetal growth. Early Hum Devel 5:243-251.

Mora JO (1983): Supplementary feeding during pregnancy: Impact on mother and child in Bogota, Colombia. In Underwood BA (ed): "Nutrition Intervention Strategies in National Development." New York: Academic Press, pp 79-90.

Mueller WH, Pollitt E (1983): The Bacon Chow study: Effects of nutrition supplementation on sibling-sibling anthropometeric correlations. Hum Biol 54:455-460.

Munro HN (1981): Nutrient requirements during pregnancy II. Am J Clin Nutr 34:679-684.

Naismith DJ (1977): Protein metabolism in pregnancy. In Philips EE, Barnes J, Newton M (eds): "Scientific Foundations of Obstetrics and Gynecology." London: Heinemann, pp 503-511.

National Research Council (1980): "Recommended Dietary Allowances." Washington: U.S. Government Printing Office.

Norgan NG, Ferro Luzzi A, Durnin JVGA (1974): The energy and nutrient intake and energy expenditure of 248 Guinea adults. Phil Trans R Soc Lond 268:309-348.

O'Laughlin B (1974): Mediation of contradiction: Why Mbum women do not eat chicken. In Rosaldo MZ, Lamphere L (eds): "Women, Culture and Society." Stanford: Stanford University Press, pp 301-318.

O'Rourke DE, Quinn JG, Nicholson JO, Gibson HH (1967): Geophagy during pregnancy. Obstet Gynecol 29:581-584.

Osgood C (1963): "Village Life in Old China." New York: Ronald Press.

Osofsky HJ (1975): Relationship between nutrition during pregnancy and subsequent infant and child development. Obstet Gynecol Survey 30:227-241.

Pharoah POD, Butterfield IH, Hetzel BS (1971): Neurological damage to the fetus resulting from severe iodine deficiency during pregnancy. Lancet I:308-310.

Picciano MF (1978): Mineral content of human milk during a single nursing. Nutr Rep Int 18:5-10.

Pitkin RM, Kaminetsky HA, Newton M, Pritchard JA (1972): Maternal nutrition: A selective review of clinical topics. Obstet Gynecol 40:773-785.

Posner LB, McCottry CM, Posner C (1957): Pregnancy craving and pica. Obstet Gynecol 9:270-272.

Potter JM, Nestel PJ (1976): The effects of dietary fatty acids and cholesterol on the milk lipids of lactating women and the plasma cholesterol of breast-fed infants. Am J Clin Nutr 29:54-60.

Prasad AS, Miale A, Farid Z, Sandstead HH, Schulert AR (1963): Zinc metabolism in patients with the syndrome of iron deficiency anemia, hepatosplenomegaly, dwarfism and hypogonadism. J Lab Clin Med 61:537-549.

Prema K, Naidu S, Neelakumari S, Ramalakshmi BA (1981): Nutrition fertility interaction in lactating women of low income groups. Brit J Nutr 45:461-467.

Prentice AM (1984): Adaptations to long term low energy intake. In Pollitt E, Amante P (eds): "Energy Intake and Activity." New York: Alan R. Liss, pp 3-31.

Prentice AM, Whitehead RG, Roberts SB, Paul AA, Watkinson M, Prentice A, Watkinson AA (1980): Dietary supplementation of Gambian nursing mothers and lactational performance. Lancet II:886-888.

Prentice AM, Whitehead RG, Watkinson M, Lamb W, Cole TJ (1983a): Prenatal dietary supplementation of African women and birth weight. Lancet I:489-492.

Prentice AM, Roberts SB, Prentice A, Paul AA, Watkinson M, Watkinson AA, Whitehead RG (1983b): Dietary supplementation of lactating Gambian women. I. Effect on breast milk volume and quality. Hum Nutr: Clin Nutr 37C:53-64.

Prentice AM, Lunn PG, Watkinson M, Whitehead RG (1983c): Dietary supplementation of lactating Gambian women. II. Effect on maternal health, nutritional status and biochemistry. Hum Nutr: Clin Nutr 37C:65-74.

Purvis R (1973): Enamel hypoplasia on the teeth associated with neonatal tetany: A manifestation of maternal Vitamin D deficiency. Lancet II:811-814.

Rajalakshmi R (1974): Reproductive performance of poor Indian women in a low plane of nutrition. Trop Geog Med 23:117-125.

Read WWC, Lutz PG, Tashijan A (1965): Human milk lipids. II. The influence of dietary carbohydrates and fat on the fatty acids of mature milk. A study in four ethnic groups. Am J Clin Nutr 17:184-187.

Reinhardt MC (1978): Maternal anemia in Abidjan—Its influence on placenta and newborn. Helv Pediatr Acta 33 (suppl 41):43-63.

Roepke JLB, Kirksey A (1979): Vitamin B_6 nutriture during pregnancy and lactation. One Vitamin B_6 intake, levels of the vitamin in biological fluids and conditions of the infant at birth. Am J Clin Nutr 32:2249-2256.

Ronaghy HS, Reingold JG, Mahloudji M, Ghavami P, Spirey Fox MR, Halsted JA (1974): Zinc supplementation of malnourished schoolboys in Iran. Increased growth and other effects. Am J Clin Nutr 27:112-121.

Rosario YP (1971): The obstetrical behavior of the anemic pregnant woman. J Obstet Gynecol India 21:4.

Rosenberg EM (1980): Demographic effects of sex differential nutrition. In Jerome N, Kandel R, Pelto G (eds): "Nutritional Anthropology." Pleasantville, NJ: Redgrave, pp 181-203.

Rush D (1983): Nutritional services during pregnancy and birthweight: A retrospective matched pair analysis. J Can Med Assoc.

Rush D, Stein Z, Susser M (1980): "Diet in Pregnancy: A Randomized Controlled Trial of Nutritional Supplements." BD:OAS Vol XVI. New York: Alan R. Liss.

Sanders TAB, Naismith DJ (1976): Long chain polyunsaturated fatty acids in the erythrocyte lipids of breast and bottle fed babies. Proc Nutr Soc 35:63A.

Sanders TAB, Ellis FR, Dickerson JN (1978): Studies of vegans: the fatty acid composition of plasma cholinephosphoglycerides, erythrocytes, adipose tissue and breast milk and some indicators of susceptibility to ischemic heart disease in vegans and omnivore controls. Am J Clin Nutr 31:805-813.

Sandstead HH, Prasad AS, Schulert AR, Farid A, Miale A, Bassily S, Darby WJ (1967): Human zinc deficiency, endocrine manifestations and response to treatment. Am J Clin Nutr 20:422-442.

Scott DE, Whalley PJ, Pritchard DJA (1970): Maternal folate deficiency and pregnancy wastage. II. Fetal malformations. Obstet Gynecol 36:26-28.

Scott, EC, Johnston FE (1982): Critical fat, menarche and the maintenance of menstrual cycles: A critical review. J Adoles Health Care 2:249-260.

Sever L, Emanuel I (1973): Is there a connection between maternal zinc deficiency and congenital malformations of the central nervous system in man? Teratology 7:117-126.

Simpson IA, Chow AY (1956): The thiamine content of human milk in Malaya. J Trop Ped 2:3-17.

Smithells RW, Shepard S, Achora C (1976): Vitamin deficiencies and neural tube defects. Arch Dis Child 51:944-952.

Sosa R, Klaus M, Urritia JJ (1976): Feed the nursing mother, thereby the infant. J Pediatr 88:668-670.

Squires BT (1952): Ascorbic acid content of the milk of the Tswana women. Trans Roy Soc Trop Med Hyg 46:95-99.

Stein Z, Susser M, Saenger G, Marolla F (1975): "Famine and Human Development: The Dutch Hunger Winter of 1944-45." New York: Oxford University Press.

Stein Z, Susser M, Rush D (1978): Prenatal nutrition and birth weight: Experiments and quasi experiments in the past decade. J Repro Med 21:287-299.

Strange L, Carlstrom K, Ericksson M (1978): Hypervitaminosis A in early pregnancy and malformations in the central nervous system. Acta Obstet Scand 57:289-291.

Svanberg B (1975): Absorption of iron in pregnancy. Acta Obstet Gynecol Scand Suppl 48:1-108.

Taggart N (1961): Food habits in pregnancy. Proc Nutr Soc 20:35-40.

Taggart NR, Holliday RM, Billewicz WZ, Hytten FE, Thomson AM (1967): Changes in skinfolds during pregnancy. Brit J Clin Nutr 221:439-451.

Tanner JM (1973): Growing up. Sci Amer 229:35-43.

Thanangkul O, Amatayakul MB (1975): Nutrition of pregnant women in a developing country—Thailand. Am J Dis Child 129:426-427.

Thomson AM (1958): Diet in pregnancy. I. Dietary survey technique and the nutritive value of diets taken by primagravidae. Brit J Nutr 12:446-461.

Thomson AM (1959): Diet in Pregnancy. 3. Diet in relation to the course and outcome of pregnancy. Brit J Nutr 13:509-525.

Thomson AM, Billewicz WZ (1957): Clinical significance of weight trends during pregnancy. Brit Med J 1:243-247.

Thomson AM, Black AE (1975): Nutritional aspects of human lactation. Bull WHO 52:163-176.

Thomson AM, Hytten FE, Billewicz WZ (1970): The energy cost of human lactation. Brit J Nutr 24:565-572.

Tompkins WT, Wiehl DG, Mitchell RMcN (1955): The underweight patient as an obstetrical hazard. Am J Obstet Gynecol 69:114-123.

Van Gelder DW, Darby FU (1944): Congenital and infant beriberi. J Pediatr 25:226-235.

Venkatachalam PS (1962): Maternal nutritional status and its effect on the newborn. Bull WHO 26:193-201.

Venkatachalam PS, Shankar K, Gopalan C (1960): Changes in body weight and body composition during pregnancy. Ind J Med Res 48:511-517.

Vermeer D (1971): Geophagy among the Ewe of Ghana. Ethnology 10:56-72.

Villar J, Smeriglio V, Martorell R, Brown CH, Klein RE (1983): Heterogeneous growth and mental development of intrauterine growth retarded infants during the first three years of life. Unpublished manuscript.

Vis HL (1976): Influence of maternal health on the volume and quality of breast milk secreted. Bull Int Ped Assoc 6:26-35.

Vuori L, Cristiansen N, Clement J, Mora JO, Wagner M, Herrera MG (1979): Nutrition supplementation and the outcome of pregnancy. II. Visual habituation at 15 days. Am J Clin Nutr 32:463-469.

Wheatley D (1977): Treatment of pregnancy sickness. Br J Obstet Gynecol 84:444-447.

WHO (1974): Handbook on human nutritional requirements. Monograph series No. 61. Geneva:WHO.

Widdowson EM (1968): Growth and composition of the fetus and newborn. In Assali NS (ed): "Biology of Gestation." Vol 2. New York: Academic Press, pp 1-49.

Winick M (1976): "Malnutrition and Brain Development." New York: Oxford Univ Press.

Winick M, Noble A (1965): Quantitative changes in DNA, RNA and protein during prenatal and postnatal growth in the rat. Dev Biol 12:451-456.

Winick M, Rosso P (1969): The effect of severe early malnutrition on cellular growth of the human brain. Pediatr Res 3:181-184.

Worthington-Roberts BS, Vermeersch J, Williams SR (1981): "Nutrition in Pregnancy and Lactation." St. Louis: CV Mosby.

Zamenhof S, Van Marthens E, Grauel L (1971): DNA (Cell number) in neonatal brain. Alteration by maternal dietary caloric restriction. Science 172:850-851.

Zuspan FP, Goodrich S (1968): Metabolic studies in normal pregnancy. I. Nitrogen metabolism. Am J Obstet Gynecol 100:7-14.

Nutritional Anthropology, pages 155-172
© 1987 Alan R. Liss, Inc.

Culture, Community, and the Course of Infant Feeding

Judith Gussler, PhD

Ross Laboratories, Columbus, Ohio 43216

INTRODUCTION

Most discussions of infant feeding begin with parturition. In fact, the feeding of an infant begins before birth, in utero, as nutrients pass through a mother's placental wall. Nutritional dependency of the infant on its mother is complete at this stage; the dependency continues after birth if the infant is breastfed. The period of breastfeeding has been called a "transitional" stage [Mead and Newton, 1967] during which the total physiologic and nutritional dependency of the fetus gradually gives way to the independency of the weaned child. This weaning process in many cases takes several years. When infants are not breastfed, the stage is terminated "when the cord is cut [ibid]."

The "infant feeding period" actually is a part of a nutritional continuum that spans an individual's entire lifecycle, and the common definition of it as birth to 12 months is arbitrary. Nevertheless, adequate and proper feeding of the young infant is critical for the survival, health, growth, and development of the individual; not surprisingly, much recent research and many recent health policies have focused on this nutritional period.

This chapter discusses several topics and issues concerning infant feeding, including characteriscs of the products and processes of breastfeeding, recent trends in infant feeding, factors affecting infant feeding practices, and common infant feeding strategies. Social and cultural context of feeding patterns is implicitly or explicitly recognized in this discussion. As in many other human behaviors, we see variety and complexity in cultural expressions of what are basic and generally uniform physiologic processes.

BREASTFEEDING AND INFANT HEALTH: PRODUCT AND PROCESS
Nutrional Properties of Breastmilk

Recent research on the composition of human breastmilk has demonstrated its complexity [Lawrence, 1985]. For purposes of this discussion, however, a detailed nutrient analysis and description of milk biochemistry are not required. A brief discussion of some important properties of human milk, however, is helpful.

Human breastmilk composition is species specific. Its compositional profile (Table I) describes a product of low nutrient density compared to that of many other mammals. Proportions of protein and fat are particularly low. Lozoff et al. [1977] suggest that human breast milk resembles that of animals such as other primates whose young are carried or otherwise kept close by and fed frequently. Thus, the nutrient profile of human milk is congruent with the pattern of biologic (ad libitum) breastfeeding recorded for many traditional societies and most hunters-gatherers [Lozoff et al. 1977; Gussler and Briesemeister, 1980].

The actual nutrient composition of breastmilk varies a great deal, depending on individual characteristics of the mother, the length of time since the infant's birth, the time of day, and how long and how much the infant has been fed at a particular feeding (whether at the beginning or end) [Lawrence, 1985:66-71]. Fat content, for example, tends to be higher at the end of a nursing session than at the beginning. (Recent research has not confirmed the

TABLE I. Mammalian Care Patterns and Breastmilk Composition[*]

| | Example of species No. of species studied | | | |
	Deer (n = 13)	Dogs (n = 18)	Goats (n = 22)	Human beings
Infant care pattern	Nest or cache	Nest or cache	Carry, follow, hibernate	???
Feeding interval	5-15 hr	2-4 hr	Continuous	???
Mean % breast milk component				
Protein	10.5	9.6	3.9	1.2
Fat	16.5	9.4	4.5	7.0
Carbohydrate	3.0	3.3	5.1	7.0
Water	67.0	76.3	86.9	87.6

[*]The mean percentage of each breastmilk component in species that hibernate, carry, or follow is significantly different (p < 0.01) from the corresponding value in species that nest or cache their young, even those which feed as frequently as every 2 to 4 hr. Calculations derived from Ben Shaul. [Lazoff et al., 1977].

hypothesis that these elevated fat levels help to satiate the nursing infant and regulate the amount of breast milk consumed [Lawrence, 1985:163]).

Human breastmilk is well-suited to meet the nutritional needs of human infants. In fact, the belief prevails that the processes of evolution would have produced a product ideally suited to promote good growth and health of infants. Not all nutrition scientists agree. While concurring that uncontaminated breast milk is the *best* product for feeding infants, some argue that the product also is deficient in several nutrients, especially vitamin K, vitamin D, and iron [Fomon, 1986].

Immunologic Factors in Breast Milk

Breast milk and, especially, colostrum contain a variety of immunologic agents, notably but not exclusively immunoglobulin secretory IgA [Sahni and Chandra, 1983:100]. The set of immunologic factors in a mother's breast milk is, in a sense, environmentally "tailored," having been produced in response to pathogens in her specific environment. The immunologic factors that pass through the placental wall to the fetus and are present at birth disappear in the early postpartal period [Sahni and Chandra, 1983:100]. The infant's immature immune system does not effectively produce its own antibodies in response to exposure to pathogens. Breastfeeding, therefore, provides infants with some protection against infectious diseases such as gastrointestinal infection, respiratory infection, and otitis media [Kovar et al., 1984, and Jason et al., 1984 review the relationships between infant feeding and morbidity/mortality].

Epidemiologic evidence suggests that this protective effect is more important in less-developed countries (LDCs) and among lower socioeconomic status (SES) groups than in developed countries and among higher SES groups (ibid). And the protective advantage of breastfeeding seems to be less pronounced in the later months of infancy. Studies such as that by Schmidt [1983] have found no significant differences in morbidity between breast- and bottle-fed older infants. Despite the superiority of breast milk as an infant food and the value of breastfeeding as a feeding mode, however, infant feeding and health statistics reveal an apparent paradox. Those areas of the world with the highest prevalence and longest duration of breastfeeding also report the highest infant mortality and morbidity. Breastfeeding, although vitally important, is alone not sufficient to maintain infant health. According to Knodel and Debavalya [1980:375], ". . . although reduced breastfeeding undoubtedly has unfavorable health consequences for children, it does not appear to be a major determinant of infant mortality levels in Thailand. Other factors are apparently more important, including access to modern health services." Insufficient and poor quality water, poor sanitation, pervasive poverty, and inadequate weaning practices often are overwhelming environmental factors that undermine the good foundation provided by breastfeeding.

Nevertheless, most health care professionals believe that breastfeeding and good weaning practices are key factors in achieving good nutritional status, especially in LDCs, and good nutritional status is important to the health and survival of infants. Therefore, as international efforts to reduce infant mortality and morbidity have increased, so have the number of programs to improve infant feeding practices [UNICEF, 1983].

HOW SHOULD INFANTS BE FED?

Health care professionals recognize that the factors underlying this loss of life and health are poverty, poor sanitation, poor education, and inadequate primary care. Nevertheless, many interventions have been planned as though the most important cause is inadequacy of feeding practices of mother and other caretakers. As health care professionals have attempted to identify these inadequate infant feeding practices, a standard of infant feeding has emerged against which actual practices are measured. This standard typically is described as follows:

Breastfeeding should be initiated immediately after birth in order to stimulate the physiologic process of lactation and establish the milk supply, to provide colostrum with its immunologic benefits, and, presumably, to promote attachment between mother and child. The infant should be carried about and nursed ad libitum to keep up milk production and provide sufficient nutrients [Jelliffe and Jelliffe, 1978].[1] Some time between the infant's third and sixth months, supplementation of the breast milk should begin in order to sustain growth and development. Good quality uncontaminated foods containing adequate amounts of protein should be added in increasing amounts until breast milk supplements the weaning foods. Sometime after the child's first year of life, breastfeeding is terminated. Throughout the weaning process, until sevrage,[2] breast milk remains an important supplement to weaning foods.[3]

---

[1]Biologic breastfeeding also is associated with high levels of prolactin production and maintenance of postpartum amenorrhea and infecundity.

[2]Sevrage refers to the termination of breastfeeding. Weaning, on the other hand, is the process during which foods other than breast milk are added to the infant's diet.

[3]Breastfeeding is a critical component of this standard feeding pattern in LDCs where good substitutes are unavailable or impossible to use safely. In developed countries, where nutritionally adequate breast milk substitutes are available, affordable, and can be safely prepared, risks of omitting the breast feeding component from the feeding pattern are reduced (Kovar et al, 1984).

HOW ARE INFANTS ACTUALLY FED?

Probably the majority of infants in the world are fed in a pattern different from this standard. The literature that has accumulated over the past decade has compiled a multitude of social, cultural, economic, and psychologic factors that interact to produce nonstandard infant feeding practices. [Forman, 1984 reviews these factors]. Much of this literature has focused on why many mothers do not breastfeed, especially in urban areas of LDCs. An array of variables associated with technologic development and urbanization of LDCs seems to negatively affect breastfeeding. During the last decade, researchers have attempted to identify the salient factors that shape infant feeding trends, in part to plan more effective interventions. Their efforts have identified several constellations of factors that can be categorized as follows [e.g., Pelto, 1981; WHO, 1981; Forman, 1984]: 1) Changing social patterns, loss of extended family supports; 2) Changing economic roles for women, incompatibility of nontraditional work with concurrent child care and feeding; 3) Increased stress, anxiety, increase in psychosocially induced lactation problems; 4) Utilization of modern medical care and facilities, especially in the perinatal period; 5) Changing values and attitudes about the body, sexuality, male-female relations, and so on; and 6) Availability of commercial infant feeding devices and products.

Urbanization and development are not the only factors adversely affecting the practice of breastfeeding. Traditional cultures also have components that shape infant feeding practices in a way that is considered by health care professionals to be less than ideal. For example, two very different cultural patterns, one a part of modern medical practice and the other traditional, delay the initiation of breastfeeding after parturition. In developed countries where most infants are born in a hospital, newborns may be taken from their mothers for "processing" and not returned for several hours. After that, the mothers may have limited access to their infants and few opportunities to nurse until they are discharged. In many traditional societies, on the other hand, infants are taken from their mothers by birth attendants to be cleaned and given a purgative. Breastfeeding may be delayed for several days, "until the milk comes in" in the common belief that colostrum is not food and could even harm the infant [Lozoff, 1983; Vemury, 1981]. In various parts of the world, colostrum is thought to be a dirty or poisoned substance, pus, or old milk left over from the previous child. Meanwhile, the newborn may be given prelacteal feeds such as honey, syrup, castor oil, herbal teas, cow or goat milk by hand, mouth, rag, or bottle. According to Vemury; "The majority of mothers [in a six-country study] . . . do not believe the infant should be given the breast immediately after birth, but rather after a mean interval of up to 34 hours in the Latin American coutries, and between approximately 46–62 hours in Tunisia, Jordan and Bangladesh (1981:177).

Whatever the reasons for the widespread practice of delayed breastfeeding, it results in waste of colostrum. Health outcomes of specific feeding practices such as delayed breastfeeding are difficult to isolate and measure. But in those communities where the loss of immunologic protection puts infants at risk of developing life-threatening infectious diseases, health outcomes of such the practices presumably could be significant.

"Nonstandard" feeding practices are also common in the use of foods other than milk. Weaning foods may be introduced very late and be deficient in both protein and energy. A common pattern of malnutrition in LDCs is the acute or chronic malnutrition of the older infant or young child who receives inappropriate weaning food or too little too late [Scrimshaw and Underwood, 1980]. Children may become underweight, stunted, or develop kwashiorkor or a combination of nutritional disorders.[4] This pattern of deprivation may be a systematic response to marginal community food resources which provide adult producers with relatively more food than nonproducers such as children. In many LDCs, beliefs rationalize the practice. Animal proteins may be thought inappropriate, unnecessary, or even harmful for young children [Vemury, 1981].

Foods other than breast milk may also be introduced to infants very early—certainly earlier than recommended by most health care professionals. In horticultural societies in Africa and the South Pacific, women are often separated from their infants while they work in their gardens. In their absensce, caretakers feed mashed, liquid, or premasticated foods to the infants. [Nerlove, 1974; Gussler, 1985]. In the Caribbean and urban Latin America and Africa, women who work or are otherwise separated from their infants frequently feed semisolids and bottle-fed products such as bush teas and porridges as early as 1 or 2 weeks postpartum. The resulting pattern of mixed breast- and bottle-feeding and early use of nonmilk foods is the norm in many communities [Marchione, 1980; Gussler and Mock, 1983; Raphael and Davis, 1985].

The foods provided these young infants may be of low nutritional value or harbor pathogens that expose infants to infectious disease. Health outcomes of early use of breast milk substitutes and mixed feeding are not well documented, but some evidence suggests that the incidence of infectious diseases

---

[4]Nutrition scientists do not agree on norms for adequate or optimal infant-child growth or on how harmful growth faltering is to health and development of the individual (Seward and Serdula, 1984: 730).

among mixed breast- and bottle-fed infants falls between those of infants exclusively breastfed and those exclusively bottle-fed [Kovar et al., 1984].

In summary, the majority of the world's infants are not fed according to the pattern recommended by most health care professionals. Some receive no breast milk at all. Others are breastfed but are introduced very early to supplements. Some are breastfed for a very short time, then fed exclusively on breast milk substitutes, Many are breastfed for a long time but are supplemented very late or inadquately. Social, cultural, psychologic, and economic factors frequently override the standard recommended feeding pattern. But health care professionals sometimes need to remind one another that most infants survive these feeding patterns and many thrive. Clearly many of these "nonstandard" courses of infant feeding are, at least, adequate.

CULTURE AND THE COURSE OF BREASTFEEDING
Starting Breastfeeding

The initial decision of a woman to breastfeed or not to breastfeed frequently is made long before the birth of her baby and is shaped by a broad range of psychologic and lifestyle factors. Recent surveys and prospective studies have demonstrated that maternal age, parity, marital status, educational level, socioeconomic status, social support system, anticipated work, and values and attitudes affect initial feeding choices (e.g., Forman, 1984).

The precise form of these factors and the ways in which they affect infant feeding practices vary from community to community. Full discussion is beyond the scope of one chapter. Two examples, however, demonstrate the complexity of the relationships.

Education and general socioeconomic status usually are reported by infant feeding researchers to be related to initial breast-, bottle-, or mixed feeding choices, but the direction of the relationship depends on the type of society. In the LDCs, the higher the educational level and SES of the mother, the less likely she is to breastfeed at all. (These factors are, of course, composites of more specific maternal characteristics.) She may consider breastfeeding the feeding mode of the old-fashioned, the poor, or the rural folk. Bottle and formula are affordable consumer items for this woman, and her infant may be more easily fed by other caretakers. In the developed world, in contrast, higher SES is strongly associated with breastfeeding. A well-educated and nutritionally well-informed mother will try to breastfeed, at least initially.

The relationship between women's work needs and infant feeding decisions is less clear cut but also varies cross-culturally. How soon after parturition a woman must return to work, how many hours a day she works, and how far away from home her work takes her all may affect the initial breast- and bottle feeding decision [e.g., Forman 1984, Marshall, 1985].

Although not all infant feeding research has found a relationship between women's work and infant feeding, anthropologists, in their holistic tradition, have generally assumed some kind of relationship must exist. Audrey Richards, for example, described the ways in which feeding patterns are embedded in the cultural and social fabric of human life [1948] as follows:

> Initially the infant is, of course, entirely dependent on its mother for the satisfaction of its hunger—at this time its most urgent physical need. But, since the nature of this nutritive relationship varies very largely according to the customs of infant feeding in each community, we have to study the methods of suckling and weaning practices, the length of the period, *and the association of the mother's nutritive function to the other social duties she has to fulfill* (emphasis added) (p. 39).

More recently, Ernestine Friedl [1975:8] referred to common assumption that women's reproductive roles are a biologic "given" and that productive economic roles will be shaped by and accommodated to them. Friedl believes that a less "sterile" and more useful perspective is to look at ways in which such reproductive roles as infant feeding are accommodated to women's other work. In fact, accommodations are usually made in both directions.

In any case, most women in most communities are allowed at least a brief period of postpartum respite from work. Thus, work plans are less likely to affect initial feeding decisions than subsequent ones. They may shorten the duration of breastfeeding, for example, or produce a pattern of mixed feeding or early supplementation. The relationship between women's work and infant feeding is discussed in greater detail below.

Maintaining Breastfeeding

Breastfeeding in traditional societies tends to be of long duration, often lasting years [WHO, 1981; Kent, 1981]. While duration varies a great deal within as well as between communities, national nutrition surveys in LDCs frequently find the mean age of sevrage to lie between 1 and 2 years [Gussler et al., 1984]. Extended breastfeeding usually is terminated because the mother has become pregnant again or has decided that the child has reached the proper size or stage of development [Guthrie, 1980:38; Marshall, 1985].

However, a very short duration of breastfeeding is observed in many developed countries and areas of LDCs undergoing urbanization. Infant feeding research in such areas suggests that the first few weeks postpartum are marked by lactation crises stemming from minor morbidity episodes and the concern of mothers for the adequacy and quality of their milk supply.

Two immediate outcomes of these lactation problems have been reported. One is early termination of breastfeeding with the introduction of exclusive bottle-feeding. The other is the maintenance of partial breastfeeding and introduction of supplementary bottle-feeds. The former pattern is common in the developed world, the latter in the urban areas of the developing world [Greiner, 1981; Gussler and Briesemeister, 1980].

In England and Wales [Martin, 1978:61], the proportion of breast feeding mothers in one study cohort dropped sharply in the early postpartum months, and nearly half of the mothers had stopped nursing by the fourth week. A study of lower income mothers in Alabama indicates that nearly one third of the mothers who tried breastfeeding at least once in the hospital had given up before their release [Jessee, 1981]. In Tucson, Arizona, half of a small sample of breastfeeding mothers had changed to bottle-feeding before their infants' 2-week checkup [Anson, 1982]. Two studies from Czechoslovakia report a mean age of sevrage of 7 weeks [Horanska, 1977; Cvengros and Stadtruck-erova, 1978]. Sjolin et al. [1979] followed a cohort of Swedish women prospectively for 6 months, or until sevrage if earlier. Through weekly phone interviews they monitored the course of lactation and breastfeeding problems. Over half of the lactation crises occurred during the first 2 months, 77% by three months.

In St. Kitts-Nevis in the eastern Caribbean, 98% of the women who bore children in 1978 initiated breastfeeding. The mean age of sevrage was 6.5 months. However, 65% of the mothers had introduced supplementary bottle-feeds by the second week. In an open-ended interview question, nearly 70% of them gave concern about milk adequacy as the primary reason for supplementation [Gussler and Briesemeister, 1980].

The immediate postpartum period is a time of physiologic, biochemical, and social transition and adaptation. The mother's body is recovering from the birth process. Lactation is stimulated by and in turn affects hormone production. Colostrum secretion gives way to transitional milk [Jelliffe and Jelliffe, 1978]. The infant grows rapidly, and sucking and hunger patterns change quickly [Illingworth and Stone, 1952]. The processes of mother–child attachment and interaction are initiated [Klaus et al., 1972; Kennell and Klaus, 1979], and mothers come to learn how and when to respond to infants' cues. Development of a contingent relationship also helps the infant learn to adjust to this early feeding environment [Gaulin-Kremer et al., 1977; Kennell and Klaus, 1979]. A mother is likely to become anxious about a crying, fussy baby that does not seem to be satisfied or calmed at the breast. Anxiety can affect the let-down reflex, inhibit lactation, and cause the mother to doubt her ability to breastfeed successfully [Newton and Newton, 1950; Raphael, 1976:69].

Such anxiety is a common reason given by women for early termination of breastfeeding [Gussler and Briesemeister, 1980].[5]

The environment in which these adaptations take place also is changing during the early postpartum period. In the nontraditional setting, obstetric care is supplanted or supplemented by pediatric care. Often a conceptual and informational gap exists between these two medical specializations. Breastfeeding information and support, belonging to both specializations and exclusively to neither, falls in the gap. The special purpural state of the mother ends as she resumes more-or-less normal activities. Women with other children and women whose duties take them away from the household must make additional adjustments. At this point, a women's kin and friends are important to the outcome of breastfeeding. Helpful and supportive individuals are significant factors in the duration and success of the breastfeeding experience [Raphael, 1976]. Finally, a woman's attitudinal set and level of enthusiasm about her choice of feeding may affect the feeding outcome [Switzky et al.,

TABLE II. Postpartum Transitional Processes Affecting Breastfeeding

Transitional realms	Specific transitional processes
Biologic–biochemical	1 Transitional milk, colostrum to mature milk
	2 Hormonal changes following parturition and initiation of suckling
	3 Changing nutritional needs of rapidly growing infant
Biobehavioral	4 Maternal-child attachment
	5 Establishment of lactation and changing sucking behavior of infant
	6 Maternal-child interaction, learning, adjustment (e.g., maternal response to hunger cues from infant)
Sociocultural	7 Availability of information about breastfeeding management
	8 Shift from prenatal to postnatal health care (obstetrical mother-centered care)
	9 Resumption of normal activities: a. other child care responsibilities b. other domestic and nondomestic roles (compatibility with breastfeeding)
	10 Impingement of social factors: a. Attitudes and support of significant others b. Internalized attitudes, emotions of mother

---

[5]Sevrage that occurs after extended breastfeeding rarely is associated with maternal anxiety and concern about milk supply.

1980]. Table II decribes a framework for understanding, at least in part, the kinds of factors that may produce early sevrage.

The interaction of factors in this framework shape breastfeeding behavior in the crucial early postpartum days. For example, changing nutritional needs of the infant may produce changes in sucking behavior resulting in sore and cracked nipples. The presence or absence of helpful kin and friends and information on breastfeeding mangement may be critical and immediate determinants of a change in infant feeding mode. The availability of such support and information varies considerably from community to community. Many traditional societies have ritualized the transitional postpartum period. Mothers in these settings are provided with help, advice, and attention (Raphael, 1976), often reinforced by a period of seclusion during which their duties are assumed by kin or neighbors. In urban areas of the developed and developing world in which nuclear family structures predominate, such measures are difficult, impractical, or impossible. With no breastfeeding tradition to guide them, women, especially if unenthusiastic about breastfeeding, are likely to be "unsuccessful."

While the biologic components of parturition and lactation are universal, the social and cultural components vary greatly within and between societies and by level of development. Infant feeding researchers should, therefore, use care when generalizing the results of one or two studies. For example, a few studies such as that by Sosa et al. [1976] suggest that the timing of initial postpartum mother–child contact and breastfeeding is a significant factor affecting duration of breastfeeding. That is, mothers who are given their newborns immediately after birth to hold and nurse are more likely to be breastfeeding several weeks later than those whose infants are "processed" and given to them several hours later. However, the traditional practice of delaying breastfeeding because of concerns about colostrum (decribed above) is usually found in those societies in which breastfeeding is universal and of long duration. Features of those social and cultural environments obviously are more important to the success of lactation than timing of first breastfeeding. Similarly, in developed countries, early supplementation of breastfeeding by bottle-feeds frequently seems to shorten the duration of breastfeeding. Yet, mixed feeding in parts of the developing world often lasts for many months, and duration of breastfeeding may not be affected [Franklin et al., 1982; Gussler and Mock, 1983]. Clearly, identifying the events that lead to early sevrage or to early supplementation of breastfeeding requires consideration of the interaction of an array of biologic, biochemical, and sociocultural factors.

Infant Feeding "Strategies"

Infant feeding practices, frequently analyzed as isolated behaviors, are intergral parts of sociocultural systems. While we speak of women making infant feeding decisions, an array of constraints in their social environment—prevailing beliefs about women's roles as nurturers and producers, social pressures from kin, restricted availability of breast milk substitutes, and so on—affect those decisions and limit options. As individual women find ways to fill all of their roles — including infant care — within these environmental constraints, infant feeding strategies develop.

The most common role accommodations are those in infant care practices and extra-household work. The process is frequently described as a "balancing act" in which women deal with their dual burden of reproductive and productive activities. The result may be early use of breast milk substitutes, as mothers reduce the nutritional dependency of their infants. Some of the more common broad strategies are outlined below. Details of these strategies vary from society to society. Since they emerge from an interplay of prevailing beliefs, practices, and social arrangements with the immediate work and social needs of individual women, they also will vary from mother to mother.[6]

Extra-household roles. In communities in which women have few if any important duties away from the household, no accommodation of work and child care is necessary. The mother and infant remain in the household together and are not separated for any significant periods of time. Such a situation has been described by Carrier for Ponam women in Oceania, a society in which the norm is that ". . . a mother should always be free to nurse her infant at any time and therefore should not leave the child's side for the first few months. . . .[1985]." Economic pursuits that can be conducted in and around the household, such as sewing, handicrafts, and kitchen gardening, may be maintained. The so-called "traditional housewife" in developed countries can be included in this category, demonstrating that these strategies cut across cultures, socioeconomic strata, and levels of development.

Extra-household roles suspended. Women may perform duties away from the household that are considered by them and their communities to be less important than child care. Their extra-household work is, therefore, discretionary and will be suspended while their infants are young and nutritionally dependent on them. Those duties may gradually be reassumed as weaning progresses and other caretakers can feed the child. Such a situation has been described by Counts [1985], also in Oceania; there women postpone their gardening activities until their infants are being weaned and are not totally nutritionally dependent upon them. The family and community can do

---

[6]Further discussion of the strategies, with ethnographic descriptions from one culture area, may be found in Marshall [1985].

without the subsistence contribution of any particular woman for several months.

Extra-household roles conducted with infant. In hunter-gatherer societies, the nutritionally dependent infant accompanies the mother on her gathering rounds [Lozoff et al., 1977]. In such societies, women's gathering activities are of such importance that they are not discretionary, and cannot be suspended for several months. But neither is breastfeeding discretionary, because, in the absence of adequate milk substitutes, the survival of infants depends on it. So infants are carried on mother's backs, fronts, or hips, and usually fed whenever they begin to fuss. No separation is necessary, nor is there a juggling of priorities and activities. Child care and other work are conducted concurrently; or as one writer says, they ". . .occupy the same time and space" in women's lives [Newland, 1980:23]. In horticultural societies, infants may accompany their mothers to their garden, sometimes with older siblings who watch the infant nearby [Lepowsky, 1985]. A few upper SES breastfeeders in North America and Europe have found ways to re-create this pattern and keep their infants with them at work.

Extra-household roles assumed by others. In many traditional communities, a system of extended families and other social supports allows women to attend to young infants without immediately having to resume other work. While the work may be considered important, husbands and other kin assume it until the weaning process is underway. Katz [1985], for example, says that in some areas of the outer Fiji Islands, the community will provision the family of a young infant for up to a year so that the mother does not have to engage in foodgetting.

Extra-household roles conducted without infant. "The impact of children," says Newland [1980:24], "is very different in a setting where formal workplaces are physically separated from the home and are age-segregated." Under these conditions, child care acquires a concrete "opportunity cost" and women must choose between staying with their child or going out to work. However, many women have no choice. In urban areas of Latin America and the Caribbean, for example, female-headed households are quite common, and an unmarried women with several children may have to leave the home to work to support them. Many of these women work outside the formal work force and are not provided with maternity leave, creches, and other supports which would allow them to focus on infant care and feeding. And the work that they do frequently is not compatible with concurrent child care and feeding. Some of these women, especially in the more developed countries, do not breastfeed at all. Their counterparts in the developing world usually breastfeed, but they introduce their infants to supplementary bottle-feeds early in life, so that other caretakers may feed them during frequent separations. In the traditional rural world, early supplementation of breastfeeding with mashed or premasticated foods is common when women must return to extra-household labors without their infants [Nerlove, 1974; Gussler, 1985].

Only the last type of strategy requires alternatives to exclusive breastfeeding. The other four produce minimal or no separation of the mother and infant and include social arrangements that provide breastfeeding opportunities. On the other hand, while exclusive breastfeeding is a *possible* part of the first four strategies, it is not inevitable. In the United States, for example, many women who stay home with their young infants choose not to breastfeed at all. Extra-household work may be an important factor in shaping the course of infant feeding in some settings, but it still is only one part of what clearly is a complex pattern of human behavior.

Infant Feeding Trends

Since infant feeding practices respond to so many environmental factors, it is not suprising that they can change rapidly. While most infants in LDCs still receive some breast milk (nearly 100% of infants in much of Africa and parts of Asia), breastfeeding duration is becoming shorter in many communities. Bottle-feeding is increasingly common in the cities of LCDs [WHO, 1981; Gussler and Mock, 1983], but exclusive bottle-feeding is common primarily in upper SES communities [Petros-Barvasian, 1983]. Bottle-fed supplements to breast milk are more common in lower SES groups.

In the developed world, infant feeding trends turned around in only a decade. In the United States, 25% of the infants born in 1970 were initially breastfed. By 1981, the proportion had increased to more than 56% [Martinez and Dodd, 1983]. Throughout most of North America and Europe, breastfeeding prevalance similarly increased [Gussler, et al., 1984]. While increases have occurred in all SES groups, the greatest percentages of breastfeeders are recorded in upper SES groups, producing an infant feeding picture in sharp contrast to that in the LDCs, where higher SES is associated with less breastfeeding.

CONCLUSION

In summary, infant feeding practices are shaped by a variety of social, cultural, economic, and psychologic factors that impinge on the lives of women. They may change very quickly, especially in areas undergoing rapid development and urbanization. Nevertheless, a great deal of breastfeeding still is practiced in the developing world, and in the more traditional rural areas duration of breastfeeding is long. Biologic breastfeeding is practiced, as infants are continually carried and fed on demand. In many of these traditional communities, breastfeeding is compatible with women's daily economic activities in and out of the household, or social accommodations are made to relieve them of those activities. Even in these communites, however, supplementation of breast milk with a variety of products may begin very early in infants' lives. Feeding bottles may be used when available. Otherwise, foods may be fed by spoon, by hand, or blown into infants' mouths.

Urbanization, changing household arrangements, work roles, lifestyles and attitudes, and the proliferation of consumer goods (including breast milk substitutes) that accompany development all affect breastfeeding behavior. The elite in developing societies often do not breastfeed at all; lower socioeconomic mothers and other caretakers frequently supplement breastfeeds early with both bottle-fed and nonbottle-fed foods.

Declining breastfeeding, however, is not an inevitable consequence of development. In the developed countries of North America and Europe, the prevalance and duration of breastfeeding are now increasing, not declining. This "renaissance" of breastfeeding is due, in part, to the re-creation of some traditional infant feeding practices, such as frequent carrying of the infant, and infant care and feeding at mother's work place.

In the urban areas of the developing world, however, prevalance and duration of breastfeeding still are declining. International health organizations are developing programs to stop the early termination of breastfeeding and the sometimes unnecessary use of supplementary bottles. Nevertheless, it is important that policy makers recognize the many environmental factors that shape the ways in which women and other caretakers feed infants. Programs and policies that are developed without recognition of these factors will very likely produce inappropriate and ineffective actions.

REFERENCES

Anson C (1982): Unpublished research report. Columbus, OH: Ross Laboratories.

Carrier AH (1985): Infant care and family relations on Ponam Island, Manus Province, Papua New Guinea. In Marshall LB (ed): "Infant Care and Feeding in the South Pacific." New York: Gordon and Breach Science Publishers, pp 189-205.

Counts DA (1985): Infant care and feeding in Kaliai, West New Britain, Papua New Guinea. In Marshall L (ed): "Infant Care and Feeding in the South Pacific." New York: Gordon and Breach Science Publishers.

Cvengros V, Stadtruckerova A (1978): A survey of breast-feeding in the District of Martin. Cesk Pediatr 33:302-305.

Fomon S (1986): Breast-feeding and evolution. J Am Diet Assoc 86:317-318.

Forman M (1984): Review of research on the factors associated with choice and duration of infant feeding in less-developed countries. Pediatrics (suppl) 74:667-694.

Franklin RR, Bertrand WE, Mock NB, et al. (1983): Feeding patterns of infants and young children in Kinshasa, Zaire. J Trop Ped 29:255-259.

Friedl E (1975): "Women and Men: An Anthropologist's View." New York: Holt, Rinehart and Winston.

Gaulin-Kremer E, Shaw JL, et al. (1977): Mother-infant interaction at first prolonged encounter: Effects of variation in delay after delivery. Presented before the Society for Research in Child Development, New Orleans.

Gussler JD (1985): Commentary: Women, work, and infant feeding in Oceania. In Marshall L (ed): "Infant Care and Feeding in the South Pacific." New York: Gordon & Breach Science Publishers.

Gussler JD (nd): Culture and the course of breastfeeding. Unpublished Resource Paper. Columbus: Ross Laboratories.

Gussler JD, Briesemeister LH (1980): The insufficient milk syndrome: A biocultural explanation. Med Anthropol 4:3-24.

Gussler JD, Mock N (1983): A comparative description of infant feeding practices in Zaire, the Philippines and St. Kitts-Nevis. Ecol Food Nutr 13:75-85.

Gussler JD, Woo-Lun MA, Smith N (1984): "International Breastfeeding Compendium," 3d ed. Columbus, Ohio: Ross Laboratories.

Guthrie GM, Guthrie HA, Fernandez TL, Estrera N (1980): Maintenance and termination of breast feeding in rural and urban Philippine communities. Ecol Food Nutr 10:35-43.

Horanska E (1977): The mother, child & breastfeeding. Cesk Pediatr 43:235-236.

Illingworth RS, Stone DG (1952): Self-demand feeding in a maternity unit. Lancet 1:683-687.

Jason JM, Nieburg P, Marks JS (1984): Mortality and infectious disease associated with infant-feeding practices in developing countries. Pediatrics 74 (suppl):703-727.

Jelliffe D, Jelliffe EFP (1978): "Human Milk in the Modern World." Oxford: Oxford University Press.

Jessee P (1981): Unpublished research report. Columbus, OH: Ross Laboratories.

Katz MM (1985): Infant care in a group of Outer Fiji Islands. In Marshall L (ed): "Infant Care and Feeding in the South Pacific." New York: Gordon & Breach Science Publishers.

Kennell J, Klaus M (1979): Early mother-infant contact. Bull Menninger Clin 43:69-78.

Kent M (1981): "Breast-feeding in the Developing World: Current Patterns and Implications for Future Trends." Reports on the World Fertility Survey. Washington, DC: Population Reference Bureau, Inc.

Klaus M, Jerauld R et al. (1972): Maternal attachment: Importance of the first post-partum days. N Engl J Med 286:460-463.

Knodel J, Debvalya N (1980): Breastfeeding in Thailand: Trends & differentials, 1969-1979. Stud Fam Plan 11:355-377.

Kovar MG, Serdula MK, Marks JS, Fraser DW (1984): Review of the epidemiologic evidence for an association between infant feeding and infant health. Pediatrics (suppl) 74:615-638.

Lawrence R (1985): "Breastfeeding: A Guide for the Medical Profession." St. Louis: CV Mosby Company.

Lepowsky MA (1985): Food taboos, malaria, and dietary change: Infant feeding and cultural adaptation on a Papua New Guinea island. In Marshall L (ed): "Infant Care and Feeding in the South Pacific." New York: Gordon & Breach Science Publishers.

Lozoff B (1983): Birth and "bonding" in non-industrial societies. Develop Med Child Neurol 25:595-600.

Lozoff B, Brittenham G, Trause MA, et al. (1977): The mother-newborn relationship: Limits of adaptibility. J Pediatr 91:1-12.

Marchione TJ (1980): A history of breastfeeding practices in the English speaking Caribbean in the twentieth century. Food Nutr Bull 2:9-18.

Marshall L (1985): "Infant care and feeding: Cases from the South Pacific." New York: Gordon & Breach Science Publishers.

Martin J (1978): "Infant Feeding 1975: Attitudes and Practice in England and Wales." Office of Population Censuses and Surveys. Social Survey Division: London: Her Majesty's Stationery Office.

Martinez GA, Dodd DA (1983): 1981 milk feeding patterns in the United States during the first 12 months of life. Pediatrics 71:166-170.

Mead M, Newton N (1967): Cultural patterning of perinatal behavior. In Richardson SA, Guttmacher AF (eds): "Childbearing—Its Social and Psychological Aspects." Baltimore: Williams and Wilkins.

Nerlove SB (1974): Women's workload and infant feeding practices: A relationship with demographic implications. Ethnology 13:125-214.

Newland K (1980): "Women, Men, and the Division of Labor." Worldwatch Paper 37. Washington DC: Worldwatch Institute.

Newton NR, Newton M (1950): Relation of the let-down reflex to the ability to breast-feed. Pediatrics 5:726-733.

Pelto GH (1981): Perspectives on infant feeding: Decision-making and ecology. Food Nutr Bull 3:17-29.

Petros-Barvasian A (1983): Prevalence and duration of breastfeeding in different parts of the world: An overview. Bull IPA 5(2):17-24.

Raphael D (1976): "The Tender Gift." New York: Schocken Books.

Raphael D, Davis F (1985): "Only Mothers Know: Patterns of Infant Feeding in Traditional Cultures." Westport, CT: Greenwood Press.

Richards AI (1948): "Hunger and Work in a Savage Tribe: A Functional Study of Nutrition among the Southern Bantu. Glencoe, IL: The Free Press.

Sahni S, Chandra RK (1983): Malnutrition and susceptibility to diarrhea, with special refernce to the antiinfective properties of breast milk. In Chen LC, Scrimshaw NS (eds): "Diarrhea and Malnutrition: Interactions, Mechanisms, and Interventions." New York: Plenum Press.

Sauls HS (1979): Potential effect of demographic and other variables in studies comparing morbidity of breast-fed and bottle-fed infants. Pediatrics 64:523-527.

Schmidt B (1983): Breast-feeding and infant morbidity and mortality in developing countries. J Ped Gastroenterol Nutr 2(suppl 1):S127-S130.

Scrimshaw N, Underwood B (1980): Timely and appropriate complementary feeding of the breast-fed infant—an overview. Food Nutr Bull 2(2):19-22.

Seward JF, Serdula MK (1984): Infant feeding and growth. Pediatrics 74 (suppl): 728-762.

Shaul B (1962): The composition of the milk of wild animals. Int Zoo Book 4:333-342.

Sjolin S, Hofvander Y, Hillervik C (1979): A prospective study of individual courses of breast feeding. Acta Paediatr Scand 68:521-529.

Sosa R, Kennell JH, Klaus M (1976): The effect of early mother-infant contact on breastfeeding, infection and growth. In: "Breastfeeding and the Mother," CIBA, Amsterdam: Elsevier, Excerpta Medica.

Switzky LT, Vietze P, Switzky HN (1979): Attitudinal and demographic predictors of breast-feeding and bottle-feeding behavior by mothers of six-week-old infants. Psychol Rep 45:3-14.

Taskforce on the Assessment of the Scientific Evidence Relating to Infant-Feeding Practices and Infant Health (1984): Pediatrics (suppl) 74:579–762.

UNICEF (1983): "The State of the World's Children, 1984." New York: UNICEF.

Vemury M (1981): "Rural Food Habits in Six Developing Countries." New York: CARE.

World Health Organization (1981): "Contemporary Patterns of Breast-Feeding." Geneva: WHO.

Nutritional Anthropology, pages 173-196
© 1987 Alan R. Liss, Inc.

Nutrition and Growth

Robert M. Malina, PhD

Department of Anthropology, University of Texas, Austin, Texas 78712

The general good health of the growing organism is dependent upon a variety of environmental conditions. Among these, nutrition is paramount though nutritional needs and influences are different at various phases of the growing years. This report addresses several aspects of the complex interrelationship between growth and nutrition. Focus is on the well child and not on the chronically under- or overnourished youngster.

Nutrition is a process that concerns the relationship of food intake to the functioning of the organism. Physiological aspects of the process include the ingestion, digestion, absorption, and transport of nutrients, the synthesis of tissue components, and the liberation of energy. Other aspects of the nutritional process relate to social and cultural conditions, including, for example, economic background, dietary habits, attitudes toward and beliefs about food, habits of physical activity, and so on. In addition, the nutritional process can have pathological consequences which are capable of altering, perhaps permanently, or even terminating the organism's functioning. Nutrition is thus broad in scope and is of prime concern throughout the life cycle, although only the developmental years are considered.

Man is a Primate and among Primates has a relatively lengthy period of growth and maturation. Assuming that the human postnatal growth period is approximately 20 years and that the human life span under reasonably favorable circumstances is about 70 to 75 years, it is immediately apparent that about two-sevenths of an individual's life span is devoted to the processes of growth and maturation with the unique nutritional needs of these stages. In addition, the prolonged immaturity of the infant and young child has an important correlate in dependency, i.e., the dependency of the child upon parents, especially the mother, and upon social institutions. Nutritionally, this dependency indicates that the nutritional environment of the developing child is not under his/her control. Rather, this environmental component is under maternal control through a long gestational period and through most of childhood. Maternal nutritional influences are both direct and indirect, e.g., maternal nutrition during pregnancy and lactation, duration of breastfeeding (direct) and maternal nutritional history, early feeding experiences, nutritional habits and attitudes (indirect). Such early nutritional experiences can perhaps have lasting effects throughout an individual's lifetime. In addition, the electronic media, especially television in developed countries, can be a significant influence on the food preferences of children and youth.

NUTRIENTS

There are six classes of nutrients: carbohydrates, proteins, fats, vitamins, minerals, and water. The last mentioned, though often taken for granted, functions primarily as a solvent and in temperature regulation, and it is perhaps the most important nutrient. Water comprises about 62% of the body weight of the young adult reference male [Brozek, 1966], and the relative water content of the body decreases from early in prenatal life through the growing years (see below).

Carbohydrates function as the main energy source for the body. Carbohydrate stores in the body are quite small, comprising about 0.4% to 0.5% of body weight during childhood and young adulthood [Fomon et al., 1982].

Fats or lipids also provide energy, but much of it is in storage form. Relative fat content of the body varies considerably among individuals, often in the range between 15 and 30% [Malina, 1969]. Two fatty acids, however, are essential in small amounts for nutritional well-being, linoleic and arachidonic acids [National Research Council, 1980].

Proteins are also a source of energy, but their primary functions are in the growth, maintenance, and repair of tissues and in the formation of enzymes, hormones, and antibodies, i.e., other proteins for specific physiological roles. Protein comprises about 16% of the body weight of the young adult reference male [Brozek, 1966], and the relative contribution of protein to body weight increases during growth. Upon hydrolysis or digestion, proteins yield amino acids. There are 22 amino acids necessary for humans, and these are divided into the essential and nonessential amino acids. The former are essential in the sense that the body cannot produce them at a rate necessary to support protein synthesis; hence, it is essential that they be provided in an individual's diet. In contrast, the nonessential amino acids can be produced by the body at an adequate rate to meet the needs of protein synthesis. Nevertheless, both are necessary to meet the body's protein needs.

Vitamins are primarily regulatory in function. They are required in very small amounts and comprise a negligible proportion of body weight. Minerals have both structural (e.g., bone, blood, hormones) and regulatory, (e.g., fluid and electrolyte balance) functions. Minerals are also required in small amounts. The precise role of many trace minerals in growth processes, among others, is only gradually being understood [Metz, 1981]. Minerals comprise about 6% of the body weight of the young adult reference male [Brozek, 1966]; the relative contribution of mineral to body weight increases during growth.

Although nutrients are generally treated individually, they do not function in isolation. Rather, nutrients are dependent upon other nutrients, on enzymes and hormones, and on the functional integrity of bodily systems. The availability and utilization of carbohydrates, for example, are dependent upon insulin (hormone), vitamins of the B complex (other nutrients), and the functional state of the gastrointestinal tract, especially the mucous membrane [Williams, 1973]. Zinc is found in high concentrations in male accessory sex organs, and testicular zinc metabolism is apparently regulated by androgens [Chan and Rennert, 1985]. In addition, the form of a nutrient in food can affect its absorption and utilization. Iron of vegetable origin, for example, has a low efficiency of absorption, while that of animal origin is better absorbed [Jacobs, 1976; Scrimshaw and Young, 1976].

Nutrients are components of food. Individuals eat food; they do not eat nutrients. Eating is a social behavior, and the food that is eaten is regulated by the cultural context within which the individual lives. What is food in one culture may be classified as nonfood in another. More importantly perhaps, there is no guarantee that knowledge of nutrients will translate into effective food-related behavior. The role of cultural influences in nutrition is thus paramount, especially when dealing with the nutrition of young individuals whose intake is regulated to a large extent by the family. In adolescence, the role of peers adds another dimension to the cultural influences affecting nutritional intake.

NUTRITIONAL REQUIREMENTS

Requirements can be viewed in terms of those necessary for the maintenance of basal metabolic states, for the support of normal growth and maturation in the young organism, for the repair and/or replacement of tissues, and for the conduct of physical activities. Nutritional requirements vary with age, sex, body size, stage of growth and maturation, level of physical activity, and physiological states, e.g.,illness and rehabilitation. Requirements are also influenced by a number of environmental factors, either directly or indirectly, for example, temperature, altitude, infectious and parasitic agents, culturally mediated dietary habits and activity patterns, and so on. There is also considerable individual variation in nutritional requirements, probably reflecting variation in actual expression of genes. In addition, genotype-nutrient and more complex genotype-environment-nutrient interactions are probably quite important in affecting individual variation in nutrient and energy requirements and utilization [Williams, 1956; Widdowson, 1962; Scrimshaw and Young, 1976; Young and Scrimshaw, 1979]. For example, given similar food intakes, individual variation in the efficiency of converting food to fat, i.e., genotypic variation, probably underlies the distribution of obesity in a population [Miller, 1979]. Individual variation in the absorption of specific nutrients under similar dietary conditions is probably likely; perhaps "'good' and 'bad' absorbers from the intestine run in families" [Widdowson, 1962:127].

Individual variation in nutritional requirements is thus considerable, which emphasizes the difficulty in specifying nutrient and energy requirements for individuals as well as groups. Further, the requirements of any one individual are not constant, and requirements of several nutrients are influenced by the rest of the diet. In the words of Young and Scrimshaw [1979:498], "It is a sad commentary that neither do we know adequately the quantitative extent of biological variation in requirements among individuals for any of the essential nutrients nor the quantitative importance of most of the factors which affect requirements in population groups." This comment applies especially to developing individuals. Considerable information on the nutrient needs of infants and young children [e.g., Fomon, 1974; Barness, 1981] and of children with clinical problems [e.g., Suskind, 1981] is available, while data on the nutrient requirements of school age children and adolescents are less extensive [Hegsted, 1976; Dwyer, 1981]. Nevertheless, there is considerable uncertainty about the nutrient needs of developing individuals.

The processes of growth and maturation obviously add another dimension to energy and nutrient requirements. These processes have their own nutritional needs. Growth and maturation are characterized by dramatic changes in overall body size. Body size, of course, is a heterogenous mass, which can be partitioned biochemically as follows: Weight = Water + Protein + Mineral + Fat [Brozek, 1966]. The components are nutrients and knowledge of changes in their contribution to body mass during growth will aid in understanding energy and nutrient requirements of the developing individual. Hence, changes in the estimated relative body composition during growth are shown in Table I. Relative body water content decreases during growth as the liquid is replaced by solids, i.e., the relative content of protein and mineral increase while the relative content of fat, though generally increasing, fluc-

TABLE I. Relative Body Composition During Childhood and in the Young Adult
Reference Male[a]

| Age | Length (cm) | Weight (kg) | Percentage of body weight | | | |
			Water	Protein	Mineral	Fat
Males						
Birth	51.6	3.5	69.6	12.9	2.6[b]　0.6	13.7
6 mo	67.6	8.0	59.4	12.0	2.3　0.5	25.4
1 yr	76.1	10.1	61.2	12.9	2.3　0.6	22.5
5 yr	109.9	18.7	65.4	15.8	3.1　0.6	14.6
10 yr	137.5	31.4	64.8	16.8	3.5　0.6	13.7
Adult		65.3	62.4	16.4	4.8　1.1	15.3
Females						
Birth	50.5	3.3	68.6	12.8	2.6　0.6	14.9
6 mo	65.8	7.3	58.4	12.0	2.6　0.5	26.4
1 yr	74.3	9.2	60.1	12.9	2.3　0.5	23.7
5 yr	108.4	17.7	64.6	15.0	2.5　0.6	16.7
10 yr	138.3	32.5	62.0	15.0	2.5　0.6	19.4

[a]Adapted from Fomon et al. [1982] and Brozek [1966].
[b]The two columns under mineral refer to osseous and nonosseous mineral, respectively.

tuates. Estimates of changes in the relative chemical composition of the body
during adolescence are not presently available for both sexes [Haschke, 1983;
Lohman, 1986].

Nevertheless, adolescence is accompanied by significant changes in body
composition, especially in males. For example, lean body mass (LBM), a
major component of which is muscle tissue, virtually doubles during male
adolescence so that by young adulthood the LBM of males is about one and
one-half times that of females. Between 10 and 20 years of age, it is estimated
that LBM increases from 27 to 62 kg in males and from 25 to 43 kg in
females, increments of 35 kg and 18 kg respectively [Forbes, 1981]. Since
LBM contains considerable nitrogen, the estimated daily increment in the
protein content of the body over this age period is about 2 g for males and 1
g for females. When related to the peak of the adolescent growth spurt, the
estimated daily increment in the protein content of the body is about twice
that estimated for the decade 10 to 20 years, i.e., 3.8 g in males and 2.2 g in
females [Forbes, 1981]. In contrast, female adolescence is accompanied by a
significant increment in body fatness, while males often experience a loss of
fatness coincident with the adolescent growth spurt. Nevertheless, males do
gain in fatness over the adolescent period of growth, but changes in fatness
are more variable than those in LBM [Malina, 1969].

Comparison of the estimated relative composition of the 10-year-old boys
and the young adult reference male would seem to suggest that chemical

maturity of the fat-free mass [FFM; Malina, 1969 discusses the difference between LBM and FFM] may be reached in early adolescence. For example, the estimated protein content of the FFM in the 10-year-old boy is 19.5% [Fomon et al., 1982], while that of the young adult reference male is 19.4% [Brozek, 1966]. Corresponding values for water are 75.1 and 73.8%, respectively. The major difference is in mineral content, specifically osseous mineral, which increases from 4.1% of the FFM in the 10-year-old boy to 5.6% of the FFM in the young adult reference male [Fomon et al., 1982; Brozek, 1966]. The gain in skeletal mineral reflects primarily the growth and maturation of the skeleton during the adolescent growth spurt. The major mineral of the skeleton is calcium. The estimated daily increment in the calcium content of the body between 10 and 20 years of age is approximately 210 mg in males and 110 mg in females, while the estimated daily increment during the peak of the adolescent growth spurt is about two times that estimated for the 10-year period, 400 mg in males and 240 mg in females [Forbes, 1981]. Hence, the adolescent growth spurt contributes significantly to the osseous mineral content of the body.

Recommendations for energy and nutrient intakes vary from one country to another and also vary over time [e.g., Miller and Voris, 1969; Truswell, 1976; Reed, 1980]. Recommended Dietary Allowances (RDA) for the United States population, which are designed to meet the energy and nutrient requirements of most of the population, have a wide margin of safety [National Research Council, 1980]. Energy needs are estimated per unit of average body size for specific age groups in infancy and childhood and for sex-specific age groups after 10 years of age. Recommendations for other nutrients, however, are set high in order to accommodate the needs of the majority of the population. In contrast, the estimated daily requirements developed by the Food and Agriculture Organization are "...estimates of actual needs with little margin of safety" [Reed, 1980:411]. Except for energy, requirements for other nutrients are based on average values augmented for variation among individuals so that the recommended intakes presumably meet the needs of nearly all persons.

ENERGY REQUIREMENTS

Caloric intake represents energy. It must be compatible with the energy needs of the organism, and it must be adequate for the efficient utilization of dietary protein and other nutrients for growth and maintenance. Protein is a source of both calories and essential amino acids and if caloric intake is inadequate, the dietary protein will be utilized for energy. It is thus not available for tissue growth and the synthesis of other proteins.

Carbohydrates, fats, and proteins are the three main energy nutrients. However, the energy value of fats is twice that of the other two nutrients. The proportion of calories in the diet derived from each nutrient usually varies with economic status. In general, the proportion of calories derived from fats increases with income status, while that derived from carbohydrates decreases. Protein-derived energy appears independent of wealth [FAO/WHO, 1973].

Calories are viewed in terms of those taken in and those expended. Hence, concern is for the balance of energy intake and output, and the concept of energy balance is important. Energy balance refers to the sum total of energy intake less energy expenditure over a given period of time. When energy intake exceeds output, chemical energy in the form of compounds is stored in tissue depots. Mobilization of these chemical compounds from tissue depots occurs when the output of energy exceeds the input. A positive energy balance, i.e., excess input over expenditure, is necessary for growth to occur over long periods of time. With a positive energy balance during growth, energy is stored in the form of accretion of protoplasm, protein and water, and to some extent in the form of accretion of adipose tissue [Cooke, 1969]. It should be noted, however, that energy intake and energy output influence each other. For example, food intake results in an increase in oxygen consumption, while an increase in physical activity is usually followed by an increase in food intake [Miller, 1979].

Energy requirements are generally given for populations defined by age, sex, body size, and physical activity. Energy requirements, "i.e., that considered adequate to meet the energy needs of the average healthy person in a specified category," suggested by the Food and Agriculture Organization (FAO/WHO, 1973:10) are given in Table II. Requirements per kilogram of body weight are greatest in infancy and decrease gradually with age during childhood and adolescence and into adulthood. After 2 years of age, energy requirements are greater in males than in females. The sex difference probably does not reflect the greater muscle mass of males as there is no sex difference in the energy requirement per unit fat-free mass [Durnin, 1976]. The difference most likely reflects physical activity, which is usually the most important factor contributing to individual variation in energy requirements, and males have higher levels of activity than females from late-pregnancy fetal activity through adolescence [Malina, 1986b; Durnin, 1976].

Energy requirements per kilogram of body weight are greatest in early infancy, reflecting the rapid growth at this time. Two estimates of the energy cost of growth are shown in Table III. Energy intake obviously increases with age and body size, but the proportion of energy intake utilized to support

TABLE II. Average Daily Energy Requirements of Children, Adolescents, and Moderately Active Adults[1]

Age (yr)	Males					Females				
	Weight (kg)	Per kg		Total		Weight (kg)	Per kg		Total	
		kcal	kJ	kcal	MJ		kcal	kJ	kcal	MJ
<1	7.3	112	470	820	3.4	7.3	112	470	820	3.4
1	11.4	103	431	1,180	4.9	11.1	106	444	1,180	4.9
2	13.6	100	418	1,360	5.7	13.4	100	418	1,350	5.6
3	15.6	100	418	1,560	6.5	15.4	99	414	1,520	6.4
4	17.4	99	414	1,720	7.2	17.5	96	402	1,670	7.0
5	20.7	91	381	1,870	7.8	20.0	90	377	1,790	7.5
6	23.2	87	364	2,010	8.4	22.4	85	356	1,900	7.9
7	25.9	83	347	2,140	9.0	25.0	80	335	2,010	8.4
8	28.6	79	331	2,260	9.5	27.6	76	318	2,110	8.8
9	31.3	76	318	2,380	10.0	30.4	74	305	2,210	9.2
10	33.9	74	310	2,500	10.5	33.8	68	285	2,300	9.6
11	36.7	71	297	2,600	10.9	37.7	62	259	2,350	9.8
12	40.2	67	280	2,700	11.3	42.4	57	238	2,400	10.0
13	45.5	61	255	2,800	11.7	47.0	52	218	2,450	10.3
14	51.7	56	234	2,900	12.1	50.3	50	209	2,500	10.5
15	56.6	53	222	3,000	12.6	52.3	48	201	2,500	10.5
16	60.3	51	213	3,050	12.8	53.6	45	188	2,420	10.1
17	62.4	50	209	3,100	13.0	54.2	43	180	2,340	9.8
18	63.7	49	205	3,100	13.0	54.6	42	176	2,270	9.5
19	65.0	47	197	3,020	12.6	55.0	40	167	2,200	9.2
Adult	65.0	46	192	3,000	12.6	55.0	40	167	2,200	9.2

[1]FAO/WHO [1973:34].

TABLE III. Estimated Energy Requirements for Growth

	Fromon [1974]			
Age	Body weight (kg)	Weight gain (kg)	Energy intake (kcal × 1,000)	Intake for growth (%)
Birth	3.5			
4 mo	7.0			
Birth–4 mo		3.5	61	32.8
12 mo	10.5			
4–12 mo		3.5	180	7.4
24 mo	13.0			
12–24 mo		2.5	365	1.6
36 mo	15.0			
24–36 mo		2.0	400	1.0
	Bergmann and Bergmann [1979]			
Age	Body weight (kg)	Weight gain (g/day)	Energy intake (kcal/day)	Intake for growth (%)
3 wk	4.0	40	475	44
4 mo	7.0	25	675	17
12 mo	10.5	10	1,050	3
2.5 yr	14.0	5	1,400	1
Adult	70.0	0	2,800	0

growth, i.e., an increase in size, decreases with age. The estimated energy cost for growth between birth and 4 months (doubling of birth weight) represents about 33% of the energy intake. This proportion then decreases markedly to 7.4% between 4 and 12 months and 1.5% between 12 and 24 months. Thus, the relative energy needs for growth are greatest early in infancy but decline rapidly during early childhood so that only a small percentage of daily energy intake is necessary to support growth during childhood and adolescence [Fomon, 1974; Bergmann and Bergmann, 1979].

Although energy requirements per kilogram of body weight decrease with age during childhood and adolescence, daily intake increases with age and especially during adolescence (Table II). Adolescent energy requirements are more closely related to biological maturity than to chronological age [Dwyer, 1981]. Peak caloric intakes of adolescents generally occur coincident with peak growth velocity [Heald et al., 1969], thus emphasizing the need to control for maturity-associated variation during adolescence in nutritional surveys and in estimating nutritional needs. Nevertheless, the estimated caloric requirements for growth in later childhood and adolescence comprise only a small percentage of energy intake, 1 to 2% [FAO/WHO, 1973].

Studies of daily energy intake of American children and adolescents illustrate qualitatively similar trends as those in Table II [Burke et al., 1959; Garn, 1968; Heald et al., 1969; Beal, 1970; National Center for Health Statistics, 1977]. Variation within and between samples of children is considerable. Median energy intakes and the 10th and 90th percentiles for a mixed longitudinal sample of Denver children are shown in Figure 1. Sex differences in average daily energy intake (Fig. 1a) are negligible during the first year of life and are clearly apparent thereafter. They increase during early childhood and persist throughout childhood into adolescence when they are magnified. Relative to body weight (Fig. 1b), males generally consume more calories than do females after 2 years of age. This sex difference per unit body weight is reasonably consistent through childhood and adolescence. However, individual variation is great and there is much overlap. For example, about 10% of the 14-year-old girls take in fewer calories than the average 4-year-old girl, while about 10% of the 16-year-old girls take in as many calories as a 1- to 2-year-old child. On the other hand, a significant percentage of young children between 2 and 3 years of age consume as many or more calories than adolescents.

There is thus considerable individual variation in energy intake and in energy intake per kilogram of body weight. There is similar variation among samples of children of the same chronological age. For example, the average daily caloric intake for 14.5-year-old Boston boys (n = 64) was 3,338 ± 674 kcal [Burke et al., 1959], that for Denver boys (n = 20) of approximately the same age was 2,640 ± 660 kcal [Beal, 1970], while that for a small sample of boys from southern Ohio (n = 9) was 2,148 kcal [Garn, 1968]. These three group means are approximately 119, 94, and 77% of the 1974 RDA for American boys 11 to 14 years of age [National Research Council, 1974]. Further, boys in these three growth studies have similar heights and weights, and do not differ in the timing of the adolescent growth spurt [Thissen et al., 1976]. Given the significant variation in energy intake and the similarity in body size and the timing of the growth spurt, it is extremely difficult to relate energy intake to growth and maturation in reasonably well nourished children and youth. More importantly, "...the general principle that people do not all eat, and do not all require, the same amount of food..." must be accepted [Widdowson, 1962:123].

ENERGY EXPENDITURE

Youngsters need energy for basal needs, for growth, for physical activity, and for special needs labeled adaptive thermogenesis, e.g., climatic conditions

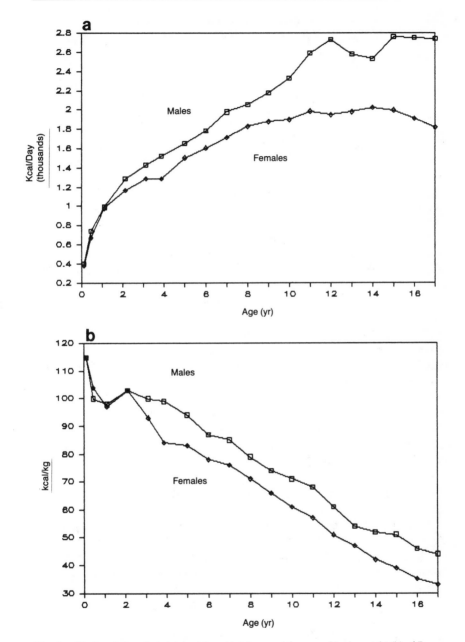

Fig. 1. Median daily caloric intake (a) and intakes per kilogram of body weight (b) of Denver boys □ and girls ◊. Drawn from the data of Beal [1970].

**TABLE IV. Components of Energy Expenditure
During Childhood and Youth**

Basal and resting metabolic rate
Dietary induced thermogenesis/thermal effect of food
Growth
Physical activity
Adaptive thermogenesis

(Table IV). Given the decline in relative energy needs for growth after infancy, a greater proportion of daily energy intake during growth is necessary for tissue maintenance and to meet the costs of daily activities. And, variation in physical activity is ordinarily the most important factor which contributes to variation in energy requirements [FAO/WHO, 1973].

The energy expended for the resting metabolic rate (basal and resting states) increases with age on an absolute basis but decreases per kg body weight. It accounts for approximately 60 to 70% of the total daily energy expenditure in sedentary young adults. The specific dynamic action of food, i.e, the thermal effect of food, accounts for about 10 to 15% of the total daily energy expenditure in sedentary individuals. It is not certain whether there is age- or sex-associated variation in this component of energy expenditure, although Poehlman et al. [1985] showed that the thermal effect of food could be increased in sedentary young adults by overfeeding. The evidence also suggested that individual variation in dietary induced thermogenesis may have a genetic basis.

The energy expended in physical activity obviously varies considerably among individuals. Using the estimates for sedentary adults cited above, it would appear that physical activity can account for approximately 15 to 30% of the total daily energy expenditure. There is, however, age- and sex-associated variation in physical activity. Further, it is a modifiable behavior so that individual behavior patterns and in turn energy expended in physical activity can be altered.

Most techniques for the measurement of energy expenditure during activity are designed for adults and have not been adequately adjusted for developing individuals (Tremblay and Bouchard, this volume). The most valid method is calorimetry, but the methods of calorimetry, direct or indirect, are complex, and the portable respirometers are not readily adaptable (e.g., too heavy and restrictive) to the diverse physical activities which characterize children and youth. Nevertheless, portable respirometers have been used in several studies of youngsters (usually 10 years of age and older) involved in a variety of activities.

The diary method of recording activities in conjunction with the measurement of oxygen consumption during the performance of several activities or in conjunction with a heart rate integrator probably provides the most satisfactory information on typical day-to-day variation in energy expenditure among children and youth [Malina, 1986b]. The use of heart rate monitors requires the establishment of individual oxygen consumption–heart rate relationships. The measures provide only estimates of daily energy expenditure and should be treated as such. They ordinarily have large errors and individual variability is great.

Data on average daily energy expenditure for several samples of children and youth are shown in Table V. Sex differences are significant, probably reflecting sex differences in levels of habitual physical activity. Compared to the daily energy requirements suggested by the Food and Agriculture Organization (Table II), the average daily energy expenditures of the Canadian children are somewhat lower, while those of Scottish youth are approximately equal. The estimates for Indian males are consistently lower and probably reflect differences in nutritional status and perhaps adaptive changes associated with chronic residence under different environmental conditions (e.g., a more tropical climate).

The contribution of energy for daily activities to total daily energy expenditure is not well documented. The Food and Agriculture Organization [FAO/WHO, 1973], for example, estimates the energy available for activity, i.e., the

TABLE V. Estimated Daily Energy Expenditure in Several Samples of School Children

Source/sample/age	Sex	kcal/day	MJ/day
Spady [1980], Canada,	M	2,164 ± 199[a]	9.05 ± 0.83
8–11 yr	F	1,716 ± 243	7.18 ± 1.02
Durnin and Passmore [1967],	M	2,800	11.72
Scotland 14 yr	F	2,300	9.62
Banerjee and Saha [1972],	M	1,811	7.61
Singapore, Indians,			
12–14 yr			
Sridharan et al. [1984], India			
11–13 yr	Mm	1,871 ± 38[b]	7.83 ± 0.16
	Ms	1,715 ± 26	7.18 ± 0.11
13–16 yr	Mm	2,326 ± 29	9.71 ± 0.12
	Ms	1,936 ± 43	8.09 ± 0.18

[a]Mean ± SD.
[b]Mean ± SEM.
m, military school; s, state school.

difference between the estimated energy cost of growth and maintenance and the observed energy intake in 9- to 10-year-old males at 640 kcal, which is 26% of the total daily energy intake. The corresponding value for 9- to 10-year-old females, using the estimated energy cost of growth and energy cost for maintenance per kilogram of body weight for male children, is approximately 525 kcal or 23% of the daily energy intake. In a sample of free-living children 8 through 11 years of age, the estimated energy needs for activity were 31% (673 kcal) and 25% (434 kcal) of the total daily energy intakes of boys and girls, respectively (Spady, 1980). Both values approximate the Food and Agriculture Organization estimates. For adolescent males 16 to 17 years of age, the estimated energy available for activity is 17% (540 kcal) of the daily energy intake [FAO/WHO, 1973], while the corresponding value for adolescent females 14 to 15 years of age (calculated as indicated above) is approximately 14% (353 kcal) of the daily energy intake.

Estimates of the energy available for activity in American youth are considerably greater than the preceding, especially for males. Among males 10 through 19 years of age, the estimated energy available for activity is about 40% of age specific mean energy intakes (962 to 1,145 kcal) and shows little age-associated variation. Among females, in contrast, the estimates decline with age: 38% (774 kcal) of mean energy intake at 10 and 11 years, 28% (548 kcal) at 12 to 14 years, and about 20% (341 to 375 kcal) at 15 to 19 years of age [Dwyer, 1981].

A question of importance is whether these estimates of energy available for physical activity are consistent with estimates of physical activity at these ages? Data from the United States National Children and Youth Fitness Study indicate a reduction in the amount of time spent in physical activity outside of school during adolescence in males, the decline from 10-11 years through 15-17 years being about 9%, 13.7 to 12.5 h per week [Ross et al., 1985] (note that the average time in school physical education combined across age and sex is 2.3 h per week). The decline in physical activity of males occurs after 14 years of age as the estimated weekly time in physical activity outside of school is virtually identical in 10-11- and 12-14-year-old boys, 13.7 and 13.8 h, respectively. Thus, if energy available for activity is stable over male adolescence and the amount of physical activity declines, the result is a positive energy balance. Since growth is largely completed by late adolescence, the excess energy will most likely be accumulated as fat.

Among females in the National Children and Youth Fitness Study the pattern differs: the estimated amount of time spent in physical activity outside of school increases slightly from 11.5 h per week at 10-11 years to 12.5 h per week at 12-14 years of age but then declines slightly to 11.8 h per week at

15-17 years [Ross et al., 1985]. Thus, the estimated amount of weekly physical activity appears to be reasonably constant over female adolescence. If the trend for physical activity is related to the decline in estimated energy available for activity (see above), many adolescent girls may be in energy balance or in a negative balance.

Presumably changing physical activity patterns during adolescence have influenced the recommended energy allowances for American youth 10 through 19 years of age. From 1942 through the 1979 revision of the Recommended Dietary Allowances, there has been a gradual reduction in the recommended energy allowance per kilogram of body weight. The reduction over 37 years amounted to 17 kcal/kg for males and 13 kcal/kg for females, but the major reduction was instituted only since the 1974 revision, 9 kcal/kg for males and 5 kcal/kg for females [Dwyer, 1981].

> The major reason for these declines is decreased physical activity among adolescents at all ages. The greater availability of automobiles and convenience devices which minimize obligatory energy expenditures in daily workaday life, the ubiquity of television sets and popularity of sedentary pursuits during leisure time no doubt all have contributed to the increasingly sedentary life styles characteristic of most American adolescents. [Dwyer, 1981:63].

This statement may be an overgeneralization, although data on activity patterns of adolescents of 40 or 50 years ago are not extensive. In an early study, Dimock [1935] reported a decrease of 36% in weekly time spent as a participant in "physical play" by boys between 12 and 16 years of age (10.5 to 6.7 h per week). These figures underestimate the amount of time spent in physical activity since walking to and from school or amusements would add significantly to the weekly time spent in physical activity. If one compares these estimates with those of the National Children and Youth Fitness Study cited earlier, recognizing of course the differences between the studies, it may be that there is not that much difference in the physical activity levels of boys over the past 40 or 50 years. The kinds of activities probably have changed. Thus, it may well be that the early recommended energy allowances for adolescent boys at least were too high to start with!

Data on energy expenditure for specific activities performed by children and youth are limited. In their comprehensive review on human energy expenditure, Passmore and Durnin [1955] listed only five studies dealing with energy expenditure during children's recreational activities, leading them to conclude: "The very limited data available at the moment are clearly insufficient to assess the energy expenditure of a normal active child's manifold activities" [Passmore and Durnin, 1955:808]. Except for cycling on an ergometer, the early data are limited largely to quiet activities. Since this classic review, several other sets of data for children and youth have become available [Moore et al., 1966; Durnin and Passmore, 1967; Seliger, 1967; Banerjee and Saha, 1972, 1982; Sridharan et al., 1984]. The results of Banerjee and Saha [1972, 1982] suggest differences in the energy expenditure of 12- to 14-year-old Indian and Chinese school boys for standard walking and running tasks. Energy costs (kcal/min) were higher in the Chinese boys, while energy cost per unit body weight (kcal/kg/hr) were higher in Indian boys. The significance of these differences is not clear and probably reflects the size and nutritional status differences between the samples, i.e., the Chinese boys were taller and heavier and from better socioeconomic circumstances. Further, many of the Chinese boys probably had experienced their adolescent growth spurts, while the Indian sample was largely preadolescent.

Energy expenditures for a variety of physical activities, including walking, running, cycling, swimming, games, physical training, and other activities, are reported by Sridharan et al. [1984] for Indian boys 11 through 16 years of age in attendance at a military school and at a state school. Estimated energy expenditures for physical activities performed during the school day (mean of the mean expenditures for each activity) were 841 kcal and 983 kcal, respectively, for 11- to 13- and 13- to 16-year-old boys at the military school, and 719 kcal and 550 kcal respectively for 11- to 13- and 13- to 16-year-old boys at the state school. As a percentage of the estimated total daily energy expenditure, these estimates were similar in the two samples of early adolescent boys, 45 and 42%. However, the estimated energy expenditure for physical activities in the older boys at the state school comprised only 28% of the total daily energy expenditure in contrast to 42% for boys at the military school. These values are greater than the estimated energy available for activity in 9- to 10- and 16- to 17-year-old boys, i.e., 26 and 17% of the daily energy intake respectively [FAO/WHO, 1973]. Clearly, the nature of the school programs influences the level of physical activity and in turn energy expenditure. Nevertheless, the observations for the boys at the state school suggest a decrease in energy expenditure in physical activities from early to later adolescence, a trend also suggested by surveys of adolescent males [Malina, 1986b].

The preceding studies of energy expenditure are limited to school age children and youth, primarily boys. Data for preschool children are limited to the observations of Torun et al. [1983] on presently adequately nourished but previously malnourished Guatemalan children 17 to 45 months of age. Compared to adults, energy expenditure of children per unit body weight is greater for a variety of tasks (Table VI). Per unit body weight, the energy costs apparently decrease with age during childhood and adolescence [Torun, 1984]. However, resting metabolic rate is highest in young children and also decreases with age. Thus, adjusting for the age-associated decline in resting metabolic rate per unit body size, the real effect of age on the energy expended in a given activity per unit body weight is probably less than suggested in Table VI. Nevertheless, the energy expended for a given task decreases with age through puberty. The differences between adolescents (about 14 years of age) and adults are quite small, so that for all practical purposes the energy costs of most activities are similar [Durnin and Passmore, 1967].

The differences in energy expenditure between children and adults while performing similar activities are related to the lower mechanical efficency of children, which is probably a function of their smaller body size and relatively shorter legs. Children generally carry out their activities more intensively, with more excitement and more associated movements, i.e., surplus activity. With increasing age and presumably greater motor skill, i.e., efficiency of movement, unnecessary energy-consuming movements are usually limited.

PROTEIN REQUIREMENTS

Protein provides amino acids for the synthesis of other body proteins and nitrogen for the synthesis of body tissue components. The first process, the synthesis of other body proteins, is the more demanding [Arroyave, 1972]. The essential amino acids, those not synthesized by mammals, are the most critical components of dietary protein. Of the amino acids comprising the body's proteins, nine are essential but all 22 are necessary to support normal growth and maturation. Nevertheless, 70% or more of the amino acids utilized in protein synthesis are provided by the breakdown of other body

TABLE VI. Estimated Energy Cost (kcal/kg/min) of Certain Activities at Different Ages[1]

Age group	BMR	Light standing	Light-to-moderate	Walking leisurely	Bicycle ergometer[2]
2–4	38		73	79	
6–8	31				110
9–11	26	47	62		85
12–14	21	44	56	70	75
14–16	20	47			
Adult	18	38	52	62	55

[1]Adapted from Torun [1984]; data from various sources.
[2]Moderately heavy load at a constant rhythm.

proteins so that dietary protein need is small relative to protein turnover in the body [Scrimshaw and Young, 1976].

The body cannot store dietary protein for long periods. That which is not immediately used for synthesis of other proteins or tissues is used for energy. On the average, about 58% of total dietary protein is reduced to glucose and then used for energy [Williams, 1973].

Protein requirements at different ages as suggested by the Food and Agriculture Organization [FAO/WHO, 1973] are shown in Table VII. These are "safe levels of protein intake", i.e., the amount "...considered necessary to meet the physiological needs and maintain the health of nearly all persons in a specified age group" [FAO/WHO, 1973:10]. Proteins vary in quality, however, so that safe levels must be adjusted for the quality of protein consumed. In addition, nitrogen and amino acid requirements vary with age, though not at the same rate (Arroyave, 1972). This would thus imply that the nutritional quality of a protein can vary with the age of the individual consuming it. Amino acid requirement information is available primarily for infants and adults, with little data for the intervening years [Arroyave, 1972].

The dietary protein requirement per unit of body weight is highest in early infancy and declines with age so that the adult requirement is, on the average, approximately 23% of the young infant's needs (Table VII). The decline in dietary protein requirement per unit body weight parallels the decline in the intensity of whole body protein synthesis with age [Scrimshaw and Young, 1976].

Whole body protein turnover and the protein dietary requirement are greatest in infancy. The estimated increment in the protein content of the body of a 3-week-old infant weighing 4 kg and gaining 40 g per day accounts for about 60% of the total protein requirement at this age. Increments in body protein content relative to the total protein requirement then decrease during infancy, i.e., they comprise about 40% of the total protein requirement at 4 months of age and 25% of the requirement at 12 months of age. By 2.5 years of age, the increment in body protein accounts for only a small percentage of the total protein requirement, about 12% [Fomon, 1974].

There is thus a large requirement for protein to support normal growth during infancy. This requirement decreases with age, and, in older children and youth, a major portion of the protein requirement is used for tissue maintenance (repair or replacement), while only a relatively small proportion is used for growth, i.e., synthesis of new tissue [Fomon, 1974].

Protein intake studies of American children (Fig. 2a) indicate increased intakes with age through adolescence, reaching a peak in the early- to mid-teen ages for girls and in the late-teen ages for boys [Burke et al., 1959; Heald

TABLE VII. Safe Levels of Protein Intake[1]

Age	Protein per kg per day
Months	
<3	2.40
3-6	1.85
6-9	1.62
9-11	1.44
Years	
1	1.27
2	1.19
3	1.12
4	1.06
5	1.01
6	0.98
7	0.92
8	0.87
9	0.85

Age (yrs)	Protein per kg per day	
	Males	Females
10	0.82	0.81
11	0.81	0.76
12	0.78	0.74
13	0.77	0.68
14	0.72	0.62
15	0.67	0.59
16	0.64	0.58
17	0.61	0.57
Adult	0.57	0.52

[1]FAO/WHO [1973; 70], expressed in terms of egg or milk protein. The suggested levels of intake ". . . are not estimates of average requirements but estimates of the upper range of individual requirements (only 2.5% of individuals might be expected to have physiological requirements above these levels." Intakes of infants <6 months of age are based on observed intakes (mean + 2 SD) of healthy infants.

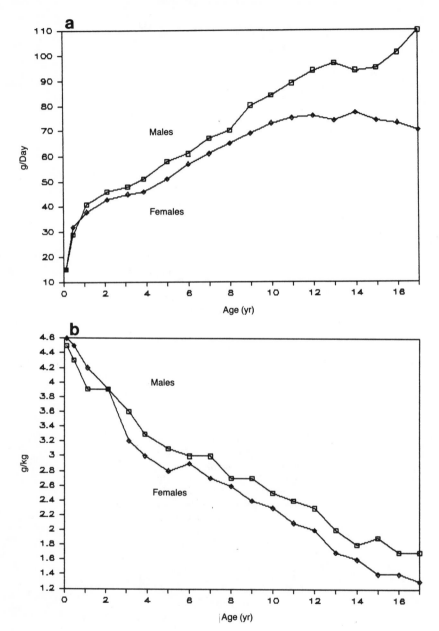

Fig. 2. Median daily protein intakes (a) and intakes per kilogram of body weight (b) of Denver boys □ and girls ◊. Drawn from the data of Beal [1970].

et al., 1969; Beal, 1970; National Center for Health Statistics, 1977]. The range of variation within and between age and sex groups is considerable. Many 2-year-old children take in more protein daily than teenagers, especially in the case of girls. Interestingly, protein accounts for about 14 to 15% of the daily energy intake in the mixed longitudinal sample of Denver children who were surveyed over a 20-year period from 1946 to 1966 [Beal, 1970]. Similar estimates are evident in the United States Health and Nutrition Examination Survey of 1971–1974, i.e., protein accounts for about 14 to 16% of the daily energy intake of children and youth.

Sex differences in protein intake, though small per kilogram of body weight, appear during early childhood and become greater with age through adolescence (Fig. 2b). Daily protein intake per kilogram of body weight in American samples is greater than that proposed by the Food and Agriculture Organization (Table VII), which would suggest that American children and youth consume, on the average, about two to four times more protein per kg of body weight than the estimated safe levels.

Although protein intake reaches a peak during adolescence, the recommended protein requirement per kilogram of body weight (Table VII) shows no increase in requirement at this time. This is perhaps related to the lack of data on the nutritional needs of adolescents emphasized by Hegsted (1976:120): "...there are so few factual data available for this age group that nearly everything we presumably know is obtained by extrapolation." On the other hand, protein requirements during adolescence are probably more closely related to biological maturity status, i.e., the timing of the adolescent growth spurt and sexual maturation and associated variation in body composition, especially muscle mass in males [Dwyer, 1981; Malina, 1986a]. Thus, as in growth studies, requirements suggested on the basis of chronological age during adolescence have a considerable degree of imprecision. As noted earlier, the estimated daily increment in the protein content of the body during the peak of the adolescent growth spurt is about two times the estimated increment in protein over the period from 10 to 20 years of age in both sexes [Forbes, 1981].

VITAMIN AND MINERAL REQUIREMENTS

In addition to energy and protein, many of the specific dietary requirements essential to support normal growth and maturation are needed in trace amounts (μg per day or only few mg per day), while others are required in more substantial portions (100 mg per day or more). Included among these dietary components are vitamins, mineral elements, and essential fatty acids.

The last mentioned was briefly considered in the discussion of fats. It is generally assumed that given a balanced diet with sufficient energy and protein, the vitamin and mineral needs of the growing individual will be adequately met.

Vitamins are required by the body in very small amounts and are largely regulatory in function. Their role in growth and maturation, though not immediately apparent in the well-nourished child, is especially evident in the stunted growth that characterizes some severe vitamin deficiency states, e.g., vitamin A and D deficiencies. Both are essential to the growth of skeletal tissues. Vitamins are also involved in the maintenance of tissues, metabolism of other nutrients, formation of red blood cells, and so on. Hence, they are essential to normal growth and maturation in a variety of ways.

Minerals have structural and regulatory functions. Of the major minerals, calcium and phosphorus are essential to bone growth and metabolism. Indeed, most of the body's calcium is contained in bone. Others are involved in cellular metabolism (magnesium), in the maintenance of fluid and electrolyte balance (sodium, potassium, chlorine), and in the synthesis, storage, and maintenance of protein (potassium, sulfur) [Williams, 1973]. All of these processes, needless to say, are essential to normal growth and maturation.

The role of trace mineral elements in growth and maturation is gradually being elaborated [Mertz, 1981]. Zinc deficiency, for example, is associated with growth depression and sexual immaturity, while copper deficiency is associated with changes in ossification in humans. Experimental studies of animals indicate growth depression and/or retardation in association with specific deficiency of silicon, vanadium, manganese, iron, cobalt, nickel, zinc, and arsenic [Mertz, 1981]. Hence, it is reasonable to assume that many trace minerals have a significant role in these processes.

REFERENCES

Arroyave G (1972): Amino acid requirements. Age and sex. Paper presented at the Symposium on Proteins and Processed Foods, Chicago, November 13-15.

Banerjee B, Saha N (1972): Energy intake and expenditure of Indian schoolboys. Br J Nutr 27:483-490.

Banerjee B, Saha N (1982): Energy cost of some common physical acitivities of Chinese school boys. Ann Nutr Metab 26:360-366.

Barness LA (1981): Nutritional requirements of the full-term neonate. In Suskind RM (ed): "Textbook of Pediatric Nutrition." New York: Raven Press, pp 21-28.

Beal VA (1970): Nutritional intake. In McCammon RW (ed): "Human Growth and Development." Springfield, Illinois: C.C. Thomas, pp 61-100.

Bergmann RL, Bergmann KE (1979): Nutrition and growth in infancy. In Falkner F, Tanner JM (eds): "Human Growth, Vol 3, Neurobiology and Nutrition." New York: Plenum, pp 331-360.

Brozek J, (1966): Body composition: models and estimation equations. Am J Phys Anthropol 24:239-246.

Burke BS, Reed RB, Van den Berg AS, Stuart HC (1959): Caloric and protein intakes of children between 1 and 18 years of age. Pediatrics 24:922-940.

Chan W-Y, Rennert OW (1985): Genetic trace mineral disturbances. J Am Coll Nutr 4:39-48.

Cooke RE (1969): Basic principles of energy balance. In Heald FP (ed): "Adolescent Nutrition and Growth." New York: Appleton-Century-Crofts, pp 177-192.

Dimock HS (1935): A research in adolescence: the social world of the adolescent. Child Dev 6:285-302.

Durnin JVGA (1976): Sex differences in energy intake and expenditure. Proc Nutr Soc 35:145-154.

Durnin JVGA, Passmore R (1967): "Energy, Work and Leisure." London: Heinemann Educational Books.

Dwyer J (1981): Nutritional requirements of adolescence. Nutr Rev 39:56-72.

FAO/WHO (1973): "Energy and Protein Requirements." Report of a Joint FAO/WHO ad hoc Expert Committee. World Health Organization Technical Report Series, no. 522.

Fomon SF (1974): "Infant Nutrition (2nd Ed)." Philadelphia: Saunders.

Fomon SJ, Haschke F, Ziegler EE, Nelson SE (1982): Body composition of reference children from birth to age 10 years. Am J Clin Nutr 35:1169-1175.

Forbes GB (1981): Nutritional requirements in adolescence. In Suskind RM (ed): "Textbook of Pediatric Nutrition." New York: Raven Press, pp 381-391.

Garn SM (1968): Food Intake of Ohio Boys and Girls During December 4-10, 1967. Yellow Springs, Ohio: Fels Research Institute.

Haschke F (1983): Body composition in adolescent males. Acta Paediat Scand, Suppl 307, 1-23.

Heald FP, Mayer J, Remmell PS (1969): Caloric, protein and fat intakes in children and adolescents. In Heald FP (ed): "Adolescent Nutrition and Growth." New York: Appleton-Century-Crofts, pp 17-35.

Hegsted D (1976): Current knowledge of energy, fat, protein and amino acid needs of adolescence. In McKigney JI, Munro HM (eds): "Nutrient Requirements in Adolescence." Cambridge: MIT Press, pp 107-122.

Jacobs A (1976): Sex differences in iron absorption. Proc Nutr Soc 35:159-162.

Lohman TG (1986): Applicability of body composition techniques and constants for children and youths. Exer Sport Sci Rev 14:325-357.

Malina RM (1969): Quantification of fat, muscle and bone in man. Clin Orthop Rel Res 69:9-38.

Malina RM (1986a): Growth of muscle tissue and muscle mass. In Falkner F, Tanner JM (eds): "Human Growth, Vol 2. Postnatal Growth (revised Ed)." New York: Plenum, pp 77-79.

Malina RM (1986b): Energy expenditure and physical activity during childhood and youth. In Demirjian A (ed): "Human Growth: A Multidisciplinary Review." London: Taylor and Francis, pp 215-225.

Mertz W (1981): The essential trace elements. Science 213:1332-1338.

Miller DF, Voris L (1969): Chronologic changes in the recommended dietary allowances. J Am Diet Assoc 54:109-117.

Miller DS (1979): Thermogenesis and obesity. Biblthca Nutr Dieta 27:25-32.

Moore ME, Pond J, Korslund MK (1966): Energy expenditure of pre-adolescent girls. J Am Diet Assoc 49:409-412.

National Center for Health Statistics (1977): Dietary intake findings, United States, 1971-1974. Vital and Health Statistics, Series 11, no. 202.

National Research Council (1974): "Recommended Dietary Allowances (8th Ed)." Washington, D.C.: National Academy of Sciences.

National Research Council (1980): "Recommended Dietary Allowances (9th revised Ed)." Washington, D.C.: National Academy of Sciences.

Passmore R, Durnin JVGA (1955): Human energy expenditure. Physiol Rev 35:801-840.

Poehlman ET, Tremblay A, Fontaine E, Despres JP, Nadeau A, Dussault J, Bouchard C (1985): Genotype and changes in body composition, fat morphology, and dietary induced thermogenesis following overfeeding. Ann Human Biol 12 (Suppl 1): 41 (abstract).

Reed PB (1980): "Nutrition: An Applied Science." St. Paul, Minnesota: West.

Ross JG, Dotson CO, Gilbert GG, Katz SJ (1985): The National Children and Youth Fitness Study; After physical education...physical activity outside of school physical education programs. J Phys Educ Rec Dance 56:77-81, (Jan.).

Scrimshaw NS, Young VR (1976): The requirements of human nutrition. Sci Am 235:50-64, (Sept.).

Seliger V (1967): "Energeticky Metabolismus u Vybranych Telesnych Cviceni." Prague: Charles University.

Spady DW (1980): Total daily energy expenditure of healthy, free ranging school children. Am J Clin Nutr 33:766-775.

Sridharan K, Mukherjee AK, Radhakrishnan U, Grover SK, Bhardwaj SK, Dimri GP (1984): Energy intake and expenditure of the boys of Indian schools governed by the state. Nutr Rep Int 29:883-902.

Suskind RM (ed) (1981): "Textbook of Pediatric Nutrition." New York: Raven Press.

Thissen D, Bock RD, Wainer H, Roche AF (1976): Individual growth in stature: a comparison of four growth studies in the U.S.A. Ann Human Biol 3:529-542.

Torun B (1984): Physiological measurements of physical activity among children under free-living conditions. In Pollitt E, Amante P (eds): "Energy Intake and Activity." New York: Alan R. Liss Inc. pp 159-184.

Torun B, Chew F, Mendoza RD (1983): Energy cost of activities of preschool children. Nutr Res 3:401-406.

Truswell AS (1976): A comparative look at recommended nutrient intakes. Proc Nutr Soc 35:1-14.

Widdowson EM (1962): Nutritional individuality. Proc Nutr Soc 21:121-128.

Williams RJ (1956): "Biochemical Individuality." New York: Wiley.

Williams SR (1973): "Nutrition and Diet Therapy (2nd Ed)." St. Louis: Mosby.

Young VR, Scrimshaw NS (1979): Genetic and biological variability in human nutrient requirements. Am J Clin Nutr 32:486-500.

Nutritional Anthropology, pages 197-221

Nutrition and Variation in Biological Aging

Cynthia M. Beall, PhD

Department of Anthropology, Case Western Reserve University,
Cleveland, Ohio 44106

Broadly defined, biological aging is "any time-dependent change that occurs *after* maturity of size, form, or function is reached and that is distinct from daily, seasonal, and other biological rhythms." [Rockstein et al., 1977:4]. Some definitions further specify that true aging phenomena are universal and irreversible under usual conditions [Kohn, 1978]. These time-dependent changes are manifest in individuals as a congeries of progressive, deleterious, morphological and functional changes that accumulate with time and underlie a loss of physiological adaptive capacity [Bourliere, 1970; Shock, 1977]. They are also reflected epidemiologically in populations as an acceleration of age-specific morbidity and mortality rates throughout adulthood [Comfort, 1979].

The influence of nutrition on human aging has received considerable attention because there are so many aspects of "nutrition" with potential relevance to the aging process. Examples include the possibility that: 1) nutritional requirements for maintaining optimal function may change as a result of aging processes [Heaney et al., 1982; Munro, 1982; Rivlin, 1981; Simopoulos, 1982; Spencer et al., 1982]; 2) nutritional factors have a prophylactic, aggravating, or therapeutic influence on the nature and severity of diseases associated with aging [Ames, 1983; NAS/NRC, 1982; Winick, 1976; Pauling, 1983; Rivlin, 1982; Stamler, 1983; Young, 1982]; and 3) nutritional factors may accelerate or delay progressive, deleterious age changes and as a result may increase or decrease age-specific mortality rates and thereby shorten or lengthen life expectancy [e.g., Bertrand, 1983; Harper, 1982; Morrison, 1983; Masoro, 1984; Walford, 1983].

This paper focuses attention on the third item—the question of whether nutrition can influence the aging processes themselves. Laboratory investigations have repeatedly demonstrated that long-term nutritional manipulations are capable of altering the aging processes of rats and mice. The finding that dietary restriction slows the aging process in some mammals encourages considering the possibility of such a phenomenon among humans. It also suggests the nature of nutritional variation likely to be influential, namely severe caloric restriction with adequate nutrient intake—undernutrition without malnutrition—beginning at weaning, young-, or midadulthood and continuing lifelong thereafter. This research also suggests that the effect of total intake is more pronounced than that of individual dietary components. Dietary restriction in laboratory rats and mice can delay the onset of and/or diminish some of the physiological changes of aging, delay the acceleration of morbidity and mortality rates, and extend the median and in some cases the maximum lifespan [Bertrand, 1983; Masoro, 1984; Ross, 1976; Walford, 1983]. Similarly, there is experimental evidence that dietary excess raises morbidity and mortality rates and thus shortens the average lifespan [Stunkard, 1983].

Using these animal models as a general guide, this chapter reviews evidence for associations between long-term nutritional variation arising from customary dietary differences and variation in the human biological aging processes. First it reviews evidence that nutritional variation is associated with variation in the timing, magnitude, and/or rate of two widely prevalent, perhaps universal, and largely irreversible physiological aging processes that are measurable in all individuals: aging bone loss and age at menopause. Then it reviews evidence that nutritional variation is associated with variation in an epidemiologic measure of aging, age-specific mortality rate, a summary measure of all aging changes, and the determinant of life expectancy.

PHYSIOLOGICAL MEASURES

Aging changes have been documented for virtually every physiological process and system. Aging bone loss and menopause are two relatively widely studied examples. Bone loss throughout adulthood appears to be a "universal phenomenon of human biology that occurs regardless of sex, race, occupation, economic development, geographical location, historical epoch, or dietary habits." [Parfitt, 1983: 1181]. The loss is substantial: American women in their eighties have 30% less compact bone in the shaft of the radius than their 20-year-old counterparts [Mazess and Cameron, 1975]. The process results in bone that is qualitatively normal but reduced in amount, i.e., less dense [Nutrition Reviews, 1983]. If bone mass decreases to a point when it is insufficient to maintain normal structural integrity, then a disease state called osteoporosis exists [Pak, 1983]. The rise in age-specific incidence of nontraumatic fractures of the vertebral column, forearm, and hip is attributed to structural weakness resulting from aging bone loss [Jowsey, 1977]. Because these are more prevalent among elderly women than men, much of the information on aging bone loss deals with women.

Aging changes are somewhat different for trabecular (spongy, cancellous bone of the flat bones, the axial skeleton, and the ends of the long bones) and compact bone (hard bone found primarily in the shafts of the long bones of the appendicular skeleton). Because it has been easier technically to measure compact bone than trabecular bone, age changes and variation in compact bone are relatively well documented while the course of trabecular bone loss remains uncertain, even though the characteristic fracture sites are largely trabecular. There is a correlation between measurements of the two types of bone. Loss of compact bone at a rate of 3% per decade begins at about age 40 in males and females and continues linearly in males. For females, however, the estrogen withdrawal at menopause is associated with an accelerated component of loss at an overall rate of 9% per decade for some years afterward [Mazess, 1982]. Loss of trabecular bone at a rate of 6-8% per decade begins by the thirties in males and females. There is conflicting evidence regarding the existence of an accelerated component of postmenopausal loss of trabecular bone [Heaney, 1982; Lindquist et al., 1981; Lindquist and Bengtsson, 1983; Mazess, 1982; Riggs et al., 1982].

Theoretically the amount of bone present at any time after maturity is a function of the maximal young adult bone mass, the age of onset of bone loss, and the rate of bone loss. If lifelong or long-term nutritional factors influence the latter two parameters, they may cause variation in the pattern of aging bone loss. However, measuring nutritional intake over a human lifespan is problematic. One approach is to measure current nutritional status using general anthropometric nutritional indices such as weight, Quetelet's (or Body Mass) Index ($QI = weight/height^2$), or triceps skinfold (see Himes, this volume). In populations in which undernutrition is not widespread, the very lean or the very obese may be viewed in a narrow sense as natural experimental examples of freely self-selected dietary restriction or excess. There is evidence for continuity in relative fatness between some stages of the life cycle, particularly for the extremes of the fatness distribution, but, there is little information spanning adulthood or extending from the growth stages of the life cycle into adulthood [e.g., Cronk et al., 1982; Garn, 1980; Hsu et al., 1977; Roche and Siervogel, 1982]. The assumption of continuity—that current nutritional status is some reflection of nutritional status earlier in life, which is implicit when using cross-sectional data—is largely untested and may be inaccurate for at least a portion of the population. General anthropometric nutritional indices of fatness are positively associated with bone mass and density and negatively associated with the prevalence of osteoporotic fractures, that is, they suggest that, in humans, caloric restriction may accelerate aging bone loss. Throughout adulthood in normal U.S. males and females there is a positive correlation between fatness measured by triceps skinfold and the amount and density of compact bone measured at the second metacarpal. Contrasting the extremes of fatness measured by triceps skinfolds in the U.S. population reveals that the fattest 15% of the sample have larger bone mass and density throughout adulthood than the leanest 15%. From the fifties onward the differences is two to three times greater than during earlier ages owing primarily to an increased difference between the obese and the rest of the sample [Garn et al., 1981]. This suggests that the pattern of bone loss may differ among the lean and the obese and that the latter may have a slower rate or later onset of loss. Longitudinal data are needed to test this hypothesis. Other comparisons of obese individuals with normal-weight, age-matched controls confirm that the former have greater bone mass through adulthood although aging bone loss does occur [Dalen et al., 1975].

Clinical samples of women who have sustained nontraumatic fractures of the vertebral column, forearm, and hip generally have a low mean bone density relative to age-matched controls. Consistent with the above epidemiological data are the findings that these osteoporotic fracture patients also have smaller skinfolds, lower weight, lower weight for height and less prevalent obesity [Brocklehurst et al., 1978; Wooten et al., 1977; Saville and Nilsson, 1966; Daniell, 1976]. Still, there is a wide and overlapping range of bone densities in both groups. Because some fracture patients have bone densities in the range of normal controls and some controls have bone densities in the range of the fracture patients, bone density must be one of several factors influencing fracture risk.

One possible explanation for the relationship between nutritional status and bone mass lies in the relationship between fatness, estrogen production, and bone metabolism. A nonovarian source of estrogen is the conversion to estrogen of a precursor secreted by the adrenal cortex, a normal process in the stromal cell of adipose tissue. The amount of estrogen produced by conversion is proportional to the degree of obesity in both males and females and increases with age [Casey and MacDonald, 1983; Kirschner et al., 1981]. Since the postmenopausal estrogen reduction is thought to play a role in female bone loss, the elevated estrogen levels of obese postmenopausal women may diminish, delay, or slow the postmenopausal acceleration component of bone loss. For males, another mechanism, presently unknown, is likely to operate also. This would help to explain the association between obesity and bone mass in males, who generally have greater bone masses and body weights but less fat and lower estrogen levels than females.

Another possible explanation for the association between body fat and bone density and mass is that people with more fat ingest more calories and in doing so obtain more of the specific nutrients involved in bone metabolism. Since the relationship between diet and aging bone loss has been the subject of recent detailed reviews highlighting the intricate nutritional, hormonal, and physiological aging interactions involved [Heaney et al., 1982; Marcus, 1982; Parfitt, 1983; Parfitt et al., 1982], only a limited aspect of this information is discussed here. Attention is directed to the role of calcium and protein.

Two studies compare residential subpopulations whose customary diets differ in calcium content. The differences were assumed to have been present throughout the lifetimes of the study participants. A Yugoslavian study documented two-to-three-fold differences in current calcium intake using recall methods [Matkovic et al., 1979]. The mean daily calcium intake in the high intake area was within the U.S. recommended daily allowance (RDA) and in the low intake area was roughly half or less. Subsistence and activity patterns and socioeconomic status were noted to be similar in the two study areas. A Japanese study compared two populations, one of which had a nutrient intake "known to be poor, especially in calcium," because of lower water calcium and lower socioeconomic status [Fujita et al., 1977]. Because these are cross-sectional samples, inferences regarding rate and age of onset of bone loss are speculative. Nevertheless, the similar shape of the published curves of age differences in bone mass and density in the Yugoslavian study and the similar slopes of the regression lines of bone density on age in the Japanese study suggest that there are no substantial differences in age of onset or rate of loss. Rather, the greater bone densities of the high calcium intake groups throughout adulthood in both the Yugoslavian and Japanese samples appear to result from maintenance of an advantage already evident in young adulthood. It should be noted that calcium intake was not measured in the Japanese study and that subsistence and activity patterns, socioeconomic status, height, and weight were noted to be dissimilar in the two study areas [Fujita et al., 1977, 1984]. Thus while the Japanese sample differences parallel those of the Yugoslavian samples, it is not clear whether this is attributable to differences in dietary calcium intake. It does appear that, within the ranges measured, variation in calcium intake does not influence the pattern of aging bone loss.

However, clinical evidence suggests a somewhat different interpretation. Women who have sustained nontraumatic fractures at the characteristic trabecular bone sites generally have low dietary calcium intake as well as low bone density [Heaney et al., 1982]. Furthermore, high doses of calcium supplementation above the U.S. RDA may slow the rate of bone loss among these women and postmenopausal women [Heaney et al., 1982]. This intervention is short-term relative to the lifespan and is given in very high doses that are more analogous to therapy than to normal diet. These data do not exclude the possibility that a very high or very low lifelong, normal dietary calcium intake could slow/accelerate the rate of aging or delay/advance the onset of bone loss. This awaits a study of the appropriate population. In the U.S. population, there is a significant but low correlation between current calcium intake and measures of bone mass and density [Garn et al., 1981]. It thus appears possible that restriction of the dietary calcium component could accelerate aging bone loss.

Variation in protein consumption may be associated with variation in the rate of compact bone loss. Comparison of Eskimo populations, whose traditional diet consists largely of meat and is therefore very high in protein, with U.S. white omnivores consuming less meat and with U.S. female Seventh Day Adventists (SDAs) avoiding meat and following a lacto-ovo-vegetarian diet for at least 10 years [Mazess and Mather, 1974, 1975; Harper et al., 1984; Marsh et al., 1980; Mazess and Cameron, 1975] reveals that the greater the meat consumption the greater the age differences in compact bone loss. Figure 1 illustrates this by plotting age differences in density of the shaft of the distal radius of these six female samples. Though studies of male vegetarians have apparently not been published, male omnivores and Eskimos exhibit the same contrast. (The differences between the two omnivorous control groups may be accounted for by differences in sample selection. The omnivore A sample is age- and height- but not smoking-matched to the lacto-ovo-vegetarians, while the omnivore B sample is a population sample.) Eskimos begin to lose bone about 10 years earlier and lose a larger percentage of bone per decade relative to the other samples. This results in interpopulation differences in bone density that increase with age. Eskimo females in their seventies have 52 to 63% of the bone density of Eskimo females in their twenties [Harper et al., 1984; Mazess and Mather, 1974] while omnivore and vegetarian women have 70 and 86%, respectively [Marsh et al., 1980; Mazess and Cameron, 1975]. Fifty-year-old Eskimos have the bone density of 80-year-old U.S. white females; in turn, U.S. white females in their late fifties have the bone density of 80-year-old vegetarians. Interpretation of these population comparisons may be confounded, mainly because inferences about dietary intake are based on the traditional or prescribed diets rather than measurement. For example, the traditional Eskimo diet is also low in calcium and vitamin D

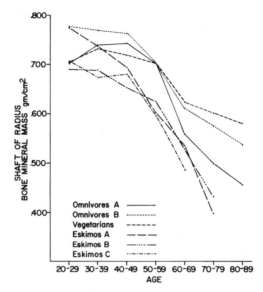

Fig. 1. Age differences in bone density measured at the shaft of the radius in six groups of females: two omnivorous samples (drawn from data in A [Marsh et al., 1980]; B [Mazess and Cameron, 1975]), one vegetarian sample (drawn from data in Marsh et al., [1980]); and three Eskimo samples (drawn from data in A [Mazess and Mather, 1974]; B [Harper et al., 1984]; C [Mazess and Mather, 1975]).

content [Draper and Bell, 1979; Harper et al., 1984] and thus the findings may not be attributable solely to protein intake. Similarly, the study of the SDA lacto-ovo-vegetarians did not measure dietary protein. Because other studies report similar protein intake for SDAs and omnivores, albeit from different sources [Schultz and Leklem, 1983], protein source or other lifestyle factors, such as the religious proscription against smoking and caffeine consumption, might account for the bone mass difference.

Experimental evidence from short-term balance studies is consistent with those interpopulation comparisons in finding an inverse relationship between nitrogen (protein) intake and calcium balance on the one hand [Heaney and Recher, 1982], while on the other hand, an intrapopulation study in the U.S. found no difference in the metacarpal bone densities of people at the high and low ends of the protein consumption distribution as assessed by 1-day recall methods [Garn and Kangas, 1981]. Considering the interpopulation comparisons in conjunction with the supportive clinical, experimental data suggests that protein excess may accelerate the process of aging bone loss. More data quantifying dietary intake and controlling for confounding factors are necessary to explore the possibility that protein restriction may slow the process.

Menopause is another biological aging event, universally experienced by surviving females, that is susceptible to nutritional influences. The median age of natural menopause in Western industrial societies is about 51, the mean recalled age at menopause is about 48, and the normal range of variation is 42 to 58 years [Gray, 1976; MacMahon and Worcester, 1966]. Variation in nutritional status assessed by body weight, relative weight, QI, and triceps skinfold is associated with variation in age at menopause. Lean women have a higher rate of undergoing menopause at any age and a lower mean recalled or median age at menopause. A number of studies report this general finding even though many rely upon self-reported current height, weight, and menopausal status. The effect of inaccurate reporting would be to reduce the strength of or distort the precise relationship. Weight reporting inaccuracies, at least, are likely to differ among the lean and obese. Prospective, retrospective, and status quo samples in the U.S., Scandinavia, and Japan agree on this relationship [Willett et al., 1983; Brand and Lehert, 1978; Sherman et al., 1981; Hoel et al., 1983; MacMahon and Worcester, 1966; Lindquist et al., 1979]. For example, in a U.S. national status quo sample, women with skinfolds of less than 3.1 cm had a median age of menopause of 48.95 compared to medians of 50.01 and 50.55 for women with skinfolds of 3.1 to 4.5 and 4.6+ cm, respectively [MacMahon and Worcester, 1966]. Lean smokers have especially high rates of undergoing menopause at all ages [Lindquist, 1979; Willett et al., 1983]. This interaction of smoking and nutrition illustrates that nutritional influences are not necessarily uniform but may be modulated by other factors. These data suggest that caloric restriction as measured by anthropometric indices of nutritional status is associated with accelerated menopause.

A postmenopausal sample of U.S. SDAs following a vegetarian diet recalled a mean age at menopause of 44.7, over 3 years younger than that recalled by a control sample of omnivores with the same QI [Armstrong et al., 1981]. Because SDA teachings proscribe smoking, it is unlikely that a higher rate of smoking accounts for the low age at menopause of the SDAs, although this was not mentioned in the study. If this finding is replicated with appropriate controls for other lifestyle and dietary influences, it suggests an investigation into the influence of protein source upon age at menopause.

These are but two among many aging processes. They were selected because of the availability of pertinent information. The influence of nutritional variation on other aging processes, such as the decline in immune system responsiveness and in memory and cognitive function, has been hypothesized but relatively little studied.

The effectiveness of the immune system declines with age. Both cell-mediated and humoral responses to foreign antigens are decreased with age and may account for the increasing susceptibility to infection and cancer throughout adulthood [Buckley and Roseman, 1976; Cohn et al., 1983; Roberts-Thomson et al., 1974; Weksler, 1982]. Trace metals may underlie some of the large variation in immune function of the elderly [Gerschwin et al., 1983; Sandstead et al., 1982). For example, a relationship between zinc nutriture and immune responsiveness is suggested by several studies. Dietary protein and zinc levels of elderly women are positively associated with humoral response to foreign antigens [Stiedemann and Harrill, 1980]. Consistent with this is the finding that zinc supplementation may enhance cellular and humoral responses of elderly people [Duchateau et al., 1981a,b; 1982]. Similarly, there is evidence that vitamin C supplementation enhances cellular immune response [Anderson et al., 1980]. Whether a sufficiently high habitual intake of these nutrients would abolish or slow the decline in immune function has not been studied. If further study confirms these relationships, then restriction of the zinc dietary component could accelerate the physiological aging process of decline in immune system responsiveness.

Cognitive function and memory tests reveal age declines and age differences. Alzheimer's Disease, the most common but not universal dementia of later life, is an irreversible brain disorder which causes impairment of memory and other cognitive functions [Shore and Wyatt, 1983]. Because there is an accumulation of aluminum in the structures that are neuropathological hallmarks of Alzheimer's Disease, there is concern that aluminum is pathogenic, although the evidence and interpretation of these data are controversial [Shore and Wyatt, 1983; Bjorksten, 1982; Hamilton, 1982; Perl, 1983]. If further study confirms the hypothesized pathogenetic role of aluminum, then its restriction could delay or prevent the deterioration in memory or cognitive function associated with Alzheimer's Disease [Leone, 1983].

EPIDEMIOLOGICAL MEASURES

The changes in biological structure and function that occur throughout adulthood create a homeostatic state that is constantly changing; one that is less able to maintain homeostasis in the face of environmental challenge and that is increasingly susceptible to disease. Disease is so common at advanced ages that it may be difficult to distinguish from aging [Kohn, 1978]. Over three-quarters of the U.S. population aged 65+ have at least one chronic disease and half have two or more chronic diseases [Hess and Markson, 1980]. However, while everyone experiences aging changes, a small proportion of people develop any given disease. For example, only about 30% of 85-year-olds have or have had cancer [Ames, 1983]. Thus, a link with nutrition is not measurable in every person and an epidemiological, population-based description is required to measure this aspect of aging. Nutritional factors influence the risk of developing many chronic diseases associated with aging in Western society. For example, cancer and coronary heart disease are leading causes of morbidity and mortality among the Western elderly and there are data, comprehensively reviewed elsewhere, relating diet to cancer [e.g., NAS/NRC, 1982; Heaton, 1983; Ames, 1983] and to coronary heart disease and its risk factors [e.g. Oliver, 1982; Stamler, 1983; Blackburn and Prineas, 1983]. Infectious disease is another leading cause of mortality among the elderly and nutritional factors may mediate the effectiveness of the immune response to infection at this stage of the life cycle as at others [Smith, 1982; Felser and Roff, 1983].

The combination of physiological aging changes and morbidity results in an exponential increase in mortality rate throughout adulthood (Fig. 2). The aging changes described in the previous section are among the many contributing to this phenomenon and illustrate these relationships.

Aging bone loss is not necessarily symptomatic, yet it may establish vulnerability to fracture because bone quantity is associated with bone strength. If nutritional factors can delay the age of attaining a skeletal bone mass so reduced that it is insufficient to maintain normal structural integrity this should be reflected in a delay in the increase in fracture rates at the characteristic sites.

The Yugoslavian and Japanese studies described in the previous section provide information on fracture rates. The Yugoslavian study measured fracture rates in the forearm and the hip and found the abrupt increase in female hip fracture rate began in the sixties in the low calcium intake study area but did not begin until the seventies in the high intake study area with the result that females in their sixties and seventies in the low calcium intake area had higher hip fracture rates [Matkovic et al., 1979]. Similarly, 60- and 70-year-old Japanese females in the low calcium intake area had higher prevalence of vertebral fractures [Fujita et al., 1984]. These data suggest that a restriction of the dietary calcium component may accelerate this epidemiological measure of aging among females but not among males.

Fractures of the hip are followed by elevated mortality risk and shortened life expectancy. The mortality rate for hip fracture patients is three to four times that expected for age–sex comparable samples [Beals, 1972; Crane and Kerneke, 1983; Gordon, 1971; Miller, 1978]. Therefore, if lifelong dietary practices can influence the pattern of aging bone loss and/or the maximal

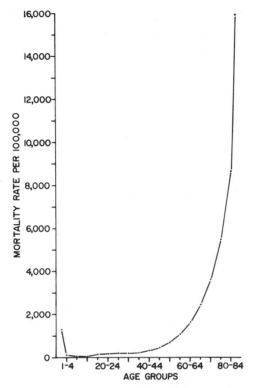

Fig. 2. Age-specific mortality rate, sexes combined, United States, 1980 (drawn from data in Monthly Vital Statistics Report [1983]).

young adult bone mass and the age-specific fracture risk, they may influence age specific mortality rates and life expectancy.

There are several ways that age at menopause could influence age-specific mortality rates and life expectancy. Theoretically, an early menopause would be expected to advance the timing of other linked aging changes. Because women with early menopause have less bone than their premenopausal peers and have less bone in later adulthood than their peers who experienced later menopause [Goldsmith, 1975; Lindquist et al., 1979; Lindquist et al., 1981; Lindquist and Bengtsson, 1983], they may form a subpopulation with an elevated age-specific risk of osteoporotic fractures and mortality. In a population in which young adults tend to have larger-than-average bone mass, the early onset of bone loss following early menopause might have less impact on subsequent fracture rate than in a population with a smaller-than-average bone mass in young adults. The size of the young adult bone mass may be a function of lifelong nutritional intake. Similarly, because postmenopausal women have higher levels of some risk factors for coronary heart disease and thus higher risks of mortality [Bengtsson and Lindquist, 1979; Gordon et al., 1978; Hjortland et al., 1976; Kannel et al., 1976; Lindquist, 1982; Lindquist and Bengtsson, 1980; WHO, 1981; Wenger, 1982], women with early menopause may experience an earlier rise in these risk factors and may form a subpopulation with elevated age-specific risk of cardiovascular disease. These two trends would result in a shorter life expectancy at any given postmenopausal age for women with younger ages at menopause relative to premenopausal women and those with later menopause.

Conversely, however, early menopause is associated with a lower risk of some causes of mortality, such as hormonally dependent tumors of the breast and endometrium, and thus a delay in the increase in their age-specific mortality rate and a higher life expectancy [Paganini-Hill et al., 1984; Sherman et al., 1981]. The overall impact on life expectancy of accelerated menopause will vary depending upon the balance between diseases whose subsequent prevalence would be enhanced and those whose prevalence would be diminished. For example, in populations in which breast cancer is a more significant cause of mortality than cardiovascular disease, the mortality risks subsequent to early menopause may be smaller than in those in which cardiovascular disease is the greater risk to health. In turn, the prevalence of breast cancer and cardiovascular disease is partly a function of nutritional influences and other lifestyle factors. These data illustrate the importance of other aspects of the environment in determining the ultimate impact on longevity of nutritional variation influencing age at menopause.

These examples follow the links between specific aging processes and causes of mortality. Often this is done at a more general level when mortality is used as an unambiguous yet nonspecific summary measure of the aging processes. In this way, relationships between nutritional status and adult mortality have been explored in a number of prospective studies. The typical research design categorizes an initial sample according to a measure of body fat, usually QI, and then calculates QI-specific mortality rates during a follow-up period (5½ to 26 years in the published literature). QI is the best simple indicator of adult total body fat [Cronk and Roche, 1982], is most useful at the extremes of the distribution of fatness [Keys, 1980], and does not show wide short-term fluctuation. Thus, it may reflect habitual consumption patterns. This study design is exemplified by a study of 1.8 million Norwegians. Figure 3 demonstrates data describing the 16-year mortality experience of 5-year cohorts of Danish males aged 20 through 89 [Waaler, 1984]. Throughout

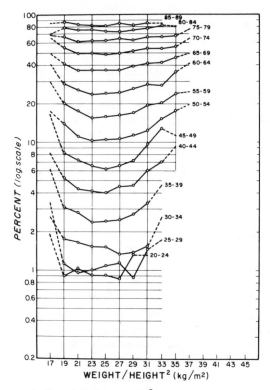

Fig. 3. Mortality rate by Quetelet's Index (wt/ht^2) in 5 year age cohorts of Norwegian males [Waaler, 1984]. (Reprinted with permission.)

adulthood, males and females exhibit U-shaped mortality curves with a broad trough of relatively low mortality in the mid range of fatness flanked by higher than average age-specific mortality rates for the leanest and most obese. This situation where intermediate values of a biological characteristic have the highest survival is termed normalizing selection. Figure 3 indicates that normalizing selection operates throughout adulthood in this population. This general relationship has been reported in numerous studies of Western adults in the U.S., France, England, and Denmark, ranging from 40 to 75+ years of age at entry to the study and followed for 5 to 24 years [Avons et al., 1983; Jarrett et al., 1982; Rhoads and Kagan, 1983; Sorlie et al., 1980; Schroll, 1981; Belloc, 1973; Dyer et al., 1975; Simopoulos and Van Itallie, 1984; Keys, 1980].

Studies of weight and mortality rate in some samples aged 60 or older upon entry to the study have found less consistent relationships. However, this inconsistency appears to be a function of study design and thus more apparent than real. One study, using a sample with an average age of 70, found elevated mortality among the lean over a 5- to 11-year period [Libow, 1974] but had screened out the obese from the starting sample. Another study, using a sample of 60-year-old women, excluded from analysis some deaths early in the 20-year follow-up period and found elevated mortality only among the obese [Cochrane et al., 1980]. Because other studies report that deaths early in the follow-up period are more likely to occur among the lean [e.g., Rhoads and Kagan, 1983; Sorlie et al., 1980], it is possible that the early, excluded deaths occurred among the lean. If so, their inclusion might restore the second tail of the U to the curve relating weight to mortality. Another study assessed survival time over a 14- to 22-year follow-up of a sample with a mean age of 77 and found no linear correlation with weight [Anderson and Cowan, 1976]. Still another analyzed the average but not the distribution of QIs among survivors and nonsurvivors of an 8-year follow-up of a sample of people aged 70+ [Burr et al., 1982]. Curvilinear analyses might have given different results in these two studies and revealed the familiar U-shaped relationship [Keys, 1980]. The data in Figure 3 do depict gradually flatter curves in the progressively older age ranges. Other studies report the same [Jarrett et al., 1982; Lew and Garfinkel, 1979]. While one interpretation of this broadening trough is a diminution of the leanness/fatness–mortality rate relationship in advanced ages, two additional factors must be considered, too.

Selective survivorship and an increasing and universally high mortality rate in the progressively older age categories may account in part for this. Individuals of advanced age are the survivors of many years of high and rising mortality rates and thus are a selected group, at least some of whom may enjoy the protection of unknown other factors lowering mortality risk. This is particularly true of studies requiring that an individual be free of coronary heart disease upon entry to the study [e.g., Lew and Garfinkel, 1979; Avons et al., 1983; Dyer et al., 1975]. In countries where this is a leading cause of mortality throughout adulthood, an individual of advanced age, particularly an obese one, who is free of this disease is somewhat unusual to begin with. Excluding people with just one disease may bias the observed relationship between mortality and weight since individuals with many other diseases are included. Furthermore, at very high mortality rates, it becomes mathematically impossible to achieve the same degree of mortality difference between intermediate and extreme fatness levels that is found among younger age categories. In the elderly categories, the lowest QI specific mortality rate is over 50% and it is not possible for the extremely lean or obese to achieve a mortality risk twice as high, something which is observed in the young adult age categories where the lowest QI specific mortality is just a few percent [Waaler, 1984]. Among Norwegians, the magnitude of the difference between highest and lowest mortality risk is roughly 7% in the 75 to 79 year age category and 3% in the 35 to 39 year category [Waaler, 1984].

The selective factors, specific causes of elevated mortality, differ at the two ends of the body fat continuum. The predominant causes of mortality among the lean include tuberculosis, obstructive lung disease, cancers, and a general "other" category (usually referring to noncardiovasular or noncancer). The predominant causes of mortality among the obese include cardiovascular and cerebrovascular disease, diabetes, and some cancers. Because virtually all these studies were designed to examine the relationship between obesity and cardiovascular disease, less attention was devoted to the lean end of the continuum and to noncardiovascular causes of mortality which are frequently lumped together simply as "other." The Norwegian study did not do this and found that mortality from virtually every disease was related to QI. The precise shape of the curve relating the two varied from disease to disease and from one age category to the next [Waaler, 1984]. This study is particularly convincing because of the huge unbiased and unselected sample.

Attempts to identify a single optimum level of fatness (or leanness), an "ideal body weight" with the lowest mortality rate, have demonstrated a complex relationship between fatness and mortality and have generated great controversy [Simopoulos and Van Itallie, 1984; Stunkard, 1983; Andres, 1980a,b; Keys, 1980]. Different studies report different "optimal" QIs and illustrate the dependence of "optimal" upon other sociocultural and physical environmental factors. For example, smokers have higher mortality rates than nonsmokers at all QI and in some samples the mortality rate of lean smokers is even more elevated than at other weights. It follows that the optimum QI is higher for smokers [Garrison et al., 1983; Lew and Garfinkel, 1979]. In another instance, the mortality rates of obese hypertensives exceeds that of all obese who have mortality above the average. Thus the optimum QI of hypertensives is lower. That is, within the population, the risk associated with a given level of fatness is influenced by other factors. These other factors may or may not be influenced in their turn by nutritional variation. Therefore, population or sample differences in the prevalence of smoking or hypertension would be expected to influence overall mortality rate as well as the shape of the curve relating QI to mortality rate and thus the "optimum" QI.

Community morbidity patterns may also influence the shape of the curve relating QI and mortality rates. This is illustrated by comparing Danish and British studies of communities in which coronary heart disease and lung disease, respectively, were the principal causes of mortality. The bronchitis mortality rate in the British community was thirty times that in the Danish community. There were so few deaths among lean Danes that a mortality rate was not even calculated for that portion of the obesity range in which a substantially elevated mortality risk prevailed in the English community. No elevated mortality risk was associated with leanness in the Danish town, but it was in the British town because of the high prevalence of bronchitis caused by cigarette smoking [Cole et al., 1974].

For all these reasons, the optimum nutritional status as measured by QI for longevity will vary from one population or subpopulation to the next in response to other lifestyle and environmental factors. As evolutionary theory predicts, optimal phenotypes differ in different environments. However, the general pattern of normalizing selection, elevated mortality at the extremes of both leanness and fatness, is found in most samples where sample selection has not eliminated one or both of the extremes of QI and when analytical methods suitable for detecting this trend have been employed. Thus caloric restriction in most human samples would be expected to be associated with high mortality rates, although the degree of elevation would depend in part upon other characteristics. An exception to this generalization could occur if the population mean and range of QI were at the very high end of the QI distribution, i.e. on the tail of the U-shaped curve. In this case, some caloric restriction might move the population into the trough of its curve relating QI to mortality rate.

The relationship between measures of the intake of particular dietary components and mortality has also been considered. Variation in dietary fats is positively associated with variation in "all causes" mortality rate in a multinational 10-year follow-up study of middle-aged European males [Anon, 1981]. Dietary cholesterol is positively and polyunsaturated fats are negatively associated with variation in mortality rate from coronary heart disease but not "all causes" in a 19-year follow-up period of middle aged (40-55) U.S. males [Shekelle et al., 1981]. An examination of the relationship between dietary fiber and mortality rate during a 10-year follow-up of middle-aged (40-59) Dutch men revealed that a low intake of dietary fiber was associated with a high mortality risk. Men in the lowest quintile of dietary fiber intake had three times higher "all causes" and cancer mortality rates than men in the highest intake quintile [Kromhout et al., 1982]. There was no indication of normalizing selection in the observed range of fiber intake in this population [Walker et al., 1982]. These data on specific dietary components suggest that restriction of the dietary fat component could delay and restricting of the fiber component could accelerate the rise in age-specific mortality rate.

SUMMARY

This chapter examines evidence for the influence of long-term nutritional variation on several measures of the human aging process. It is evident that simple relationships may not be forthcoming because of the complex ways that human diets vary and interact with other population characteristics. Taking the most generous interpretations of the incomplete picture and making the simplifying assumption that it might be possible to vary just one nutrient at a time, the data suggest the following. Caloric restriction, the most effective at extending life expectancy in laboratory animal experiments, might accelerate human aging bone loss, lower age at menopause, and raise age-specific mortality rates. Similarly, calcium restriction might accelerate aging bone loss while dietary fiber restriction might raise age-specific mortality rate. In contrast, restriction of dietary fats might lower age-specific mortality rates and restriction in dietary protein might slow aging bone loss. At the same time, caloric excess might slow bone loss and delay menopause but also raise the age-specific mortality rate. Excess dietary fats might raise age-specific mortality rate and protein excess might accelerate bone loss. These data suggest that general dietary restriction may be unlikely to delay the human aging process and this may be particularly so for women. It is noteworthy that many of the well-known animal experiments restricted males only [e.g., Ross, 1976; Masoro et al., 1980; Weindruch and Walford, 1982]. Nor is dietary excess likely to delay the aging process. Instead, normalizing selection appears to be operating to select for varying intermediate levels of intake with relatively favorable age-specific mortality rates.

Perhaps it is not surprising that the laboratory findings on dietary restriction are not replicated in the real world. After all, the dissimilarities between the laboratory and the real world of humans are numerous [Harper, 1982; Morrison, 1983; Ross, 1976]. Yet the ways in which the experimental animal and the quasi-experimental human studies and results differ are instructive. Animal studies directly monitor intake of carefully composed diets. Human population studies are unable to do this. Indeed, a large number of the studies reviewed here either omit measurement of intake or rely on self-reported information. The problem of conveniently summarizing lifelong intake is difficult. The common practice of relying on general nutritional assessments that summarize many things may confound results. To illustrate, QI and body weight are actually measures of the balance between energy intake and expenditure and the latter is almost never measured. The same QI in a 70- and a 40-year-old probably reflects different degrees of fatness because changes in body composition throughout adulthood in Western industrial societies include stature and bone mass decrease and fat increase. Another consideration is the degree of "tracking" or continuity in these measures throughout adulthood and back into earlier stages of the life cycle. It is of interest to understand to what degree the 70-year-old with a high QI had a relatively or absolutely high QI at ages 45, 20, etc. Measurements' appropriateness or accuracy at different stages of the life cycle must be determined. Answers to these questions require longitudinal data, perhaps obtained by extending existing child growth studies into midadulthood and beyond.

Most laboratory dietary restrictions are severe—restricted animals consume 20 to 50% fewer calories than do controls [Weindruch and Walford, 1982]. Body weights are so low that they are well outside the normal range of variation maintained by normalizing selection. For example, a human analogy has been drawn as "comparable to a fully grown woman being the size of an 8- to 10-year-old girl." [Harper, 1982: 743]. The environmental conditions required to maintain animals with biological characteristics outside the normal range of variation are equally extraordinary. These experiments require very special protected environments: pathogen-free, climate controlled, asexual socially isolated housing conditions, precisely regulated and unvarying diets. Little could be more unlike the human environment, full of stresses and social, biological, and cultural interactions that vary widely from time to time and from population to population. Studies conducted using less extreme conditions, for example, using self-selected diets found that heavier rats and rats that ate more died sooner [Ross and Bras, 1975] and indicate that a relationship between intake and length of life may exist across a broad range of dietary intake. (However, not all experimenters would agree on this interpretation [Walford, 1983]). This is justification for continuing to examine nutrition and aging in humans eating, freely, self-selected diets. There is a relative abundance of information in the Western literature dealing with the negative consequences of extremely high intake and the information reviewed here suggests negative consequences of extremely low intake, i.e., normalizing selection may occur.

The paucity of information on the aging processes from the lesser developed countries (LDCs) is noteworthy. The possible liabilities of undernutrition, accompanied by malnutrition, as is too frequently the case, indicate that it is timely to investigate the nutrition–biological aging process interaction in such settings. For example, consider the age at menopause.

The few studies of menopause in LDCs report generally lower mean and median ages of menopause than found in Western samples. Mean recalled ages at menopause in samples of women from India and Nepal range from 39.6 to 48.4 [Beall, 1982; Singal and Sidhu, 1981], while median ages at menopause of status quo samples from rural India, Nepal, and New Guinea range from 43.6 to 48.9 [Beall, 1982; Flint, 1974; Gray, 1976]. Women in these countries are generally leaner than women in the developed countries and nutritional differences might account partially for these findings, although they differ in many other characteristics. One report provides evidence for nutritional influence on the timing of menopause within these countries. Median ages at menopause of 43.6 and 47.3 are reported for "poorly" and "adequately" nourished New Guinea samples; the former had the smaller QI [Gray, 1976]. In contrast, mean recalled ages at menopause of 43.2 and 45.1 are reported for two samples of Indian women, but the younger had the larger QI [Singal and Sidhu, 1981; Singh and Ahuja, 1980]. Perhaps these contradictions are due to inaccurately recalled ages. It is important to find out what is occurring in such settings. If there is nutrition-associated variation around a low median age at menopause then a sizable proportion of women may experience accelerated menopause by Western standards. A case was made above that early onset of menopause could be detrimental to female longevity. If the sequelae of accelerated menopause are similar in the two environments, there are serious implications for female health and longevity.

Nutrition clearly plays a role in human biological aging, as a piece of the kaleidoscope of the complex human environment including physical environment, cultural practices, personal lifestyles, and so on. Attempts to identify *the* role of an isolated specific nutrient seems unrealistic. Restriction of one dietary component probably means restriction of others and excesses of still others. Human diets rarely differ in just a single nutrient alone. Similarly, one physiological system influenced by nutritional variation may have a cascade effect on others. From the anthropological and the evolutionary perspectives, the attempts to identify a single optimum nutritional status seem naive. As discussed above, a given QI carries different mortality risks depending upon other factors. In countries with good medical care, similar life expectancies at birth have been obtained with diets as different as the Scandinavian, Far Eastern, Mediterranean, and North American, each accompanied by great differences in major causes of death [Harper, 1983]. These are consistent with predictions from evolutionary theory that different environments will select for different phenotypes. It is the study of the interaction of nutrition with other apsects of the environment and their impact on human biological aging that is likely to provide research excitement for the future.

REFERENCES

Ames BN (1983): Dietary Carcinogens and Anticarcinogens. Science 221:1256-1264.

Anderson R, Oosthuizen R, Techron DP, Van Rensburg AJ (1980): The effects of increasing weekly doses of ascorbate on certain cellular and humoral immune functions in normal volunteers. Am J Clin Nutr 33:71-76.

Anderson F, Cowan NR (1976): Survival of healthy older people. Br J Prev Soc Med 30:231-232.

Andres R (1980a): Effect of obesity on total mortality. Int J Obes 4:381-386.

Andres R (1980b): Influence of obesity on longevity in the aged. In Borek C, Fenoglio CM, King DW (eds): "Aging, Cancer and Cell Membranes." New York: Verlag, Adv Pathobiol 7:238-246.

Anon (1981): The diet and all causes death rate in the seven countries study. Lancet 2:58-61.

Armstrong BK, Brown JB, Clarke HT, Cooke DK, Hahnel R, Masarei T, Ratajczak T (1981): Diet and reproductive hormones: a study of vegetarian and nonvegetarian postmenopausal women. JNCI 67(4):761-767.

Avons P, Ducimetiere P, Rakotovao R (1983): Weight and mortality. Lancet 1(8333):1104.

Beall CM (1982): Ages at menopause and menarche in a high-altitude Himalayan population. Ann Hum Biol 10:365-370.

Beals RK (1972): Survival following hip fracture. J Chronic Dis 25:235-244.

Belloc NB (1973): Relationship of health practices and mortality. Prev Med 2:67-81.

Bengtsson C, Lindquist O (1979): Menopausal effects on risk factors for Coronary Heart Disease. Maturitas 4:165-170.

Bertrand HA (1983): Nutrition-Aging Interactions: Life-Prolonging Action of Food Restriction. Rev Biol Res in Aging 1:359-378.

Bjorksten JA (1982): Dietary Aluminum and Alzheimer's Disease. Sci Total Environ 25:81-84.

Blackburn H, Prineas R (1983): Diet and hypertension: anthropology, epidemiology and public health implications. Prog Biochem Pharmacol 19:31-79.

Bourliere F (1970): "The Assessment of Biological Age in Man. Public Health papers no. 37." Geneva: WHO, ch 1, pp 11-23.

Brand PC, Lehert H (1978): A new way of looking at environmental variables that may affect the age at menopause. Maturitas 1:121-132.

Brocklehurst JC, Exton-Smith AN, Barker SML, Hunt LP, Palmer MK (1978): Fracture of the femur in old age: a two-centre study of associated clinical factors and the cause of the fall. Age Ageing 7:7-15.

Buckley CE, Roseman JM (1976): Immunity and Survival. J Am Geriatr Soc 24:241-248.

Burr ML, Lennings CI, Milbank JE (1982): The Prognostic Significance of weight and Vitamin C status in the elderly. Age Ageing 11:249-255.

Casey ML, MacDonald PC (1983): Origin of estrogen and regulation of its formation in post-menopausal women. In Buchsbaum HJ (ed): "The Menopause." New York: Springer-Verlag, pp 1-8.

Cochrane AL, Moore F, Baker IA, Hally TJL (1980): Mortality in two random samples of women aged 55-64. Br Med J 280:1131-1133.

Cohn JR, Hohl CA, Buckley CE (1983): Relationship between cutaneous cellular immune responsiveness and mortality in a nursing home population. J Am Geriatr Soc 31(12):803-809.

Cole TJ, Gilson JC, Olsen HC (1974): Bronchitis, smoking and obesity in an English and a Danish town. Male deaths after a 10-year follow-up. Bull Physiol-Path Resp 10(5):657-677.

Comfort A (1979): "The Biology of Senescence." New York: Elsevier.

Crane JG, Kerneke CB (1983): Mortality associated with hip fractures in a single geriatric hospital and residential health facility: a ten-year review. J Am Geriatr Soc 31:472-475.

Cronk CE, Roche AF (1982): Race- and sex-specific reference data for triceps and subscapular skinfolds and weight/stature^2. Am J Clin Nutr 35:347-354.

Cronk CE, Roche AF, Chumlea WC, Kent R (1982): Longitudinal trends of weight/stature^2 in childhood in relationship to adulthood body fat measures. Hum Biol 54:751-764.

Dalen N, Hallberg D, Lamke B (1975): Bone mass in obese subjects. Acta Med Scand 197:353-355.

Daniell HW (1976): Osteoporosis of the slender smoker. Ann Intern Med 136:293-304.

Draper HH, Bell RR (1979): Nutrition and osteoporosis. Adv Nutr Res 2:79-106.

Duchateau J, Delespesse G, Kunstler M (1982): Influence of supplemental oral zinc on the immune response of old people. In Fabris N (ed): "Immunology and Aging." The Hague: Martinus Nijhoff, pp 220-229.

Duchateau J, Delespesse G, Vrijens R, Collet H (1981a): Beneficial effects of oral zinc supplementation on the immune response of old people. Am J Med 70:1001-1004.

Duchateau J, Delespesse G, Vereeke P (1981b): Influence of oral zinc supplement on the lymphocyte response to mitogens of normal subjects. Am J Clin Nutr 34:88-93.

Dyer AR, Stamler J, Berkson DM, Lindberg HA (1975): Relationship of relative weight and body mass index to 14-year mortality in the Chicago Peoples Gas Company study. J Chronic Dis 25:109-123.

Felser JM, Roff MJ (1983): Infectious disease and aging: immunologic perspectives. J Amer Geriatr Soc 31(11):802-807.

Flint MP (1974): Menarche and Menopause of Rajput Women. Ph.D. Dissertation, New York: City University of New York.

Fujita T, Okamoto Y, Sakagami Y, Ota K, Ohata M (1984): Bone changes and aortic calcification in aging inhabitants of mountain vs seacoast communities in the Kii Peninsula. J Am Geriatr Soc 30(2):124-128.

Fujita T, Okamoto Y, Tomito T, Sakagami Y, Ota K, Ohata M (1977): Calcium metabolism in aging inhabitants of mountain vs seacoast communities in the Kii Peninsula. J Am Geriatr Soc 25(6):254-258.

Garn SM (1980): Continuities and Change in maturational timing. In Brimm OG, Kagan J (eds): "Constancy and change in Human Development." Cambridge: Harvard University Press.

Garn SM, Kangas J (1981): Protein intake, bone mass and bone loss. In DeLuca HF, Frost HM, (eds): "Osteoporosis: Recent Advances in Pathogenesis and Treatment." Baltimore: University Park Press, pp 257-263.

Garn SM, Solomon MA, Friedl J (1981): Calcium intake and bone quality in the elderly. Ecol Food Nutr 10:131-133.

Garrison RJ, Feinleib M, Castelli WP, McNamara P (1983): Cigarette smoking as a cofounder of the relationship between relative weight and long-term mortality. JAMA 249:2199-2203.

Gerschwin ME, Beach R, Hurley L (1983): Trace metals, aging and immunity. J Am Ger Soc 31(4):216-222.

Goldsmith NF (1975): Normative data from the osteoporosis prevalence survey, Oakland, CA, 1969-1972. In Mazess RB (ed): "International Conference on bone mineral measurement." Washington, D.C.: DHEW Publication no. (NIH) 75-683.

Gordon PC (1971): The probability of death following a fracture of the hip. Can Med Assoc J 105:47-51.

Gordon T, Kannel WB, Hjortland MC, McNamara PM (1978): Menopause and coronary heart disease. Ann Int Med 89:157-161.

Gray RH (1976): The menopause—epidemiological and demographic considerations. In Beard RJ (ed): "The Menopause. A Guide to Current Research and Practice." Baltimore: University Park Press.

Hamilton EI (1982): Aluminum and Alzheimer's Disease—A comment. Sci Total Environ 25:87-91.

Harper AE (1982): Nutrition, aging and longevity. Am J Clin Nutr 36:737-749.

Harper AE (1983): Coronary heart disease—an epidemic related to diet? Am J Clin Nutr 37:669-681.

Harper AB, Laughlin WS, Mazess RB (1984): Bone mineral content in St. Lawrence Island Eskimos. Hum Biol 56:63-77.

Heany RP (1982): Nutritional Factors and Estrogen in age related bone loss. Clin Inv Med 5(2-3):147-155.

Heany RP, Gallagher JC, Johnston CC, Neer R, Parfitt AM, Whedon GD (1982): Calcium, nutrition and bone health in the elderly. Am J Clin Nutr 36:986-1013.

Heany RP, Recker RR (1982): Effects of nitrogen, phosphorous and caffeine on calcium balance in women. J Lab Clin Med 99:46-55.

Heaton HW (1983): Dietary fiber in perspective. Hum Nutr Clin Nutr 37:151-170.

Hess BB, Markson EW (1980): "Aging and Old Age." New York: MacMillan, pp 79-118.

Hjortland MC, McNamara PM, Kannel WB (1976): Some atherogenic concomitants of menopause: The Framingham Study. Am J Epidemiol 103:304-309.

Hoel DG, Wakabayashi T, Pike MC (1983): Secular trends in the distribution of breast cancer risk factors—menarche, first birth, menopause and weight—Hiroshima and Nagasaki, Japan. Am J Epidemiol 118:78-89.

Hsu PH, Mathewson FAL, Rabken SW (1977): Blood pressure and body mass index patterns—A longitudinal study. J Chronic Dis 30:93-113.

Jarrett RJ, Shepley MJ, Rose G (1982): Weight and Mortality in the Whitehall Study. Br Med J 285:535-537.

Jowsey J (1977): "Metabolic Diseases of Bone." Philadelphia: W.B. Saunders, ch 29.

Kannel WB, Hjortland MC, McNamara PM, Gordon T (1976): Menopause and risk of cardiovascular disease: the Framingham Study. Ann Intern Med 85:447-452.

Keys AB (1980): W.O. Atwater Memorial lecture: Overweight, obesity, coronary heart disease and mortality. Nutr Rev 38:297-307.

Kirschner MA, Ertel N, Schneider G (1981): Obesity, hormones and cancer. Cancer Res 41:3711-3717.

Kohn RR (1978): "Principles of Mammalian Aging." Englewood Cliffs: Prentice-Hall.

Kromhout D, Bosschieter EB, de La Coulander C (1982): Dietary fiber and 10 year mortality from coronary heart disease, cancer and all causes. The Zutphen Study. Lancet 2:518-521.

Leone A (1983): The prophylactic reduction of aluminum intake. Food Chem Toxicol 21:103-109.

Lew EA, Garfinkel L (1979): Variations in mortality by weight among 750,000 men and women. J Chronic Dis 32:563-576.

Lindquist O (1979): Menopausal age in relation to smoking. Acta Med Scand 205:73-77.

Lindquist O (1982): Influence of menopause on ischemic heart disease and its risk factors and on bone mineral content. Acta Obstet Gynecol Scand (suppl) 110:1-32.

Lindquist O, Bengtsson C (1980): Serum lipids, arterial blood pressure and body weight in relation to menopause results from a population study of women in Goteburg, Sweden. Scand J Clin Lab Inv 40(7):629-636.

Lindquist O, Bengtsson C (1983): Changes in bone mineral content of the axial skeleton in relation to aging and the menopause. Results from a longitudinal study in Goteburg Sweden. Scand J Lab Clin Inv 43(4):333-338.

Lindquist O, Bengtsson T, Hansson T, Roos B (1979): Age at menopause and its relation to osteoporosis. Maturitas 1(3):175-181.

Lindquist O, Bengtsson C, Hansson T, Roos B (1981): Bone mineral content in relation to age and menopause in middle aged women. Scand J Clin Lab Inv 41:215-223.

MacMahon B, Worcester J (1966): Age at menopause, United States 1960-62. USDHEW Pub. no 1000, series 11, no. 19. Washington, D.C.: Vital and Health Statistics.

Marcus R (1982): The relationship of dietary calcium to the maintenance of skeletal integrity in man—an interface of endocrinology and nutrition. Metabolism 31(1):93-102.

Marsh AG, Sanchez TV, Mickelsen O, Keiser J, Mayor G (1980): Cortical bone density of adult lacto-ovo-vegetarian and omnivorous women. J Amer Diet Assoc 76:148-151.

Masoro EJ (1984): Food Restriction and the aging process. J Am Geriatr Soc 32(4):296-300.

Masoro EJ, Yu BP, Bertrand HA, Lynd FT (1980): Nutritional probe of the aging adolescents. Hum Biol 48:693-711.

Matkovic V, Kostial K, Simonovic I, Buzina R, Brodarec A, Nordin BEC (1979): Bone status and fracture rates in two regions of Yugoslavia. Am J Clin Nutr 32:540-549.

Mazess RB (1982): On aging bone loss. Clin Orthop 165:239-252.

Mazess RB, Cameron JR (1975): Bone mineral content in normal U.S. Whites. In Mazess RB (ed): "International Conference on Bone Mineral Measurement." DHEW Pub. No. (NIH) 75-683, pp 228-238.

Mazess RB, Mather WE (1974): Bone mineral content of North Alaskan Eskimos. Am J Clin Nutr 27:916-925.

Mazess RB, Mather WE (1975): Bone mineral content in Canadian Eskimos. Hum Biol 47:45-63.

Miller CW (1978): Survival and ambulation following hip fracture. J Bone Jt Surgery 60A:930-934.

Monthly Vital Statistics Report (1983): Advance Report of Final Mortality Statistics, 1980. Monthly Vital Statistics Report 32 (suppl): 10.

Morrison SD (1983): Nutrition and longevity. Nutr Rev 41(5):133-142.

Munro HN (1982): Nutritional requirements in the elderly. Hosp Pract 17:143-154.

NAS/NRC Committee on Diet Nutrition and Cancer (1982): "Diet, Nutrition and Cancer." Washington, D.C.: National Academy Press.

Nutrition Reviews (1983): Osteoporosis and calcium balance. Nutr Rev 41(3):83-85.

Oliver MF (1982): Diet and coronary heart disease. Hum Nutr Clin Nutr 36(6):413-427.

Paganini-Hill A, Krailo MD, Pike MC (1984): Age at natural menopause and breast cancer risk: the effect of errors in recall. Am J Epidemiol 119(4):81-85.

Pak CYC (1983): Postmenopausal osteoporosis. In Buchsbaum HJ (ed): "The Menopause." Springer-Verlag, New York, pp 9-20.

Parfitt AM (1983): Dietary risk factors for age-related bone loss and fractures. Lancet 2:1181-1185.

Parfitt AM, Gallagher JC, Heaney ROP, Johnston CC, Neer R, Whedon GD (1982): Vitamin D and bone health in the elderly. Am J Clin Nutr 36:986-1013.

Pauling L (1983): Vitamin C and longevity. Aggressologie 24(7):317-319.

Perl DP (1983): Pathological association of aluminum in Alzheimer's Disease. In Reisberg B (ed): "Alzheimer's Disease." New York: The Free Press, pp 116-127.

Rhoads GG, Kagan A (1983): The relation of coronary disease, stroke, and mortality to weight in youth and in middle age. Lancet 1:492-495.

Riggs BL, Wahner HW, Seeman E, Offord KP, Dunn WL, Mazess RB, Johnson KA, Melton LJ III (1982): Change in bone mineral density of proximal femur and spine with aging. Differences between the postmenopausal and senile osteoporosis syndromes. J Clin Inv 70(4):716-723.

Rivlin RS (1982): Summary and concluding statement: evidence relating selected vitamins and minerals to health and disease in the elderly population in the United States. Am J Clin Nutr 36:1083-1086.

Rivlin RS (1981): Nutrition and aging: some unanswered questions. Am J Med 71:337-340.

Roberts-Thomson IC, Whittingham S, Youngchaiyud U, MacKay IR (1974): Ageing, immune response, and mortality. Lancet 2:368-370.

Roche AF, Siervogel RM (1982): Serial changes in subcutaneous fat thicknesses of children and adults. Basel: Karger Monographs in Paediatrics, vol 17.

Rockstein M, Chesky J, Sussman R (1977): Comparative biology and evolution of aging. In Finch CE, Hayflick L (eds): "Handbook of the Biology of Aging." New York: Van Nostrand Reinhold, pp 3-34.

Ross MH (1976): Nutrition and longevity in experimental animals. In Winick M (ed): "Nutrition and Aging." New York: John Wiley and Sons, pp 43-57.

Ross MH, Bras G (1975): Food preference and length of life. Science 190:165-167.

Sandstead HH, Henriksen LK, Greger JL, Prasad AS, Good RA (1982): Zinc nutriture in the elderly in relation to taste acuity, immune response, and wound healing. Am J Clin Nutr 36:1046-1059.

Saville PD, Nilsson BER (1966): Height and weight in symptomatic postmenopausal osteoporosis. Clin Orthop 45:49-54.

Schroll M (1981): A longitudinal epidemiological survey of relative weight at 25, 50 and 60 in Glostrup population of men and women born in 1914. Dan Med Bull 28(3):106-116.

Shekelle RB, Shryock AM, Paul O, Lepper M, Stamler J, Liu S, Raynor WJ (1981): Diet, serum cholesterol and death from coronary heart disease. The Western Electric Study. New Engl J Med 304:65-70.

Sherman B, Wallace R, Bean J, Schlabaugh L (1981): Relationship of body weight to menarcheal and menopausal age: implications for breast cancer risk. J Clin Invest 52(3):488-493.

Shock NW (1977): System integration. In Finch CE, Hayflick L (eds): "Handbook of the Biology of Aging." New York: Van Nostrand Reinhold, pp 639-665.

Shore D, Wyatt RJ (1983): Aluminum and Alzheimer's Disease. J Nerv Ment Dis 171:553-558.

Shultz TD, Leklem JE (1983): Nutrient intake and hormonal status of premenopausal vegetarian Seventh Day Adventists and premenopausal nonvegetarians. Nutr Cancer 4:247-259.

Simopoulos AP, Van Itallie P (1984): Body weight, health and longevity. Ann Intern Med 100:285-295.

Simopoulos AP (1982): The role of the federal government in research on nutrition and aging. J Am Coll Nutr 1:11-15.

Singal P, Sidhu LB (1981): Age changes in weight and linear measurements of the two communities of Punjab (India) with special reference to senescence. Anthropol Anz 39:116-128.

Singh L, Ahuja S (1980) Trend of menopause among the women of Punjab. Anthropol Anz 38:297-300.

Sorlie P, Gordon T, Kannel WB (1980): Body build and mortality. The Framingham Study. JAMA 243:1828-1831.

Spencer H, Kramer L, Osis D (1982): Factors contributing to calcium loss in aging. Am J Clin Nutr 36:776-787.

Stamler J (1983): Nutrition related risk factors for the atherosclerotic diseases: present status. Prog Biochem Pharmacol 19:245-300.

Stiedmann M, Harrill T (1980): Relation of immunocompetence to selected nutrients in elderly women. Nutr Rep Int 21:931-940.

Stunkard AJ (1983): Nutrition, aging and obesity: a critical review of a complex relationship. Int J Obes 7:201-220.

Waaler HT (1984): Height, weight and mortality. The Norwegian experience. Acta Med Scand (suppl) 679:1-56.

Walford RL (1983): "Maximum Life Span." New York: W.W. Norton & Co.

Walker ARP, Segal I, Hathorn S (1982): Dietary Fibre and Survival. Lancet 2:980.

Weindruch R, Walford RL (1982): Dietary Restriction in mice beginning at 1 year of age: effect on life-span and spontaneous cancer incidence. Science 215:1415-1418.

Weksler ME (1982): Age-associated changes in the immune response. J Am Geriatr Soc 30:718-723.

Wenger NK (1982): Coronary disease in women: myth and fact. Hosp Pract 17:114a-x.

WHO (1981): Research on the menopause. WHO Technical Report Series 670:1-120.

Willett W, Stampfer MJ, Bain C, Lipnick R, Spelzer FE, Rosner B, Cramer D, Hennekens CH (1983): Cigarette smoking, relative weight and menopause. Am J Epidemiol 117:651-658.

Winick M (ed) (1976): "Nutrition and Aging." New York: John Wiley and Sons.

Wooten R, Bereton PJ, Clark MB, Hesp R, Hodkinson HM, Klenerman L, Reeve J, Slavin G, Levich MT (1977): Fractures of the neck-of-femur: an attempt to identify patients at risk. In Barzel US (ed): "Osteoporosis." New York: Grune and Stratton, pp 238-239.

Young EA (1983): Nutrition, aging and the aged. Med Clin North Am 67(2):295-313.

Young EA (1982): Evidence relating selected vitamins and minerals to health and disease in the elderly population in the United States: Introduction. Am J Clin Nutr 36:979-985.

SECTION IV:
ANTHROPOLOGY, NUTRITION, AND ECOLOGY

Nutritional Anthropology, pages 225–254
© 1987 Alan R. Liss, Inc.

Effects of Iron Deficiency on Mental Development: Methodological Considerations and Substantive Findings

Ernesto Pollitt, PhD

School of Public Health, The University of Texas Health Science Center, Houston, Texas 77225

Many conceptual and methodological problems faced in the last three decades by studies on the effects of protein-energy malnutrition (PEM) on mental development [Brozek and Schurch, 1984; Galler, 1984] are currently faced by studies on the effects of iron deficiency (sideropenia) on cognitive development [Pollitt and Leibel, 1982; Ross Laboratories, 1983]. Barret [1984] in a cogent review of such problems concerning PEM, considered four validity criteria that must be met before reaching at any conclusions regarding the effects of undernutrition on behavior: 1) statistical-conclusion validity; 2) internal validity; 3) external validity; and 4) construct validity of putative causes and effects.

These four criteria are used in the first part of this chapter to discuss conceptual and methodological issues relevant to the research on the effects of iron deficiency on cognitive development. This initial discussion provides working tools to evaluate critically, in the second part of the chapter, available studies on infants and preschool children. An attempt is made at the end to integrate this body of knowledge by deriving specific conclusions of significance to public health and educational policies.

Ernesto Pollitt's present address is Department of Applied Behavioral Sciences, University of California, Davis, California 95616.

CONCEPTUAL AND METHODOLOGICAL ISSUES
Statistical Conclusion Validity

This criterion refers to the quality (e.g., reliability) of the data collected which will influence the robustness of the inferences made from the statistical associations observed among independent and outcome variables. Confounding factors or variables, which might condition the probabilities of rejecting or accepting the null hypothesis, threaten statistical conclusion validity. These factors include, among others, low reliability in the measurements of independent and outcome variables and heterogeneity of subjects in relationship to the sampling criterion. In the specific case of studies on the functional consequences of iron deficiency, statistical conclusion validity is threatened because of problems in the sensitivity and specificity of the tests used to measure iron status in man.

Up to the mid-70s, most studies on the behavioral effects of iron deficiency focused on iron deficiency anemia [Pollitt and Leibel, 1976]. Accordingly, the diagnosis was generally based on hemoglobin (Hgb) or hematocrit (Hct) values. Anemia, however, is an extreme form of this micronutrient deficit [Cook and Finch, 1979]. Body iron stores, iron transport, and even tissue levels of essential heme-containing enzymes can be exhausted or markedly diminished before the circulating mass of red cells is affected [Bothwell et al., 1979; Dallman et al., 1978; Oski, 1979; International Nutritional Anemia Consultative Group (INACG), 1979]. Diagnoses of these milder conditions require direct biochemical measures of body iron [Cook and Finch, 1979; Finch and Cook, 1984].

Serum ferritin (SF) is one parameter measured to assess levels of iron stores. Low values (i.e., 10 to 12 ng/ml) of SF are indicative of low iron storage, which constitutes the earliest stage of sideropenia. A second stage is defined by low levels of iron transport, which is generally measured by transferrin saturation (TS), the ratio of serum iron to total iron binding capacity. Ideally, low SF and TS ($<$ 16 to 20%), should be strongly correlated with low iron stores and transport. However, in the presence of infection iron-deficient subjects present normal SF values, while iron replete subjects have low TS values [Bothwell et al., 1979; Worwood, 1980]. Depletion in the supply of transport iron influences erythropoiesis. If there is insufficient iron to form heme, erythrocyte protoporphyrin (EP) is elevated in the red blood cells. Thus, high EP is evidence of more advanced stage of iron deficiency and an immediate antecedent of anemia. However, EP is also elevated in the presence of infection and in cases of lead intoxication which is generally accompanied by anemia [Dallman et al., 1981; Dallman, 1982].

Low hemoglobin (Hgb) is a marker of anemia, but its diagnostic efficiency varies with the degree of severity of the depletion [Kim et al., 1984]. Hgb has a high level of diagnostic accuracy solely in cases of severe anemia. In mild to moderate anemia the diagnostic power of the test is thwarted because of an overlap between normal low Hgb values among iron replete subjects and comparatively high Hgb values among some iron depleted subjects [Federation of American Societies of Experimental Biology (FASEB), 1984; INACG, 1979]. In addition, there are significant age-related changes in Hgb concentration [Yip et al., 1984]. Accordingly, substantive errors can occur in the estimation of prevalence of anemia within populations whenever the cut-off points used as diagnostic criterion are not age appropriate [Dallman et al., 1984].

The problems noted above with the diagnostic tests of body iron status in man establishes a certain degree of risk in selecting heterogeneous subjects within a sample, in reference to a given criterion (i.e., iron depletion). This methodological risk is particularly high in those studies on the functional consequences of iron deficiency that base their sampling criteria on a single diagnostic test (e.g., SF) [Leibel et al., 1982]. Each diagnostic test reflects changes in body iron at different stages of depletion; and no single test monitors the entire spectrum of iron status [Cook and Finch, 1979]. Also, as already noted, infection and inflammation influence the values of the biochemical tests of iron status in the presence or absence of sideropenia. This will result in similar problems of sample heterogeneity [Crosby, 1979].

An additional problem faced by all the diagnostic tests of iron deficiency defined above is the selection of cut-off points which accurately discriminate between deficient and sufficient cases among populations with different prevalence rates. Normal biological variability, measurement error, and confounding factors such as inflammation influence the diagnostic efficiency of these tests [FASEB, 1984]. This is illustrated in the discrepancy that often exists between the generally accepted definition of iron deficiency and anemia and epidemiological observations among specific population samples. The World Health Organization (WHO), for example, has proposed that a Hgb < 11 g/dl, or a Hct < 33% be used to identify anemia in children between the ages of 6 months and 6 years. However, this definition underestimated the prevalence of iron depletion in two samples of children in the United States [Marner, 1969; Moe, 1965].

An effective method to determine in the field the truly anemic is by an assessment of the response of Hgb to iron treatment [Beaton, 1974; Garby, 1970; Kim et al., 1984]. A substantive increase in Hgb (e.g., > 1 g/dl) following the intervention, independent of the original Hgb value, is indication of anemia; conversely, lack of Hgb response points to a nonanemic state. This approach is used to establish the sensitivity and specificity of the iron indicators and the magnitude of the change in these two diagnostic parameters as a function of changes in the cut-off points. For example, on the basis of data from an experimental intervention Kim et al. [1984] showed in a group of 3-to-6-year-old rural Guatemalan children that the sensitivity of EP was higher than that of SF and TS. The highest EP sensitivity was achieved at 100 ug/ml.

In conclusion, among studies on iron and cognition the probabilities of making Type I (rejecting a null hypothesis when it should be accepted) or Type II errors (accepting a null hypothesis when it should be rejected) are partly determined by the sensitivity and specificity of the diagnostic tests used to establish body iron status. The definition of the values of these two test parameters is critical to determine sample size. These statistics will in part establish the magnitude of the differences in test performance that must be observed between groups to avoid the probabilities of equivocal inferences.

Internal Validity

This criterion refers to the nature of the evidence required to prove that a statistical association between independent and outcome variables genuinely reflect a cause–effect relationship. A critical issue in this regard is the availability of evidence showing a covariation between changes in body iron status and changes in test performance. Thus, on the one hand, double blind clinical trials yield the strongest evidence to meet the requirements of internal validity. On the other hand, static group comparisons fail to meet the conceptual and methodological requirements to establish a cause–effect relationship between independent and outcome variables [Campbell and Stanley, 1963; Cohen and Cohen, 1975]. A single comparison between the mental test scores of iron deficient and iron sufficient subjects cannot determine whether any differences between groups are solely determined by the differences in iron status. The following is a discussion of the weaknesses of this latter type of research design in the context of studies on the functional consequences of iron deficiency.

Two strategies generally used to avoid or prevent problems derived from static group comparisons are selective matching and statistical control of confounding effects[1]. The former calls for the identification of potentially nui-

---

[1]Confounding variable: a factor that distorts the apparent magnitude of the effect of a study variable.

sance variables (e.g., socioeconomic) and matching the subjects accordingly. The latter is best illustrated in the use of regression or covariance analyses that attempt to partial out the variance of the outcome variable accounted for the confounding variables [Cohen and Cohen, 1975]. As discussed below, however, neither approach satsifies the needs of internal validity; in fact they might augment the differences between samples.

The association between iron anemia and short stature illustrate the threats against internal validity in studies using static group comparisons. Studies on the functional consequences of iron deficiency in developing countries reported that iron deficient anemic children are smaller and lighter than normal controls [Lozoff et al., 1982a; Pollitt et al., 1984; Guarda, 1984]. One explanation for this association is that iron deficiency generally coexists with a history of PEM [Baker and DeMaeyer, 1979], which is a cause of physical growth faltering [Martorell et al., 1982]. The association of iron deficiency and short stature is therefore due to their common relationship with PEM. Accordingly, it appears logically sound to control for the confounding effect of PEM by matching body sizes of the iron deficient and the so-called controls. If this were not logistically possible or if it were too costly, the confounding effects of PEM might be statistically controlled by partialling out the association between body size and the outcome variables.

However, although a causal relationship between body size and iron status has not been conclusively demonstrated, there is some evidence to suggest that iron depletion slows growth velocity [Oski, 1979; Guarda, 1984]. If this were the case then selective matching for size increases rather than decreases the differences among confounding factors between groups. Likewise, partialling out statistically the effect of size through regression or covariance analyses would in fact decrease the power of the iron variable to account for a significant portion of the variance in the outcome variable.

This example can be extended to the confounding effects of demographic or socioeconomic variables, particularly among low income rural communities in developing countries. The parents of children with iron deficiency anemia as compared to those of normal controls have been reported to have lower income and less education [Macia, 1983; Palti et al., 1983]. Family income and parental education are generally associated with children's mental test performance. Thus, the possible confounding effect of these variables should be controlled in an assessment of the relation between iron and cognition. Matching, however, immediately implies that the iron-anemic children are not compared with a representative sample of the population. Because iron-deficient children are atypical as compared to average children within the communities where they live, selective matching would lead to the sampling of nonanemic children who are also atypical insofar as their socioeconomic and demographic characteristics are concerned. Matching might therefore lead to the selection of a comparison group that differs systematically from the average family within the community. Moreover, given the similar socioeconomic status of both samples, why is it that in only one and not both groups were there children with iron-deficiency anemia? Differences in the underlying family dynamics not captured by the socioeconomic and demographic variables assessed may be implicated in the differences in nutritional status of the children. These intrafamilial differences may have other parallel developmental effects, and the possible differences between groups which may be found in the outcome variables may be one other illustration of such effects.

External Validity

The extent to which the results obtained in one sample and research setting can be generalized to other samples and settings defines external validity. At least two interrelated conditions must be met to fulfill the requirements of this criterion: 1) the nature of the independent and outcome variables remain invariant; and 2) the nature of the intervening (or confounding) variables is similar between populations. Between group differences in the ecology and causality of iron deficiency work against the generalization of findings from studies on the effects of iron deficiency on cognition.

Inadequate iron absorption and blood loss are the two major causes of iron deficiency [Bothwell et al., 1979; Baker, 1978; Baker and DeMaeyer, 1979]. Iron deficiency and anemia are generally associated with poor iron absorption among populations in which health indicators, such as low infant mortality or prevalence of low birth-weight infants, point to a healthy population. This is generally the case in developed countries. In contrast, in low-income populations in developing countries, particularly in the tropics, iron-deficiency anemia results in part from blood loss secondary to parasitic infestation and from low iron absorption [Bothwell et al., 1979; Baker and DeMaeyer, 1979]. There is an inverse relationship between hookworm load and Hgb levels in rural communities [Layrisse and Roche, 1964]. In fact, it has been estimated that bleeding from the gut due to hookworm affects approximately 450 million people [Farid et al., 1969]. Among these populations iron treatment raises the Hgb levels among the iron-anemic children; however, anemia is reinstated once the treatment is discontinued. A high incidence of gastrointestinal and respiratory infections, among others, are also observed among anemic children [Chandra, 1976; Chandra and Saraya, 1975].

Differences in the etiology of iron deficiency and anemia and in the general health picture of children in developed and developing countries has important implications for studies on cognition. Parasitic infestations and infection can confound the relationship between body iron status and cognition among children selected from populations whose health and general nutritional status is poor [Crosby, 1979]. Poor cognitive test performance among iron-deficient children who are undernourished and in poor health may fail to improve following iron repletion therapy. This lack of improvement can be strictly determined by the morbid conditions that covary with iron anemia [Pollitt, 1983].

Generalizations from the behavioral or cognitive test performance of children whose iron anemia is secondary to blood loss and poor iron absorption to children whose iron anemia is strictly of a nutritional origin are questionable. The converse is also true. Behavioral generalizations from one situation to another require equivalence in the nutritional and health status of the children in both places or comprehensive and valid information relevant to these issues to implement adequate methodological controls. Currently, the external validity of some studies (particularly those in developing countries) on the cognitive effects of iron deficiency is limited by the differences in the nature and number of confounding variables in different populations.

Construct Validity of Causes and Effects

The degree of fitness between the underlying construct of the study and the measurements used define this criterion. A corollary is the extent to which the nature of the relationships observed between measurements match the theoretical constructs involved in the hypotheses tested. There are at least two critical and interrelated issues that need to be examined in studies on iron and cognition: 1) the nature of the tests used to assess cognitive function and 2) the nature of the underlying mechanisms behind the relation of iron deficiency and anemia and deficits in cognition. At issue is whether the effects observed are secondary to depletion of iron in enzymatic functions of brain tissue or to hematological changes [Sourkes, 1982; Scrimshaw, 1984; Dallman et al., 1978; Finch et al., 1976].

Infant development scales such as the Gesell Schedule or the Bayley Scale of Mental and Motor Development or intelligence scales such as the Stanford Binet or the Wechsler Scale for Children provide aggregate scores of performance. These are represented by a developmental or intelligence quotient (DQ and IQ, respectively), which define the overall performance of a subject as compared to a reference standard. An IQ or DQ provides no information on the different abilities tapped by the tests. However, detailed analyses of the subject's performance in the different subtests (or items) provide information on particular mental abilities.

Once the normative and construct validity of an IQ test is established, it can be inferred that this test taps some abilities that are an important part of human cognition. It can also be assumed that test performance is influenced by motivational and personality variables [Zigler and Seitz, 1982]. However, the IQ by itself will not indicate the independent contributions of mental competence and motivation of the subject to the test performance.

These psychometric problems are even more critical in the case of infant developmental scales such as the Gesell Schedule or the Bayley Scale [Pollitt, 1984; Pollitt et al., 1978]. These scales which measure development in the first 24 months of life do not measure the mental abilities and skills tested at a later age by IQ tests. At best, they measure the bases or precursors of later mental development [Honzik, 1976]. Moreover, even within the first 24 months of life these scales measure different abilities at different ages. For example, at 4 months of age about 45% of the items in the Gesell Schedule measure motor skills, while only 3% tap language development. Conversely, at 24 months, the motor items are limited to about 11% of the Schedule while language includes about 25%. This difference in the abilities tested at different ages partially explains why, when the time differential between test and retest is spread out over months, the magnitude of the test-retest correlations is small, often statistically not different from zero. There is almost no predictive power in scale scores obtained during the first 12 months of life. Significant developmental transformations occur in the functions assessed by these tests during infancy [Lewis and McGurch, 1972; McCall, 1976, 1983; McCall et al., 1972].

The issue of predictive power of infant scales with a normal population might be considered relevant in connection with studies on undernutrition and cognition if these scales accurately predicted developmental retardation. At issue is whether it is possible to predict from early infancy those children who will have developmental abnormalities or to identify subnormal intelligence in childhood and adulthood [McCall, 1983]. The limited body of data currently available shows that for "at risk" samples (e.g., low birth weight; early neurological trauma), the predictive power of infant developmental assessment is only slightly higher than that for the normal population. McCall [1983] reported that these test-retest correlations are not "usefully" higher than for normal individuals.

Further evidence that iron deficient infants and children obtain lower developmental or intelligence test scores than normal controls contribute little to our understanding of the putative effects of iron deficiency. There is a need to specify the locus of the effects of iron deficiency on the information-processing chain in human cognition and to evaluate the role played by motivation. This type of data could provide insights or guidelines as to the nature of the underlying biochemical or hematological mechanisms involved. Lastly, it should be pointed out that the measurements of specific cognitive processes can be validly accomplished among populations with different cultural backgrounds and ecological contexts [Pollitt et al., 1984].

A critical issue in connection with the putative effects of iron deficiency on cognition is whether they have a nonhematological basis. This assumption has been prompted by observations of clinicians that patients with iron anemia displayed more somatic and psychic symptomatology (weakness, irritability, pica, etc.) than individuals with equivalent reductions of Hgb from other causes. In some instances, these symptoms were alleviated within days of the initiaton of iron therapy, before any substantial augmentation of Hgb mass could occur [Beutler, 1957; Fairbanks et al., 1971; Harris and Kellermeyer, 1970]. A possible explanation for these clinical observations is that iron depletion may produce alterations in iron-linked enzymes in the brain which, in turn, may have behavior-functional consequences [Pollitt and Leibel, 1976; Sourkes, 1982].

Table I identifies areas of possible central nervous system (CNS) impact of iron deficiency. This is summary information originally presented by Leibel et al. [1979]. None of these putative effects are accompanied with conclusive experimental evidence. The areas of possible CNS impact presented are

TABLE I. Areas of Possible CNS Impact of Iron Deficiency[a]

General biochemical	Specific sites	Impact
Heme synthesis	1. Porphyrin synthesis	Toxic or intracellular deficiency
	2. Mitochondrial cytochromes (ck oxidae)	Respiratory oxidative phosphorylation
	3. Microsomal cytochromes	Toxic
Krebs cycle	Succinate dehydrogenase	Respiration
Fe-flavoprotein	NADH-ubiquinone reductase α-GP dehydrogenase	Respiration, oxidative phosphorylation
Nucleic acid	DNA synthesis, mitosis	Brain growth
Catecholamines	Phenylalanine hydroxylase, tyrosine hydroxylase, MAO oxydase	Neurotransmitter levels
Serotonin	Tryptophan pyrrolase, tryptophase hydroxylase, aldehyde oxidase	Neurotransmitter levels
Folic acid/B_{12}	Formimino transferase, THF methyltransferase	

[a]Leibel et al. [1979].

strictly hypothetical mechanisms that might eventually explain the relationship between iron deficiency and poor cognitive test performance.

Two main avenues of research have been followed to assess the nonhematological effects of iron deficiency on cognition. One has been assessment of the cognitive function of iron deficient subjects without anemia. The other approach has been the assessment of changes, within relatively short periods of time (e.g., 1 week) in the intellectual test performance of iron-deficient anemic subjects treated with iron.

The next section reviews the studies available on iron deficiency and anemia and mental test performance among infants and preschool children. The four validity criteria previously discussed provide a methodological and conceptual basis from which to evaluate critically the data currently available. This will lead us to some general conclusions on the putative effects of iron deficiency on cognition.

EFFECTS OF IRON DEFICIENCY AND ANEMIA ON COGNITIVE FUNCTION

A comprehensive and critical review of research published up to the mid-70s on the effects of iron deficiency and anemia on mental development was published by Pollitt and Leibel [1976]. The following is a critical assessment of the most recent research on infants and young children (3 to 7 years of age). Three studies [Cantwell, 1972; Howell, 1971; Sulzer et al., 1973] included in this review were published before 1976. Criteria for their inclusion were the experimental nature of the research design and their contribution to our understanding of the relationship between iron deficiency and specific cognitive processes (e.g., attention).

The review is restricted to studies that focused on mental test measurements as outcome variables. Research on other aspects of behavior, such as work productivity and activity, is excluded. A distinction is also made between studies on iron deficiency with and without anemia.

Infancy

Iron deficiency. A study by Deinard et al. [1981], using a static group comparison design, included infants from 11 to 13 months of age with Hct > 33%. The infants were classified into three groups (G1, G2, G3) according to a single iron parameter, SF levels: G1 < 9 ng/ml; G2 from 10 to 19 ng/ml; and G3 > 20 ng/ml. The Bayley Infant Scale of Mental and Motor Development (BSMMD) [Bayley, 1969], the Uzgiris-Hunt Ordinal Scale, and a habituation measure of attention formed the battery of psychological tests used. There were no statistically significant differences between any of the groups in the scores of the BSMMD. Likewise, SF and the other cognitive and attention measures were independent of each other.

The static-group comparison used in this study precluded the investigators from certifying that, except for SF, the groups compared were equivalent in other factors relevant to the infants' performance in the battery of psychological tests used. Likewise, as noted in part one, the choice of a single iron indicator (i.e., SF) to establish the criterion for sampling is not a reliable approach to case selection. It is likely that within each of the three samples, the subjects were heterogeneous in reference to the iron criterion.

Oski et al. [1983] compared the developmental performance in the BSMMD of ten iron replete infants with that of three groups of infants having different levels of iron depletion without anemia before (T1) and after (T2) an iron-therapeutic intervention. This treatment consisted of 50 mg of iron as 1 ml of iron–dextran (imferon) by intramuscular injection. The mean age and values for Hgb, SF, EP, and mean corpuscular volume (MCV) for the four groups are presented in Table II. The change scores (T2 − T1) in the BSMMD of the normal (G1) and iron-depleted (G2) infants were not statistically significant. In contrast, a 20.1-(SD 13.1) and a 23.6-(SD 11.2) point improvement in the Bayley scale of mental development of the two other groups (63, 64) with iron deficiency (with and without cellular evidence) were statistically significant.

TABLE II. Characteristics of Four Study Groups[a]

	1: Normal (n = 10)	2: Iron depleted (n = 10)	3: Iron deficient (n = 10)	4: Iron deficient (n = 8)
Age (mo)	10.7 ± 0.7	11.0 ± 0.8	11.0 ± 0.8	11.4 ± 0.9
Sex: M/F	5/5	5/5	5/5	4/4
Color: B/W	6/4	6/4	6/4	4/4
Hemoglobin (g/dl)	11.9 ± 0.4 (11.0-12.6)	12.7 ± 0.4 (11.7-13.3)	11.9 ± 0.5 (11.2-13.1)	11.3 ± 0.4 (11.0-12.7)
Ferritin (ng/ml)	31.2 ± 16.6 (14.0-49.2)	10.4 ± 1.4 (7.8 ± 12.0)	10.2 ± 1.3 (8.8-11.9)	9.8 ± 2.0 (6.6-11.9)
Erythrocyte porphyrin (μg/dl)	20.4 ± 6.9 (8-29)	17.5 ± 7.5 (8-29)	40.6 ± 11.3 (32-60)	41.8 ± 7.1 (33-55)
Mean corpuscular volume (fl)	77.3 ± 3.6 (74-84)	75.9 ± 3.0 (70-80)	74.7 ± 1.9 (73-79)	68.3 ± 1.8 (64-69)

[a]Values are mean ± SD; range is shown in parentheses. From Oski et al. [1983].

There were no statistically meaningful differences between the performance of the iron-deficient and control infants at T1 and at T2 in the mental
and motor scores. Thus, there is no evidence of an association between iron
deficiency without anemia and developmental delay. A problem against
statistical criterion validity in this study is the sample size. None of the groups
included more than ten subjects. Accordingly, the confidence limits of the
statistical differences between T1 and T2 scores (for G3 and G4) must be
broad. There is, therefore, a risk of falling into a Type II error: accepting the
hypothesis of an improvement in test performance following iron therapy
when, in fact, it should be rejected.

A similar experimental study, with a similar problem of sample size and
statistical criterion validity, was conducted by Walter et al. [1983] in Santiago,
Chile. The samples in this study included iron-deficient infants with and
without anemia; the results on the anemic infants are reviewed in the section
on iron deficiency and anemia. The diagnosis for iron deficiency was based
on a Hgb > 11 gm/dl, with one or more of the following criteria: TS <
10%; SF < 10 ng/ml; EP > 100 μg/dl; MCV > 3 fl. Infants with a Hgb
response to the iron treatment of 1 g/dl or more but whose original Hgb
values were > 11 g/dl were also included in this group. The controls had to
meet all the biochemical criteria suggestive of an iron-replete state.

The BSMMD was administered at T1 to 15 controls and 12 iron-deficient
15-month-old infants. Once this evaluation was completed they received for
15 days orally administered ferrous sulphate at a dose of 3 to 4 mg/kg/day.
They were then reevaluated with the BSMMD. The mean MDI of the control
and iron-deficient children at T1 was 113 and 108, respectively; this difference was not statistically significant (p > .05). At T2 the means for the
groups were 112 and 113, respectively; again this difference was not statistically significant. Moreover, the change in the mean scores (delta) from T1 to
T2 (108 to 113) in the iron-deficient children was not significant.

An analysis restricted to a subgroup of six (out of twelve) infants within
the group with "two or more biochemical measures or response to therapy"
did show a statistically significant (p < .05) delta in the mean MDI from T1
to T2(108 to 118). The motor scale and the Bayley Infant Behavior Record
did not discriminate between groups at a statistically significant level.

In summary, three developmental studies [Deinard et al., 1981; Oski et
al., 1983; Walter et al., 1983] focused on iron-deficient infants without
anemia (mean ages ranged from 10 to 15 months old) and found no statistically significant differences between their performance on the BSMMD and
that of normal controls before or after iron treatment. One of these studies
[Oski et al., 1983] did show, however, a statistically significant increase (p <

.05) in the MDI of the iron-deficient infants after an iron-therapeutic intervention.

The three studies used the Bayley Scale as a criterion for mental development. As pointed out in the section on construct validity, the BSMMD yields an aggregate measure of development (MDI). This score does not discriminate between the particular contributions made to the final score by each of the abilities tested or by motivation. The iron-deficient infants might have specific cognitive disabilities that remained undetected by the global developmental measures. This is most likely to be the case if the effects of mild iron deficiency are restricted to subtle changes in particular cognitive processes.

Iron deficiency and anemia. Cantwell [1972] reported one of the first iron intervention studies using a longitudinal research design beginning in the infancy period. The study included a follow-up assessment when the subjects were of school age. A working hypothesis was that hypoxemia from anemia causes brain damage. Unfortunately, the report on the research was limited to an abstract, and the absence of complete information on the measurements and study design makes it impossible to assess it critically. The study is nevertheless reviewed because of its significant anecdotal importance.

Sixty-one full-term infants from comparable socioeconomic groups represented the complete sample. At 6 to 18 months of age, 32 of the infants exhibited iron-deficiency anemia (Hgb ranged from 6.1 to 9.5 g/dl). Twenty-nine infants had received neonatal iron dextran injections and were not anemic (Hgb ranged from 11.5 to 12.9 g/dl). Neurologic examinations were done at 6 to 7 years of age, and the examiners had no knowledge of the presence or absence of previous anemia. The anemic group had a higher incidence of soft neurologic signs, such as clumsiness in balancing on one foot, tandem walking, and repetitive hand or foot movements. They were also less attentive and more hyperactive than control subjects. The author does not report statistical comparisons between groups but noted that the average IQ scores of the nonanemic and anemic groups were 98 and 92, respectively. The author claims that, in the absence of protein energy malnutrition, anemia in infancy is one cause of possible permanent minimal brain dysfunction.

Oski and Honig [1978] were probably the first to assess the nonhematologic effects of iron deficiency by measuring the short-term effects of iron treatment on the developmental test performance of iron-anemic infants. Twenty-four iron-anemic subjects were equally divided into two subgroups; one received intramuscular iron for 7 to 9 days, while the other received a placebo. The mean ages of these two groups were 14.3 and 16.3 months, respectively.

Criteria for inclusion were a Hgb < 10.5 g/dl; a TS < 12%, and a serum iron concentration < 50 ng/dl. The Bayley Behavioral Profile was used jointly with the BSMMD. At T1 neither the mean mental scores (experimental, 96.2; control, 90.5) nor the mean motor scores (experimental, 96.4; control, 93.1) discriminated between groups at a statistically significant (p < .05) level. However, the upward change (13.1 points) of the mean MDI from T1 to T2 was statistically significant (p < .05) in the experimental group. Conversely, the upward delta in the control group (6.5 points) was not statistically signifi- cant (p > .05). In the motor scale there was an increment in both groups, but neither of these changes was statistically significant. There was a statistically significant negative correlation between the magnitude of the increase in the MDI and the Hgb values at T1 in the iron-treated group. The MDI and the initial Hgb values were independent of each other in the control group.

This study [Oski and Honig, 1978] did not include a group of infants with normal body iron levels. Accordingly it is impossible to determine whether the performance of the iron-anemic children was statistically different and poorer than that of iron-replete infants. Moreover, the size of each sample was small (12 infants), and infants ranged from 9 to 26 months of age. If, as noted in the first part of this chapter, infant developmental scales test different functions at different ages, then the BSMMD in this study might have tested different abilities in different infants both within and between samples. The reasons for the salutary effect of the iron treatment on a wide and heterogeneous range of abilities are far from clear. These issues were discusssed in a published critique of this study [Pollitt et al., 1978]. Honig and Oski [1979] responded: "The fact that iron deficiency results in a disturbance in catecholamine metab- olism with resultant elevations in epinephrine and norepinephrine levels could easily produce alterations in a wide spectrum of seemingly unrelated skills and abilities" [Honig and Oski, 1979: 239]. Currently, there are no experimental data to support these provocative hypotheses.

Johnson and McGowan [1983] published a study based on a static group comparison design on anemic and control infants with a mean age of 13 months. This study is a secondary analysis of data on the BSMMD collected from a longitudinal behavioral intervention study at the Houston Parent-Child Development Center. The medical records of the children were reviewed and those cases whose records included Hgb determinations were chosen as potential subjects for inclusion in the study sample. Anemia was defined by a Hgb < 10.5 g/dl; and the cut-off point for the controls was > 11.5 g/dl. Besides the BSMMD the behavioral protocol also included evaluations of mother-infant interactions. Analyses of the BSMMD showed that there were no statistically significant differences (p > .05) between these two groups in their mean mental and motor development scores. Likewise, the observations on the mother-infant interactions yielded no evidence of differences in the social behavior of these two groups. A more specific analysis restricted to controls and severely anemic children (Hgb < 8 g/dl) also yielded no significant difference between groups. Given that the only diagnostic criterion used was Hgb it is impossible to conclude that the anemic children represented a homogenous sample. Conceivably, there might have been significant differences in the causes of the hematological disorder between subjects within the sample.

Lozoff et al. [1982a, 1982b] conducted a study in Guatemala that included both an anemic and a control sample of infants whose ages ranged from 6 to 24 months. These samples were, in turn, divided into an iron- and a placebo-treated group. The infants were recruited from a socioeconomically deprived population in a settlement in Guatemala City. The iron-anemic children were defined by a Hgb < 10.5 g/dl, plus two out of three of the following criteria: TS < 10%; EP > 100 μg/dl; and SF < 12 ng/ml. The selection criterion for the controls was Hgb > 12.0 g/dl. Psychological evaluation, as in most studies already reviewed, was based on the BSMMD. At T1 there was a 14-point difference (p < .05) between the MDI means of the two original groups (control, 100.4; anemic, 86.8). In the motor scale there was a 9-point difference (control, 94.4; anemic, 85.6) which was also statistically significant (p < .05).

Fifteen and nineteen subjects of the anemic and control groups, respectively, were placed on iron (ferrous ascorbate) therapy at a dosage of 5 mg/kg/day, for a period of approximately 7 to 10 days. The remaining infants were placed on placebo. The mean scale scores for all groups at T2 were higher than those at T1; but none of these changes were statistically significant. Lozoff et al. [1982b] also investigated the influence of age on the differences in performance between groups. The subjects were divided into three main age groups; 6 to 12, 13 to 18, and 19 to 24 months. There were no differences between the performance of the iron-anemic and control groups in the two youngest age subgroups. The between group differences were restricted to the older infants whose ages ranged from 19 to 24 months. Thus, the performance in the oldest explained the differences between iron-anemic and control infants across ages. Older anemic infants also weighed less than nonanemic controls and had smaller arm circumferences.

The positive correlation between age and differences in test performance between groups supports the hypothesis that certain test items may be more sensitive to the effects of iron anemia. In the mental development scale there is a progressive increase in the number of social and language items as a function of age; while sensorimotor items are targeted to the younger infants. The authors noted that the older infants had particular difficulty with the language items of the mental scale. This age hypothesis, however, is not fully satisfactory because it is somewhat discrepant with data reported by Oski et al. [1983]. These authors found significant improvements in the developmental test performance of 10 to 11-month-old iron deficient infants following iron-repletion therapy.

One other hypothesis to be considered is that within the anemic group the overall nutritional and health status of the older infants was poorer than that of the younger infants. This hypothesis is of direct relevance to the issue of external validity raised in the first section of this chapter. General nutrition and health differences between samples might mediate the differences in test performance. The older anemic children weighed less and had smaller arm circumference than the control infants. This finding suggests that, at least among the older infants, there were other nutritional differences between groups besides iron status. A related observation is that breast feeding is also likely to vary as a function of age and that breast milk has important immunological properties [Jellife and Jellife, 1978]. Because of this phenomenon and because weaning is associated with a greater exposure to vectors of infection [Gordon et al., 1963], the incidence of morbidity was likely to be higher among the older as compared to the younger infants.

The age related differences in nutritional status and health is in keeping with the notion of a cumulative deficit. This proposition contends that as children grow older up to about 36 months of age, growth faltering (an index of health status) tends to increase. This cumulative deficit has also been observed in the area of cognitive function among Guatemalan rural preschool children [Saco-Pollitt et al., 1985].

Accordingly, the lack of significant improvement in the MDI following the experimental intervention among the older infants might have been determined by nutritional and health factors which did not respond to iron therapy. This, however, does not negate the fact that iron deficiency has an adverse influence on cognitive function, which is reversible following iron repletion among otherwise healthy children. In any event, it becomes apparent that the nature of the problem among these Guatemalan infants is different from that of the infants assessed by Oski and Honig [1978]. Thus, the study designs that might be appropriate in one context may be inappropriate in another.

The study by Walter et al. [1983] in Santiago, Chile, which was previously cited, also included a group of iron-deficient anemic infants. The criteria for iron deficiency was already reported; the criterion for anemia included a Hgb < 11 g/dl. The mean MDI of the ten anemic infants was 98 and 108 at T1 and T2, respectively. This 10-point MDI delta was statistically significant (p < .05). Moreover, the difference in the first evaluation between the mean MDI of the anemic (98) and controls (108) was statistically significant (p < .05). The motor scale score did not discriminate between groups at a significant level.

The improvement in test performance among iron-anemic children observed by Walter et al. [1983] and by Oski and Honig [1978] support the hypothesis that there is a nonhematologic basis for the adverse effects of iron deficiency on mental test performance. The short time interval between the baseline and the post-treatment behavioral evaluation makes it unlikely that the iron intervention has had a significant effect on Hgb mass. The data reported by the investigators, however, does not address itself to the possible underlying mechanisms behind the behavioral observations.

In summary, three [Oski and Honig, 1978; Lozoff et al., 1982a; Walter et al., 1983] of the four studies reviewed agree with the hypothesis of a positive association between body iron level and developmental test performance. Two studies [Lozoff et al., 1982a; Walter et al., 1983] showed statistically significant (p < .05) differences between the performance of the anemic and control children in the Bayley Scale of mental development. However, only one [Walter et al., 1983] of these two studies showed an improvement in the performance of the anemic subjects following iron repletion therapy. This finding agrees with the developmental improvement observed in the study by Oski and Honig [1978] on iron-anemic infants, which excluded a control group of normal subjects. In one study [Lozoff et al., 1982a] the iron therapeutic trial had no detectable effects on the MDI of the iron deficient anemic infants. Finally, the fourth study with anemic infants [Johnson and McGowan, 1983] did not find any differences in the Bayley Scale performance between 13-month-old infants with mean Hgb of < 10.5 g/dl and > 11.5 g/dl, respectively. However, in this study there is no way of assessing the etiology of the anemia in the subjects sampled.

Preschool Children

Iron deficiency. A study on preschool iron-deficient children (3 to 6 years old) without anemia was conducted in Cambridge, Massachusetts by Pollitt et al. [1983]. It included a pre- and post iron-treatment evaluation of cognitive test performance. Fifteen subjects were defined as iron deficient. The diagnostic criterion was based on a change (delta) of TS, after a 3-month period of oral iron therapy. The TS change required was from one SD below the mean for the 110 subjects recruited for the study (T1) to 1.5 SD above the mean for only those subjects whose TS at the end of the study (T2) was above 20%. The mean Hgb and TS of these index children were 11.2 g/dl (SD, .80) and 11.0% (SD, 2.0), respectively. The criteria for the selection of the controls were children having TS > 20% and a Hgb > 11 gm/dl, both at T1 and T2. At T1 their mean Hgb was 12.1 g/dl (SD, .50) and their mean TS was 26.1% (SD, 7.6).

The battery of psychological tests included the Stanford-Binet Intelligence Scale and measures of attention (discrimination learning), conceptual learning (oddity learning), and short-term recall. There were no IQ differences between groups at either T1 or T2. However, as observed in Figure 1 there were statistically significant differences at T1 between the experimental and control subjects in the number of trials to reach the learning criterion in the three discrimination learning tasks. The experimental subjects took more trials to learn to discriminate between two visual stimuli than the controls. There were no significant between group differences at this time in either the oddity learning or the memory tasks. At T2 there were no significant differences between groups in two of the three discrimination learning tasks in the

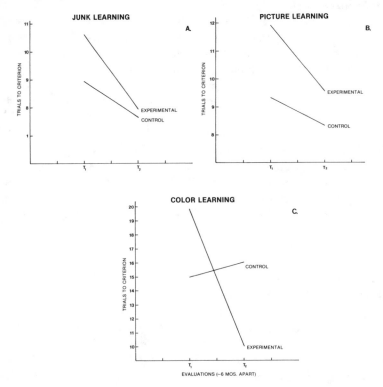

Fig. 1. Mean scores of iron deficient and iron sufficient preschool children in three discrimination learning tasks before and after iron treatment (see Pollitt et al., 1983).

post-treatment evaluation. In the remaining task the experimental group required fewer trials to reach the learning criterion than did the control group.

Differences in discrimination learning were taken as evidence among the iron-deficient preschool children of a deficit in the capacity to attend to relevant information in problem-solving situations. However, this deficit did not represent an obstacle in the oddity-learning tasks, which taps conceptual learning, and is considered to be more difficult than discrimination learning. Thus, when the children were challenged by a complex problem-solving situation they responded as well as the iron-replete children. Moreover, the deficit in discrimination learning was reversed following iron therapy.

This study used TS as a single body iron indicator for the selection of the index cases, while Hgb and TS were used to select the controls. This diagnostic problem of using a single iron measure to define the experimental cases was amended in part because the selection criteria included a substantive change in TS from T1 (before treatment) to T2 (after treatment). However, this post-hoc dynamic definition of iron depletion does not preclude the possibility that the sample of iron-deficient cases represented a heterogeneous group of subjects in reference to their iron status. Some were likely to be iron-anemic, while others were strictly iron deficient.

Iron deficiency and anemia. Probably the first study on preschool iron-deficient anemic children was conducted in Philadelphia by Howell [1971]. Unfortunately, the data from this study have only been published in the proceedings of a conference. The report provides brief description of the subjects and methods used; thus, it is difficult to assess the scientific rigor of the research and the precise nature of the study protocol. Yet this study is included in this review because of the large pool of subjects used to select the sample. It also points to some specific deficits in the cognitive function of anemic children that are diagnostically important.

The study included 8,744 low-income black children, 3 to 5 years of age, enrolled in a Headstart Program. In this population the prevalence of anemia was defined by a Hgb < 10 g/dl and a Hct $< 31\%$ was 1.9%. The prevalence increased to 5% when anemia was defined by a Hgb < 10.5 g/dl.

Eighty-three children with Hgb ranging from 9 to 10.5 g/dl constituted the final sample. All hematologic disorders other than hypochromic mycrocytic anemia were excluded from the study. The sample was then randomly divided into two groups. Forty-two children received intramuscular iron at a dose calculated to bring their Hgb to 12 g/dl. The remaining cases received the same volume of saline intramuscularly. A psychological evaluation was conducted before (T1) as well as 2 and 4 months after this injection. The battery of psychological tests included the Goodenough Draw-a-Man test and the Stanford Binet Intelligence Scale. In addition, two aspects of attention were measured: field articulation and scanning. Field articulation was defined by finding an embedded figure within a picture; while scanning was operationalized by the ability of a child to inspect a total picture and evaluate differences within it.

The report did not include data on the statistical comparisons but identified differences in test performance whenever present. After the iron treatment there were no differences between anemic and nonanemic children in the intelligence quotients obtained. However, as indicated by the attentional tasks, the anemic girls exposed to the placebo treatment displayed more aimless manipulation, a narrower attention span, and less complex purposeful activity than the nonanemic girls. Likewise, the anemic boys perceived significantly fewer stimulus objects in the visual field than nonanemic boys when a dominant stimulus was present. Howell interpreted this to mean that anemic boys were more passive and less able to respond to nondominant features of the environment when a dominant stimulus overshadowed the visual field. In summary, the author indicated that children with mild iron-deficiency anemia had normal IQs but showed markedly decreased attentiveness, more aimless manipulation, less complex and purposeful activity, narrower attention span, and perceived fewer stimuli in the presence of dominant stimuli.

Sulzer et al. [1973] conducted a study on over 230 male and female, 4 to 5-year-old black children enrolled in a Head Start Program in Louisiana. This study based on a static group comparison design focused on anemia. It illustrates many of the problems discussed in connection with statistical criterion and internal validity, in the first part of the chapter. Moreover, it should also be noted that the independent variable (i.e., anemia) is solely defined by the level of Hgb, and there are no data on the body iron status of the subjects within the sample (see discussion on the study by Johnson and McGowan [1983] in the review on infancy).

Of the original pool of subjects 11.7% had Hgb values < 10.5 g/dl. Two batteries of psychological tests were used. The first included a global, allegedly culture-free IQ test, a vocabulary test, and measures of moral development and grouping behavior. The other battery comprised reaction time, attentive recall, and cranking tasks.

When compared with control subjects the performance of anemic subjects (Hgb < 10 g/dl) was significantly poorer on the vocabulary tests and showed similar, but not significant, trends on all other measures. The score differential between groups become more statistically evident when the cutoff point in Hgb values was 10.5 g/dl, which increased the sample size of anemic subjects.

Compared with the control group the anemic subjects had significantly lower scores on the IQ measure, the vocabulary test, and the latency and associative reactive measures. An important finding was that younger anemic children were unable to integrate effectively experience accumulated during different steps of the associative reaction test. The authors suggested that the younger group may have been more vulnerable to the possible effects of iron-deficiency anemia on cognition.

Recognizing that the nutritional history of the child (independent of current anemia) might have contributed to the observed results, the investigators compared the test scores of tall and short children (see the discussion on the conceptual and methodological problems of controlling for body size in studies on the functional consequences of iron deficiency in the first section of this chapter). When the age variable was controlled, differences (the authors do not specify which tests differed) between tall and short children were small. The data did indicate, however, that the combination of a history of inadequate nutrition and current low Hgb value was the best predictor of inferior performance.

Education of the father was the only social factor that distinguished anemic from nonanemic children; the educational level of the fathers of children in the anemic group was lower. Family size, occupation of the head of the household, housing characteristics, health, and many other social characteristics failed to differentiate the groups.

Because of the problems in research design and many uncontrolled confounding variables, the investigators considered the results inconclusive. However, the data were used to develop relevant hypotheses for subsequent testing. Two alternatives were presented to explain the better performance of the nonanemic children: better learning ability and higher motivation. The investigators add that their observations excluded the possibility that the differences in the psychological test performance were caused by attentional factors.

A study of the performance of 25 iron-deficient anemic and 25 iron-replete three- to six-year-old Guatemalan children was conducted in a series of attention, memory, and learning tasks before and after 11 to 12 weeks of iron treatment [Pollitt et al., 1986]. A preliminary report on this study was published in 1982 [Pollitt et al., 1982]; the most recent analysis optimizes accuracy of the diagnostic classification of subjects as anemic or iron replete. The field was carried out in two lowland villages, Las Guacas and Los Llanitos, 85 km south of Guatemala City. The inhabitants are exclusively ladino, a mixture of Mayan Indian and Spanish.

The selection criteria were: a gestational age of 38 weeks or more; birthweight of 2,500 g or more; and no evidence of any chronic illness, severe malnutrition, or primary hematologic disorder that could adversely affect body hemoglobin mass. One hundred fifty-three children, ranging in age from 30 to 72 months, represent the total sample of the study. The present analysis is concerned with 50 of the 153 subjects originally selected. These 50 subjects were equally divided into two groups according to their body iron status. The experimental design called for evaluations of cognitive test performance before and after an iron/placebo intervention. Treatment lasted for an average of 11 weeks and it consisted of a daily dosage of ferrous sulfate of 3 mg/kg/day.

The response of Hgb concentration to oral iron administration was used a priori as an operational definition of iron deficiency and as the referent to which other indicators of systemic iron status were compared (see the discussion on the diagnosis of iron deficiency in connection with statistical crieterion validity in first section of chapter). Optimal cut-off points for each iron indicator were selected by intentionally varying the diagnostic cut-off point and observing the resulting changes in sensitivity and specificity. These estimates can be carried out systematically with the use of so-called Response Operator Curves (ROC) as illustrated in Figure 2. In this particular case iron deficiency was operationally defined as a delta Hgb > 2 g/dl in response to oral iron therapy.

Table III presents the criteria used for the selection of the experimental and comparison children. The mean values of four indicators for both groups of subjects before treatment are presented in Table IV. The post-treatment mean values on these same biochemical and hematological parameters are included in Table V. After 11 weeks of treatment there were no between-group differences in transferrin saturation and ferritin. However, the substantive changes in Hgb and EP from T1 to T2 in the experimental group, did not eliminate statistically significant differences between the experimental and control groups in these two iron parameters. Moreover, it should also be noted that at T1 the children in the experimental groups were smaller and lighter than those in the control group (p $<$ .05).

The battery of psychological tests was similar to the battery used in the study in Cambridge, Massachusetts [Pollitt et al., 1983]. The tests used were derived from a theoretical model [Fisher and Zeaman, 1973] relating attention, learning, and memory processes. The structure of the test battery which relies on visual discrimination skills, minimizing verbal behavior, allows measurements of cognitive processes developing in the preschool child in a manner that appears to reduce cultural bias. Data on the normative and construct validity of these tests in the context of cross cultural comparisons has been reported [Pollitt et al., 1984].

At T1 the total number of trials to criterion in the three tasks of discrimination learning (measures attention) were 33.3 (SE, 2.69) and 26.6 (SD, 1.46)

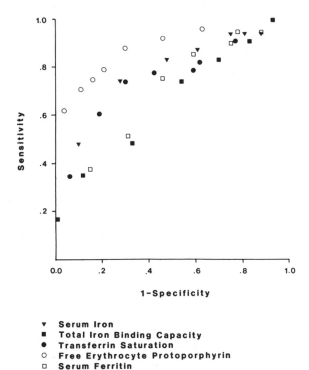

Fig. 2. Receiver operator curves for various indicators of iron nutrition. Iron deficiency is operationally defined as a Hb delta > g/dl in response to oral iron therapy (see Kim et al., 1984).

for the experimental and control groups, respectively. This difference is statistically significant (p < .05). Further, the score differences (T2 − T1) in the iron-deficient children were statistically significant (p < .05); conversely, the control group did not show any significant change in performance (M T2 = 26.2; SE, 1.52) from T1 to T2. The difference between groups in trials to criterion in the second evaluation is not statistically significant.

In comparison to the performance of the anemic children the control children obtained a higher number of correct responses across the four tasks in oddity learning (measures conceptual learning) both at T1 and T2. However, this difference was statistically significant in the second but not in the first evaluation. In fact, at T2 the differences between groups (5.39) was as large as two standard errors of the mean in the experimental group (5.34). Both groups improved their performance from T1 to T2; however, the delta in the

TABLE III. Selection Criteria Used for Experimental and Control Cases

Time	Experimental cases	Controls
T1	Hb ≤ 10 g/dl and FEP > 100 μg/dl	Hb ≤ g/dl and FEP ≤ 150 μg/dl
T2	I. Hb > 11 g/dl and (FEP ≤ 175 μg/dl or ΔFEP ≤ − 70 μg/dl or II. FEP ≤ 100 μg/dl and (HB > 10 g/dl or ΔHB > 2.0 g/dl)	HB < 11 g/dl and FEB ≤ 150 μg/dl

TABLE IV. Experimental and Control Groups: Means and SD for Biochemical
Determination Before Iron Treatment

		Experimental		Control		
	N	Mean (SD)	N	Mean (SD)	t	P
Transferrin saturation (%)	25	11.08 (10.25)	24	20.25 (9.67)	3.38	.001
Free erthyrocyte protoporphyrin (μg/nl)	25	291.38 (154.35)	25	65.98 (27.74)	7.19	.000
Hemoglobin (g/dl)	25	8.96 (0.98)	25	12.39 (0.81)	13.47	.000
Serum ferritin (mg/nl)	21	7.86 (6.05)	22	19.15 (13.57)	3.49	.000

control group (9.95) was larger ($p < .05$) than that of the experimental group
(6.70). Finally, in the memory test there were no differences between groups
in either of the two evaluations.

The differences between groups in oddity learning observed at T2 suggest
that iron therapy did not have a salutary effect on the iron-deficient children
across all the different cognitive processes tapped by the test battery. The
treatment was associated with an improvement in attention, but it did not
prevent the differences in conceptual learning. Note that at T2 there were still
differences between groups in both Hgb and EP. Moreover, the weight and
height of the experimental group were 13.5 kg and 94.4 cm; while those of
the controls were 15.2 kg and 99.2 cm, respectively ($p < .05$). It is therefore
possible that the general nutritional and health status of these two groups of
children was not equivalent at the completion of the study. Accordingly, the

TABLE V. Experimental and Control Groups: Mean and SD for Biochemical Determinations After Iron Treatment

	Experimental		Control			
	N	Mean (SD)	N	Mean (SD)	t	p
Serum ferritin (ng/ml)	21	26.41 (17.49)	22	22.75 (18.16)	.67	NS
Transferrin saturation (%)	25	18.80 (6.92)	25	21.42 (7.69)	1.27	NS
Free erythrocyte protoporphyrin (μg/nl)	25	107.09 (53.14)	25	67.76 (23.17)	3.39	.000
Hemoglobin (g/dl)	25	11.86 (1.11)	25	12.67 (0.93)	2.79	.004

differences in test performance between groups might not have been determined by iron but by related biological factors. However, strictly speaking, there is no way of testing this alternative hypothesis with the available data (see the discussion on confounding factors in connection with external validity in the first section of chapter).

In summary, all the studies that have focused on iron deficiency with and without anemia among preschool children have shown a statistically significant covariation between body iron levels and cognitive test performance. Three of these studies [Pollitt et al., 1983; Pollitt et al, 1985; Howell, 1971] support the contention that attention (or the reception of information) is the cognitive process most sensitive to the effects of iron deficiency. One study [Pollitt et al., 1983] that focused on preschoolers with iron deficiency without anemia showed that the differences between the experimental and control groups were reversible following an 11-week period of iron therapy. Conversely, another study [Pollitt et al., 1985] conducted in two rural communities in Guatemala did not show any significant therapeutic effect from the iron intervention. All studies, however, have substantive methodological and conceptual gaps that preclude conclusive inferences.

CONCLUSIONS

A review of studies published after 1976 on the effects of iron deficiency on cognition among infants and preschool children shows significant methodological improvements as compared to those published before that date. Some of the important changes are: 1) a shift from study designs using static group comparisons to experimental manipulations of the body iron status of the subjects under study; 2) the addition of biochemical measures of iron storage (serum ferritin), transport (transferrin saturation), and erythropoiesis (erythrocyte protoporphyrin), which increased the sensitivity of the diagnosis of body iron status; 3) an increased focus on the possible functional effects of iron deficiency without anemia; and 4) a greater degree of specificity in the hypotheses regarding the underlying mechanisms on the effects of iron on cognition. However, there are still significant methodological and conceptual gaps in the studies published that threaten one or more of the validity criteria that must be met before conclusive inferences regarding the effects of iron on cognition may be reached. Some of these problems are: 1) small sample sizes (e.g., 10 to 15 subjects per group); 2) the use of aggregate measures of mental development which impede analyses of specific cognitive processes (i.e., attention), or motivational factors, likely to be affected by iron depletion; 3) lack of data on the health history and other nutritional deficiencies of subjects selected from populations with a high prevalence of undernutrition and infectious diseases.

However, although no conclusive inferences are yet warranted, it is still possible to make some tentative generalizations based on the data from most of the robust studies published:

1) In comparison to infants without signs of sideropenia, infants with iron deficiency with and without anemia tend to score lower in the Bayley Scale of Mental Development.

2) There is no substantive evidence of an association between iron deficiency and delayed infant motor development.

3) Iron repletion therapy implemented over a period of 7 to 10 days is likely to result in an improvement in the performance in the Bayley Scale of Mental Development among infants with iron deficiency with and without anemia.

4) There is no evidence yet available on the specific mental abilities and skills that may be affected among iron-deficient infants which may explain their comparatively low performance in the Bayley Scale of Mental Development.

5) In comparison to preschool children without signs of sideropenia, preschool children with iron deficiency with and without anemia are less likely to pay attention to relevant cues in problem-solving situations.

6) Among populations in which there is a high prevalence of protein-energy malnutrition, iron-deficient infants and preschool children tend to be smaller and lighter than children without signs of iron deficiency.

7) Among these populations iron-deficiency anemia in preschool children is likely to be associated with selective deficits in attention and higher order cognitive functions, such as conceptual learning.

8) Among these populations the iron deficient infants and preschool children are not likely to improve their performance in mental development scales and specific measures of cognitive function following iron repletion therapy.

Finally, it should be noted that most of the evidence already accumulated strongly supports the proposition that iron deficiency is associated with cognitive deficits. Because these deficits are likely to occur in attention processes it seems reasonable to infer that learning may be in jeopardy among iron-deficient infants and young children. This conclusion should be a major public health concern even in countries, such as the United States, in which the prevalence of iron deficiency and anemia among young children is about 4% [FASEB, 1984].

REFERENCES

Baker, SJ (1978): Nutritional anemia: a major controllable public health problem. Bull WHO 56:659-674.

Baker, SJ, DeMaeyer EM (1979): Nutritional anemia: its understanding and control with special reference to the work of the World Health Organization. Am J Clin Nutrit 32:368-417.

Barrett DE (1984): Methodological requirements for conceptually valid research studies on the behavioral effects of malnutrition. In Galler J (ed): "Nutrition and Behavior." New York: Plenum Press, pp 9-36.

Bayley N (1969): The Bayley infants scale of development. New York: The Psychological Corp.

Beaton GH (1974). Epidemiology of iron deficiency. In Jacobs A, Worwood M (eds): "Iron in Biochemistry and Medicine." New York: Academic Press, pp 437-476.

Beutler E (1957): Iron enzymes in iron deficiency. Am J Med Sc 234:517-527.

Bothwell TH, Charlton RW, Cook JD, Finch CA (1979): "Iron metabolism in man." London: Blackwell publications.

Brozek J, Schurch B (eds) (1984): "Critical issues in malnutrition research: methodology and findings." Lausanne, Switzerland: The Nestle Foundation.

Campbell DT, Stanley JC (1963): Experimental and quasi-experimental designs for research. Chicago: Rand McNally.

Cantwell RJ (1972): The long term neurological sequelae of anemia in infancy. Pediatr Res 8:342 (abstr).

Chandra RK (1976): Iron and immunocompetence. Nut Rev 47:863-866.

Chandra RK, Saraya AK (1975): Impaired immunocompetence associated with iron deficiency. J Pediatr 86:899-902.

Cohen J, Cohen P (1975): Applied multiple regression/correlation analysis for the behavioral sciences. New Jersey: Lawrence Erlbaum.

Cook JD, Finch CA (1979): Assessing iron status of a population. Am J Clin Nutr 32:2118-2129.

Crosby WH (1979): Iron deficiency anemia in a nutritionally complex situation. Am J Clin Nutr 32:715-716.

Dallman PR (1982): Biochemical and hematologic indices of iron deficiency. In Pollitt E, Leibel RL (eds): "Iron deficiency: brain biochemistry and behavior." New York: Raven Press, pp 63-77.

Dallman PR, Beutler E, Finch CA (1978): Annotation: effects of iron deficiency exclusive of anemia. Br J Haemat 40:179-184.

Dallman PR, Reeves JD, Driggers DA, Lo EYT (1981): Diagnosis of iron deficiency: The limitations of laboratory tests in predicting response to iron treatment in one-year-old infants. J Pediatr 99:376-381.

Dallman PR, Yip R, Johnson C (1984): Prevalence and causes of anemia in the United States. Am J Clin Nutr 39:437-445.

Deinard A, Gilbert A, Dodds MA, Egeland B (1981): Iron deficiency and behavioral deficits. Pediatr 68:828-833.

Fairbanks VF, Gahey G, Beutler E (1971): "Clinical Disorders of Iron Metabolism." New York: Grune & Stratton.

Farid Z, Patwardhan VN, Darby WJ (1969): Parasitism and anaemia. Am J Clin Nutr 22:498-503.

Federation of American Societies for Experimental Biology. Life Science Research Office (1984): Assessment of the iron nutritional status of the U.S. population based on data collected on the second national health and nutrition examination survey, 1976-1980. Bethesda, Maryland.

Finch CA, Miller LR, Inamdar AR, Person R, Seiler K, Mackler B (1976): Iron deficiency in the rat. Physiological and biochemical studies of muscle dysfunction. J Clin Invest 58:447-453.

Finch CA, Cook JD (1984): Iron deficiency. Am J. Clin Nutr 39:471-478.

Fisher MA, Zeaman D (1973): An attention-retention theory of retarded discrimination learning. In NR Ellis (ed): "International Review of Research in Mental Retardation, Vol 6." New York: Academic Press.

Galler J (1984): "Nutrition and Behavior." New York: Plenum Press.

Garby L (1970): The normal haemoglobin level. Brit J Nutr 19:429-439.

Gordon JE, Chitkara ID, and Wyon JB (1963): Weanling diarrhea. Am J Med Sc 245:345-377.

Guarda-Peragallo N (1984): Severity of iron deficiency anemia and its relationship to growth and morbidity in a population of pre-schoolers in rural Guatemala. Dissertation submitted to the School of Public Health of the University of Texas, Houston for the doctoral degree in Public Health. Houston, Texas.

Harris JW, Kellermyer RW (1970): "The Red Cell." Cambridge, MA: Harvard University Press.

Honzik MP (1976): Value and limitations of infant tests: An Overview. In Lewis M (ed): "Origins of Intelligence." New York: Plenum Press, pp 59-96.

Honig AS, Oski FA (1979): Reply to Pollitt et al. Inf Behav Developm 2:239-240.

Howell D (1971): Significance of iron deficiencies. Consequences of mild deficiency in children. Extent and meaning of iron deficiency in the United States. Summary Proceedings of the Workshop of the Food and Nutrition Board. Washington, D.C.: National Academy of Sciences.

International Nutritional Anemia Consultative Group (1979): Iron deficiency in infancy and childhood. Washington, D.C.: The Nutrition Foundation.

Jellife DB, Jellife EFP (1978): Human milk in the modern world. New York: Oxford University Press.

Johnson DL, McGowan RJ (1983): Anemia and infant behavior. Nutr and Behav 1:185-192.

Kim I, Pollitt E, Leibel RL, Viteri FE, Alvarez E (1984): Application of receiver-ooperator analysis to diagnostic tests of iron deficiency in man. Pediatr Res 18:916-920.

Layrisse M, Roche M (1964): The relationship between anaemia and hookworm infection. Am J Hyg 79:279-287.

Leibel RL, Greenfield DB, Pollitt E (1979): Iron deficiency: Behavior and brain biochemistry. In Winick M (ed): "Nutrition, Pre- and Postnatal Development." New York: Plenum Press, pp 383-439.

Leibel RL, Pollitt E, Kim I, Viteri F (1982): Studies regarding the impact of micronutrient status on behavior in man: iron deficiency as a model. Am J Clin Nutr 35:1211-1221.

Lewis M, McGurck H (1972): The evaluation of infant intelligence: Infant intelligence scores—true or false? Science 178:1174-1178.

Lozoff B, Brittenham GM, Viteri FE, Wolf AW, Urrutia JJ (1982a): The effects of short-term oral iron therapy on developmental deficits in iron-deficient anemic infants. J Pediatr 100:351-357.

Lozoff B, Brittenham GM, Viteri FE, Wolf AW, Urrutia JJ (1982b): Developmental deficits in iron-deficient infants: Effects of age and severity of iron lack. J Pediatr 101:948-952.

Macia N (1983): Social and biological determinants of short-term growth velocity among pre-schoolers of rural Guatemala, a path analysis approach. Dissertation submitted to the school of Public Health of the University of Texas, Houston for the doctoral degree in Behavioral Sciences, Houston, Texas.

Marner F (1969): Haemoglobin, erythrocytes and serum iron values in normal children 3-6 years of age. Acta Paedr Scand 58:363-370.

Martorell R, Habicht JP, Kelin RE (1982): Anthropometric indicators of changes in nutritional status in malnourished populations. In Underwood B (ed): "Methodologies for Human Population Studies in Nutrition Related to Health." Washington, D.C.: NIH Publication No. 82-2462, pp 99-110.

McCall RB (1976): Toward an epigenetic conception of mental development in the first three years of life. In Lewis M (ed): "Origins of Intelligence." New York: Plenum Press.

McCall RB (1983): Predicting developmental outcome. Resume and redirection. In Brazelton TB, Lester BM (eds): "New Approaches to Developmental Screening of Infants." New York: Elsevier.

McCall RB, Hogarty PS, Hurlburt N (1972): Transitions in infant sensorimotor development and the prediction of childhood IQ. Am Psychol 27:728-748.

Moe PJ (1965): Normal red blood picture during the first three years of life. Acta Paedtr Scand 54:69-75.

Oski FA (1979): The nonhematological manifestations of iron deficiency. Am J Dis Child 133:415-422.

Oski F.A., and Honig A.S. (1978): The effects of therapy on developmental scores of iron deficient infant. J Pediatr 92:21-25.f

Oski FA, Honig AS, Helu B, Howanitz P (1983): Effect of iron therapy on behavior performance in nonanemic, iron deficient infants. Pediatr 71:877-80.

Palti H, Pevsner B, Adler B (1983): Does anemia in infancy affect achievement on developmental and intelligence tests? Hum Biol 55:183-194.

Pollitt E (1983): Morbidity and infant development: A hypothesis. Int J Behav Devel 6:461-475.

Pollitt E (1984): Methods for the behavioural assessment of the causes of malnutrition. In Sahn DE, Lockwood R, Scrimshaw NS (eds): "Methods for the Evaluation of Food and Nutrition Programs." United Nations University Food and Nutrition, Supplement 8. Cambridge, Mass.

Pollitt E, Greenfield DB, Saco-Pollitt C, Joos S (1984): A validation of attention-retention tests in studies on malnutrition and behavior in two cultures. In Brozek J, Schurch B (eds): "Critical Issues in Malnutrition Research: Methodology and Findings." Lausanne, Switzerland: The Nestle Foundation.

Pollitt E, Leibel RL (1976): Iron Deficiency and Behavior. J Pediatr 88:372-381.

Pollitt E, Leibel RL (eds) (1982): "Iron Deficiency: Brain Biochemistry and Behavior." New York: Raven Press.

Pollitt E, Leibel RL, Greenfield DB (1978): Significance of Bayley Scale score changes following iron therapy. J Pediat 92:172-178.

Pollitt E, Leibel RL, Greenfield DB (1983): Iron deficiency and cognitive test performance in preschool children. Nutr & Behav 1:137-146.

Pollitt E, Saco-Pollitt C, Leibel RL, Viteri FE (1986): Iron deficiency and behavioral development in infants and preschool children. Am J Clin Nutr 43:555-565.

Pollitt E, Viteri F, Saco-Pollitt C, Leibel RL (1982): Behavioral effects of iron deficiency anemia in children. In Pollitt E, Leibel RL (eds): "Iron Deficiency: Brain Biochemistry and Behavior." New York: Raven Press, pp 195-208.

Ross Laboratories (1983): Behavioral manifestations of iron deficiency in infants and children. Columbus, Ohio: Ross Laboratories.

Saco-Pollitt C, Pollitt E, Greenfield D (1985): The cumulative deficit hypothesis in the light of cross cultural research. Int J Behav Devel 8:75-97.

Scrimshaw NS (1984): Functional consequences of iron deficiency in human populations. J Nutr Sc Viatminol 30:47-63.

Sourkes TL (1982): Transition elements and the nervous system. In Pollitt E, Leibel RL (eds): "Iron Deficiency: Brain Biochemistry and Behavior." New York: Raven Press, pp 1-29.

Sulzer JL, Wesley H.H, Leonig F (1973): Nutrition and behavior in head start children: results from the Tulane study. In Kallen DJ (ed): "Nutrition, Development and Social Behavior." Washington, D.C.: DHEW Publication No. (NIH) 73-242.

Walter T, Kovalskys J, Stekel A (1983): Effect of mild iron deficiency on infant mental development scores. J Pediatr 68:828-838.

Worwood M (1980): Serum ferritin. In Jacobs A, Worwood, M (eds): "Iron in Biochemistry and Medicine, Vol. II." New York: Academic Press, pp 204-244.

Yip R, Johnson C, Dallman PR (1984): Age related changes in laboratory values used in the diagnosis of anemia and iron deficiency. Am J Clin Nutr 39:427-436.

Zigler E, Seitz V (1982): Social policy and intelligence. In Sternberg RJ (ed): "Handbook of Human Intelligence." New York: Cambridge University Press, pp 587-640.

Nutritional Anthropology, pages 255-276

Obesity

Manuel Peña, MD, PhD, Manuel Amador, MD, PhD, and Jorge Bacallao

Instituto Superior de Ciencias Médicas de La Habana, Havana 16, Cuba

Obesity is one of the most prevalent nutritional disorders in developed countries. It is characterized by an excessive amount of body fat which reflects an imbalance in energy intake with respect to energy expenditure.

We believe that this energy imbalance is the crucial aspect in an approach to the study of obesity. Thus we will not refer in this context to other frequently invoked factors of genetic or environmental origin.

Obesity is considered as a predisposing factor to a large number of disorders such as ischemic heart disease, hypertension, diabetes mellitus, gallstones, skeletal abnormalities, and psychosocial problems, among others, all leading to increased morbidity and mortality.

Despite the prevalence of obesity and the considerable amount of research this has stimulated, very little is known so far about its etiology and pathogenesis. Moreover, the results of different therapeutic measures in the treatment of obesity are somewhat contradictory and disheartening. Preventive actions and investigation of the multiple factors involved are imperative and must be approached in a multidisciplinary way.

In this chapter we will discuss the importance of anthropometric aspects for the assessment and characterization of obesity, the impact of excess body fat upon the physical fitness of obese individuals, and, finally, the principal bases to be taken into consideration in the treatment of obese subjects.

METHODS

One of the basic problems in biomedical research is the adequate choice of a metric system, that is, a set of variables providing a good characterization of individuals. The classic inferential and descriptive methods of univariate statistics are insufficient because they do not take into account the complex pattern of interactions among variables. These shortcomings are, to a great extent, overcome by multivariate methods which have developed extensively with advances in computational facilities. The characterization of an obese individual is clearly a typical multivariate problem, since an objective assessment of a subject calls for the use of anthropometric, functional, and other types of attributes.

We view the problem from two vantage points: 1) data or dimension reduction and 2) variable selection.

The first goal can be achieved by means of factor analysis or principal component techniques which yield a set of uncorrelated variables, each of which is responsible for a given amount of the total variability [Mueller, 1982].

Variable selection can be approached by different statistical methods, among which discriminant analysis and principal component techniques play an important role.

We believe that the main efforts should be directed toward the projection of the individuals into factor space. The time fluctuations or changes in individuals due to treatment or to the natural progress of their condition could be assessed objectively by studying the location of the point-individual in the factor space.

This approach makes it absolutely irrelevant to attach labels to the individuals such as obese, nonobese, overwieght, and so on, which depend on controversial criteria. The whole problem is reduced to searching for the factors, interpreting them and studying the position of the individuals in the aforementioned space. Individuals may be grouped together if a proper distance or similarity measure is defined in this space.

Anthropometric Criteria of Obesity

Inspection is the easiest and cheapest of all procedures for diagnosing obestiy and has its own importance. Generally, the obese-looking subject has excess fat and this method has been used as a reference system [Rauh and Schumsky, 1969]. However, the diagnosis of obesity is most often based on anthropometric measurements, single or combined, as indices of diverse complexity.

Single anthropometric measurements. Excess body weight beyond given cut-off lines has been widely used and is still the criterion most commonly employed in daily practice. Hence, body weight for age or, better, body weight for height above 20% of the median can be used, taking into account that the former can be misleading because different heights for the same body mass result in different degrees of corpulence. Body weight for height avoids this eventuality, although, as it measures total body mass, it does not take into account variations of the different components: body weight could increase not only because of increased body fat but also as a consequence of water retention or muscle hypertrophy. Thus, a given subject could be overweight without being overfat (Figs. 1 and 2).

Another issue that arises involving body weight as a criterion of obesity is that, since body weight is not normally distributed, it is not advisable to use percentage values of the median to establish cut-off points. Instead, the use of percentiles has been advocated.

Arm circumference has been used as a rapid and reliable method for nutritional assessment, mainly in screening for undernutrition. Values above the 97th percentile are consistent with the diagnosis of obesity, although the development of muscle mass can also play a role in the increase of arm circumference.

The terms "overweight" and "obese" commonly used to define two different degrees of excessive weight are misleading because they mix two different criteria and distort the concept of obesity. By definition, obesity is the increase of body fat above certain limits and can only be diagnosed with accuracy if the degree of adiposity can be measured. We can say in agreement with Roche et al. [1981] that given suitable reference data "excess body fat" can be defined as the attribute of any subject having values above a particular percentile, say the 90th, for a measure of body fatness.

The simplest means of measuring body fat is through fatfolds obtained by means of a caliper at different sites of the body. The proportion of body mass that is fat varies with age and sex (Fig. 3); the proportions between subcutaneous and visceral fat are also different and there is an individual constitutional pattern to the distribution of fat and thickness of subcutaneous layers in different sites of the body [Garn, 1955, Garn et al., 1975; Yuhasz, 1980; Siervogel et al., 1982]. All of this leads to a degree of inaccuracy in appraising the magnitude of overfatness.

If we take fatfolds as single measure of adiposity, we can etablish a cut-off line at the 90th percentile for triceps and subscapular fatfolds, which are the most reliable because of their closer correlation with total body fat [Bogin and MacVean, 1981; Amador et al., 1984]. Suprailiac and calf fatfolds and some others less often employed show greater interindividual variability and therefore are not recommended for this purpose.

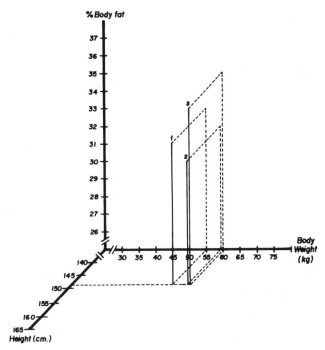

Fig. 1. Three obese boys with the same heights and different weights are plotted. Subject 2 is heavier than subject 1, however he is less obese since his body fat is lower. Subjects 2 and 3, with practically the same weight and height, exhibit obvious differences in their percentage of body fat.

Composite indices. Different indices for the assessment of obesity have been described that combine two or more anthropometric measurements. Ponderal Index ($HT/\sqrt[3]{BW}$) BW/HT, BW/HT^2 (Quetelet's or Body Mass Index), and BW/HT^3 (Rohrer Index) have been employed, mainly in adults.

Quetelet's Index (or the BMI) has been found suitable for application in children, but the different stages of growth and changes in body composition must be taken into account when assessing adiposity [Rolland Cachera et al., 1982]. The same authors have used this index to predict the development of adiposity rebound and final adiposity. The earlier the rebound, the higher the adiposity level reached [Rolland Cachera et al., 1984].

McLaren and Read [1975] introduced the weight/length classification of nutritional status, considering as overweight those subjects above 110%. This ratio increases gradually with age from values of 60 to 65 at birth to above 310 at 19 years of age.

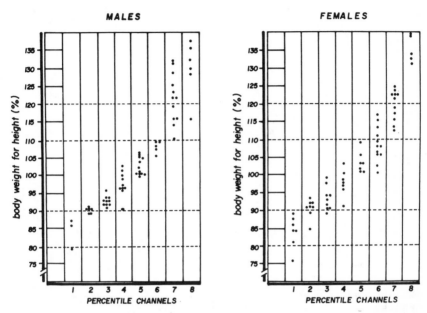

Fig. 2. A comparison between different criteria of weight for height is made in 66 girls and 64 boys aged 9-14 years. In both sexes a number of children above 120% weight for height are between the 90th and 97th percentile (channel 7). Moreover, among girls four cases are classified as overweight in percentiles between 75 and 90 (channel 6). Hence, weight for height in percent tends to overestimate obesity.

Edwards [1978] has used the so-called Weight Index (WI), which is based on weight/height ratios, to measure weight changes in children. BW/HT seems to be more reliable in women [Watson et al., 1979], while BW/HT^3 has the lowest correlations with other adiposity indices [Rolland Cachera et al., 1982].

The use of indices which include fatfolds permits a closer assessment of adiposity. Fat areas of the mid-upper arm obtained through the expression

$$FA = \frac{T(AC \times 10)}{2} - \frac{T^2}{4\pi}$$

[Gurney and Jelliffe, 1973] where T is triceps fatfold and AC is arm circumference, have been used for assessing obesity [Himes et al., 1980]. The advantages of considering the cross-sectional area of the limb instead of the fatfolds (biceps or triceps) alone are based on the influence of the underlying muscle mass of the area of the surrounding fat ring, so that in subjects with

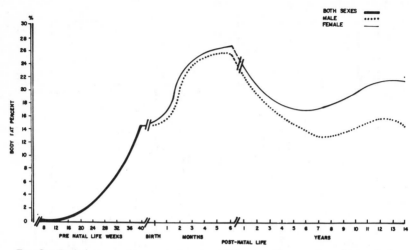

Fig. 3. Body fat percent in pre- and post-natal life up to 14 years of age (both sexes).

the same fatfold thickness, the one with a larger area will be the more muscular.

Himes et al. [1980] stressed the usefulness of fat areas in describing age changes or sex differences in adiposity, taking into account that the tendencies in some periods of life may be opposite: fat areas may increase while fatfolds decrease. The same authors found a significant correlation between body fat in kg and fat areas but not with percentage fat or body density.

Energy/Protein Index (E/P) is the ratio between transformed fatfold at triceps and the logarithm of mid-arm muscle circumference [Amador et al., 1975].

$$E/P = \frac{\text{Transformed T}}{\text{Log}_{10}\text{ AMC}}, \text{ where AMC} = AC - \pi T.$$

The usefulness of E/P in nutritional assessment has been demonstrated [Amador et al., 1980] and higher values have been found in overweight subjects than in lean ones [Amador, 1978]. A significant correlation has been found between percent of body fat and E/P [Amador et al., 1981]. Hence, values of E/P above the 90th percentile are consistent with the diagnosis of obesity.

Body Composition

The determination of body composition is the most exact way of measuring adiposity. The degree of acccuracy in the determination of the amount of body fat depends on the methods employed. Such methods should preferably be used for individual assessment because most of them are expensive, time-consuming, and require special equipment, and therefore they are not suitable for field or community studies. Reference values for obesity based on body fat in children have not been established, but it is generally accepted that a fat content above 25% of body weight for males and 30% for females is excessive [Bray et al., 1972]

Obviously, the amount of body fat can be determined in cadavers with relatively more exactness than in living subjects. When the study of body composition in vivo is needed, several methods can be used: dilution techniques for determination of total body water, cell mass, or body fat; detection of K^{40}; electrical conductivity; roentgenometry; measurement of body density, or anthropometric measurements.

Total body water (TBW) can be determined using the method of isotopic dilution by oral or intravenous administration of isotopes of hydrogen, sodium or potassium, the first being the only one currently in use, either with deuterium or with tritium [Cheek, 1979].

Dilution techniques using uptake of fat soluble gases such as cyclopropane have been employed [Lesser et al., 1971] but are technically very complex and expensive.

More commonly used is the detection and quantification of the naturally existing isotope of potassium (K^{40}) which has a long physical half-life, emits a strong gamma ray, and is found in sufficient quantity in the body to allow its determination by special scintillation counters. Since the isotope is not bound to neutral fat, the lean body mass can be estimated by a simple calculation [Forbes, 1981] and body fat can be obtained by subtracting this value from total body weight. This noninvasive method, though requiring expensive equipment, needs little cooperation from the subject and can be applied even in small children.

The neutron activation method has been used for measuring total body nitrogen [Cohn et al., 1983]. The relationship between total body nitrogen and total body potassiuim has proved to be an expression of the relationship of body cell mass to lean body mass, total body potassium being the more sensitive and reliable indicator of changes in body cell mass.

The estimation of body composition by electromagnetic methods is based on the differences existing in electrical conductivity and dielectric properties of body components, primarily muscle and fat [Harrison and Van Itallie, 1982]. The actual merit of this method is still subject to evaluation.

The measurement of muscle or bone widths can be made by X-ray examinations or ultrasound. Computer tomography has also been used as a means of studying bone, muscle, and fat cross-sectional areas of the limbs [Heymsfield et al., 1979].

The study of body composition by measuring body density is based on the differences in density existing between fat and lean tissues. The body fat compartment is anhydrous and has a fairly constant density of about 0.90 g/m^3, while the fat-free compartment has a density of about 1.10 g/m^3 and a water content of about 720 g/kg. Thus, measurement of body density allows calculation of the relative proportion of these two body compartments and, therefore, of the total fat content as well.

Body density can be calculated by the technique of underwater weighing as the ratio of subject weight in air and in water immersion. Previous correction for factors such as water temperature and residual capacity of the lung, among others is necessary. This method is laborious and requires cooperation from the subject. Its advantage, however, is that the mathematical expression starts from the assumption that the compositon and density of fat-free mass is constant and, thus, fat content may be under- or overestimated in subjects with a relatively high or low proportion of bone, a tissue which has a low water content but a high density compared with other lean tissues [Durnin and Womersley, 1974].

The introduction of anthropometric measurements for studying body composition is a consequence of the search for simpler techniques that could have more extensive application.

The finding of a fairly uniform relationship between body density and subcutaneous fat leads to the development of regression equations based on densitometric data [Parizková, 1961; Durnin and Rahaman, 1967; Parizková and Roth, 1972; Boileau et al., 1981], who combined five skinfolds, five circumferences, and six skeletal widths in different equations.

Similar correlations were found between fatfolds and lean body mass obtained by whole body counting by Forbes and Amirhakimi [1970], Burmeister and Fromberg [1970], and Dugdale and Griffiths [1979], who combined in several regression equations body weight; height; and one, two, or four fatfolds.

Undoubtedly, the calculation of body fat using regression equations that combine different anthropometric measurements had the advantages of its low cost and ease of application even in field studies. Moreover, the highly significant correlation existing between body weight for height and body fat or percent body fat obtained from regression equations that use only body weight and height allows an approximation of adiposity when only these two measurements are availalbe [Amador et al., 1982a].

Nevertheless, the use of such equations has the disadvantages of a lower level of precision, variability among subjects in subcutaneous tissue thickness at various body sites, limitations of measuring only subcutaneous fat, which represents no more than 40 to 45% of total adipose tissue of the body, and the technical hazards of measuring fatfolds with the different types of calipers, which can lead to errors of unknown magnitudes in the hands of unskilled personnel. Hence, it is not advisable to apply regression equations obtained from populations other than the original ones and special care must be taken in the training of measuring staffs and selection of equipment.

The selection of methods for assessing obesity depends on the purpose of the study: for the screening or surveillance of a given population, the simplest methods are best; if knowledge of the body composition or degree of fatness of a single subject is needed in details, more sophisticated methods should be used [Johnston, 1981].

The most frequently used criteria of obesity are summarized in Table I.

A particular situation occurs when an increase of body fat is suspected and cannot be determined with accuracy. A subject could be constitutionally heavy or stocky without being fatty and a decision on therapeutic intervention must be based on a differentiation between these two states (Fig. 4). In such "marginal" cases, a combination of several criteria could be used.

According to our own experience with overweight children, if E/P Index values are below the 90th percentile, the probabilities of the subject being obese are very low; and, conversely, if the E/P is above that cut-off line, the overweight child is very likely to be overfat [Amador et al., 1982b].

Precise evaluation allows better care of the subject and prevents misdiagnosis and iatrogenic interventions.

PHYSICAL FITNESS IN OBESITY

Physical fitness has become a major field of interest for physiologists, sports scientists, and clinicians. Response to excercise is now considered a very important tool for a comprehensive evaluation of health or its impairment.

TABLE I. Anthropometric Criteria of Obesity Summarized

Indicator	Criterion
Body weight for age	Above 120% of median
Body weight for height	Above 120% of median More than 2 SD above the median Above the 97th percentile
Arm circumference	Above 97th percentile
Triceps fatfold	Above 90th percentile
Subscapular fatfold	Above 90th percentile
Energy/Protein index	Above 90th percentile
Body composition	Above 25% of body weight in fat (males) Above 30% of body weight in fat (females)

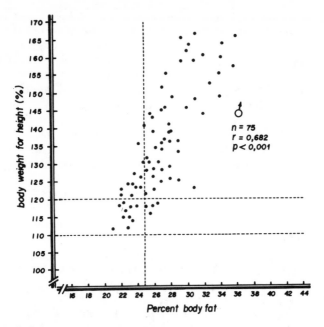

Fig. 4. Correlation between body fat percent and body weight for height in 75 boys between 9 and 14 years of age. It may be seen that 11 children with an overweight greater than 120% show a body fat percent below the generally accepted cut-off point of 25%. Conversely, four children with a body fat percent above that line exhibited a weight for height between 110 and 120%.

Malina [1980] has stated that any consideration of growth and development should concern itself with physical performance and those factors that influence it. Indeed, for the biological characterization of any population or specific samples of it, assessment of functional capacity is of great importance.

Multiple factors are involved in the physical fitness of an individual: hereditary, physical, organic, and social determinants, but it seems that individual endowment and habitual physical activity are the most important. [Dedoyard and Ghesquiere, 1980].

Cross-sectional Studies

Obesity has been linked to a low level of physical fitness and considered a handicap from the functional point of view. The validity of this assertion is clouded by problems in design and interpretation frequently encountered in most studies of this sort (Table II).

Obese subjects have been characterized as poor performers with a low aerobic capacity.

TABLE II. Difficulties in Design and Interpretation of Epidemiologic Studies Relating Physical Activities to Obesity

1) Self-selection for different types of physical activity

2) The classification of "active" or "less active" occupational activities may be due to health-related causes

3) The assessment of physical activity level has different methodological approaches and limits the comparisons among different studies

4) Limitation and heterogeneity of the criteria of obesity

Vamberová, as cited by Parizková [1977], found that when obese and lean individuals performed the same work, the obese consumed more oxygen than the nonobese. Parizková [1977] measured the oxygen consumption during a maximum work-load ($\dot{V}O_2$ max) and detected no differences between normal and obese boys. Nevertheless, the relative values of $\dot{V}O_2$ max were poorer in the obese while, conversely, the lean were able to perform significantly more work [Sprynarová and Parizková, 1965]. They concluded that obese children exhibited a reduced work economy.

Peña et al. [1982] studied the physical work capacity (PWC_{170}) and the $\dot{V}O_2$ max of a selected sample of 60 Cuban boys ranging from 10.0 to 14.9 years of age. They were divided into three groups: swimmers, obese, and controls. The swimmers, as might be expected, had the highest scores for aerobic capacity. There were no differences between the obese and the controls but, when the relative values of these variables (body weight or lean body mass) were compared, the obese yielded the lowest results.

The correlation between percent body fat and the PWC_{170} per kg of body weight logarithm (Fig. 5) showed that the higher the percent of body fat the lower the aerobic capacity. This confirmed that an excess of fat produces a negative influence upon physical fitness and in fact contributes to an elevation of the energy cost of external work.

An attempt was made to determine how much oxygen the subjects consumed per kilogram-meter of work done during one submaximal workload. Both swimmers and controls did not differ in thier results, but the obese consumed significantly more oxygen per unit of work than the other groups. This result agrees with previous findings [Vanberová et al., 1971 in Parizková, 1977].

Moreover, it has been suggested by several authors [Apfelbaum et al., 1971; Goldman, 1975] that the work efficiency of the obese is reduced, a controversial assertion. The relationship between oxygen consumption and work rate for obese and nonobese subjects during exercise on a cycle ergometer was studied in young men by Bray et al. [1977]. They found an upward

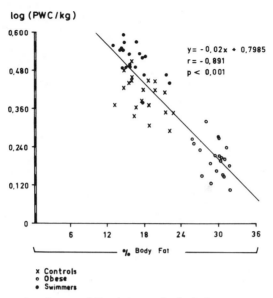

Fig. 5. Shows a negative correlation between the body fat percent and log-transformed PWC_{170}. The highly significant correlation coefficient is a proof of the strong relation between excess body fat and physical fitness.

and parallel displacement of oxygen consumption at each work rate for the obese as compared to the lean.

This is consistent with the greater leg mass of the obese subjects while pedalling. Similar findings were also reported by Peña [1982] in children between 10 and 14 years of age. Hence, it is essential to correct for differences in energy expenditure related to moving legs when there is no external load [Bray, 1983].

These results confirm that excess weight may impair work capacity but does not mean that work efficiency is altered in obese individuals. Thus, the handicap of the obese when performing physical activity is mainly due to the excess of mass (overfatness) rather than to an actual impairment of work efficiency.

Poor physical fitness in obese individuals may also result from a lowered acitvity level as reported in studies of obese high school girls [Johnson et al., 1956] and boys [Waxman and Stunkard, 1980]. These two factors interact, thus producing a positive feedback process in which the factors complement each other, creating the well-known cycle of overfatness–sedentarism. Still other factors may play an important role in the impaired fitness of obese subjects.

During physical activity, internal body temperature rises with the increasing intensity of excercise. This elevation of core temperature provides the central stimulus to sweating and cutaneous vasodilation [Gisolfi, 1983]. There is evidence that some obese subjects exhibit a reduced heat tolerance during excercise, probably related to a decrease in blood flow between skin and working muscle, as reported by Vroman et al. [1983].

Effect of training on Obese Subjects

Longitudinal studies. Only a few studies document the effect of weight loss on fitness levels in obese individuals. Most of them have a relatively short duration, a fact that makes it difficult to draw definite conclusions.

Franklin et al. [1979] studied 36 sedentary women who attended a 12-week physical conditioning program. Thirteen subjects were initally classified as lean and twenty-three as obese. Among the physiological changes resulting from that program for normal and obese, respectively, were increases of 12.7 and 18.9 percent in $\dot{V}O_2$ max, decreases of 0.4 kg and 2.56 kg in body weight, and a decrease of 0.8 and 1.8 in percent body fat.

Peña and Bacallao [1983] studied the changes of body composition and physical fitness in obese children undergoing four different trials during 4 weeks, in which either a fiber diet or a physical training program or both were involved. The energy content of the diet was 4.18 MJ in all groups.

The authors found significant reductions of body weight and body fat with the four therapeutic regimens. Those groups on the physical exercise program showed a greater total body mass reduction, lost more fat, and spared more lean body mass than the other groups.

The aerobic capacity, measured through PWC_{170} and $\dot{V}O_2$ max, improved significantly within each of the regimens, mainly in those in which exercise was involved. The authors concluded that the predominant influence upon the changes of aerobic capacity, as well as on body composition, was clearly excercise, although the fiber content of the diet had a systematic benefical effect which was not always significant.

In another paper, Epstein et al. [1983] reported that weight losses in obese children are strongly related to improvements in fitness. This study was performed with 113 obese preadolescents participating in a 6-month behavioral weight control program. They stressed that "the combination of effective weight loss and an initally moderate degree of overweight combined to produce the greatest fitness changes."

The performance enhancements in these studies in which physcial training was involved could be explained by different mechanisms: 1) improvement of the adaptive function; 2) development of better skills while exercising; and 3) the reduction of total body mass and fat and, consequently, a reduction of the work necessary to move a lighter body.

These observations notwithstanding, no definite conclusions can be drawn as to a cause-effect relationship in experiments yielding an improvement in physical fitness. It is extremely difficult to identify isolated factors as the cause of the observed changes in physical capacity, as is generally true with other biological phenomena. Experiments are usually not designed with this purpose in mind, for obvious reasons, so the researcher is left with several varying factors and conditions and no precise criteria as to causes and effects.

For example, the question remains open as to what should be expected concerning physical fitness if a group of individuals—obese or not—undergoes a training program while maintaining a constant body weight; or alternatively, if they experience a weight reduction at the expense of, say, a controlled diet with no changes in their everyday physical activity.

PRINCIPAL BASES IN THE TREATMENT OF OBESITY

The regulation of body mass and body composition is dependent on energy intake, energy expenditure, and on the behavior of numerous, complex and still not well understood regulating mechanisms. The first two factors are susceptible to control and their combination seems the most natural way to reduce fat.

Furthermore, the treatment should be supported by substantial changes in incorrect habits relating to nutrition and lifestyle. Hence, the main aspects in the comprehensive treatment of obesity are: 1) reduction of energy intake; 2) increase of energy expenditure by increased physical exercise; and 3) induction of behavioral changes in the nutritional habits and physical acitvity pattern of the obese individual.

In the ensuing paragraphs we will devote our attention to the first two aspects since the third one is beyond the scope of this chapter.

Dietary Aspects

The oldest and most widely used approach in treating obesity deals with dietary restriction. A great number of diets have been described, but the most frequently employed are briefly summarized.

Total fasting and semistarvation diets. These diets induce great weight loss, mainly at the beginning of the treatment. But this weight loss results from the breakdown of lean rather than adipose tissue. Moreover, a lack of carbohydrate ingestion promotes substantial water and mineral excretion. Hence, the results obtained are not successful since the goal in the treatment of obese subjects is to reduce body fat. These diets are not indicated in children and adolescents because the course of growth and development could be seriously impaired and severe nutritional deficiencies could result.

In addition, many deleterious effects have been reported: functional impairment of glomerular filtration and hepatic function, disturbances of acid-base equilibrium, increased uric acid excretion, alteration of endocrine functions, arrhythmias [Pringle et al., 1983], and also the risk of sudden death [Spencer, 1968] have been described.

Protein-sparing modified fast. These diets were in vogue two decades ago. Calloway and Spector stated in 1954 that energy restriction is associated with nitrogen loss. Several authors [Apfelbaum et al., 1970; Genuth et al., 1974; Baird et al., 1974]. observed that when protein intake was increased, a better nitrogen balance was achieved in spite of low energy intakes.

The protein-sparing modified fast was developed in an attempt to minimize negative nitrogen balance and had, therefore, a sparing effect upon the lean body mass [Blackburn et al., 1975]. Archibald et al. [1983] assessed the effect of a 3-month period on this diet in 17 obese adolescents. They found that the weight loss was 15% of the inital body weight and a nonsignificant total nitrogen loss was observed. However, the change in lean body mass was high—determined from skinfold thicknesses—and contributed approximately 44% of the toal weight loss.

Pencharz et al. [1980] stuided the effect of a protein-sparing modified fast on the protein metabolism of five growing adolescents. They reported a preservation of the nitrogen balance during each dietary interval; nevertheless, significant individual differences with the treatment were seen. The authors concluded that energy restriction in obese adolescents does not interfere with their whole-body protein turnover provided that they receive an adequate protein intake.

Flatt and Blackburn [1974] and Jourdan et al. [1974], suggested the biochemical basis of the diet. Garrow [1978] and Wadden et al. [1983] have commented on the optimum amount of protein to be given.

This diet should be supplemented with vitamins and minerals. More recently, Heraief et al. [1983] proposed supplementation also with tryptophan in order to restore the plasma tryptophan/large neutral amino acid ratio. In any event, as reported by Newmark [1981], the protein-sparing modified fast should still be considered an experimental diet.

Fiber diets. Over the last two decades, fiber has been considered a nutrient of importance and the role it plays in nutrition and health has been stressed [Trowell, 1976; Burkitt et al., 1980]. Many diseases and symptoms, such as constipation, diverticulosis, ischemic heart disease, diabetes mellitus, colon cancer, and obesity have been related to some extent to poor fiber consumption [Burkitt, 1979].

The term "fiber" has not yet been well classified. It has been defined as a residue of plant cells resistant to digestion by alimentary enzymes [Trowell, 1976; Van Soest, 1978]. The main components are cellulose, hemicellulose, pectins, and lignins present in the plant cell walls. To these the interior indigestible polysaccharides such as guar gums and other leguminous galactomannans must be added. Nonetheless, many authors are not fully satisfied with the current criteria for digestibility of fibers, use of the term calls for futher discussion.

A variety of nutritional effects have been attributed to dietary fibers. However, two presumably similar dietary fibers coming from the same source can exert distinctly different metabolic effects [Schweizer et al., 1983]. The underconsumption of fiber and overconsumption of sugars and fats have been linked with the greater prevalence of obesity in the 20th century [Beyer and Flynn, 1978; Lee and Lawler, 1983].

The possible mechanisms by which a fiber intake of about 40g/day may contribute to the prevention or treatment of obesity have been discussed. [Heaton, 1973; van Itallie, 1978]. They are: 1) reduction of energy density of the diet; 2) promotion of chewing; the rate of ingestion is reduced and the increased secretion of saliva and gastric juice contributes to satiety; 3) larger residue of undigested material in the intestine whose bulking effect promotes abdominal distension; and 4) slight reduction of the absorption efficiency of the intestine.

High fiber content in the diet, however, may adversely affect mineral balance [Kelsay, 1981; Peña and Bacallao, 1983]. Hence, mineral supplementation is suggested during prolonged treatment.

The present-day approach to diet emphasizes eating a balanced diet provided by fresh fruits and vegetables as well as whole-grain cereals and breads.

Physical Exercise as a Therapeutic Procedure

The role physical exercise plays in the reduction of body weight is still a matter of discussion. Dempsey [1964] studied the effect of vigorous exercise in obese and nonobese young men. He found significant losses of body weight and body fat and increases in lean body mass. Similar results were also obtained by Franklin et al., [1979] and Ylitalo [1981].

Peña et al. [1980] assessed the influence of physical exercise upon body composition in obese children. They compared two groups subject to similar amounts of energy intake, differing only in a physical training program. They observed no differences in total body weight though the exercising group reduced significantly more fat than did the other one. Furthermore, exercise itself minimizes the loss of lean body mass that usually accompanies dietary restriction [Peña and Bacallao, 1983].

Wilmore [1983] provided information regarding the changes in body composition with physcial training obtained in numerous studies. Exercise appears to result in moderate losses in body weight, moderate reducton in body fat, and small increases in lean body mass. However, these relatively small changes are accompanied by important benefits to health and should be "the first line of treatment in children and adolescents" [Bray, 1983].

Exercise can produce important changes in blood cholesterol levels and in certain lipoprotein fractions. The effect of exercise on these variables was assessed by Vu Tran et al. [1983] in studies conducted during 26 years, using the metanalysis technique. They found a reduction in total cholesterol and triglycerides, an increase in high density lipoprotein cholesterol, and a decrease in low density lipoprotein cholesterol. They advise caution due to the very likely interaction of exercise and several other factors.

It is well known that prolonged exercise promotes profound changes in peripheral circulation and metabolism. Bülow [1982], among other researchers, demonstrated that adipose tissue blood flow increases during excercise. This fact has physiological significance since the supply of a free fatty acid carrier to the tissue facilitates the mobilization of free fatty acids from adipose tissue to the working muscles.

The proportion of energy supplied by lipid oxidation gradually increases with the duration of exercise, reaching more than 80% after 3 hours of activity [Pirnay et al. 1977]. Therfore this type of prolonged exercise induces lipid mobilization and facilitates the reduction of body fat depots.

In obese subjects, as compared to lean ones, free fatty acid mobilization is reduced during exercise [Klein et al., 1965; Minuk et al., 1980]. In a recent paper, Scheen et al. [1983] related the impairment of the free fatty acid mobilization to a significantly higher insulin level and a lack of glucagon increase. They suggested an increased contribution of carbohydrates to the energy supply. This fact could represent metabolic limitations of prolonged exercise in obese individuals.

Moreover, exercise influences the insulin response to glucose load [Björntorp, 1981], resulting in a lowering of plasma insulin and an improvement of glucose tolerance [Krotkiewsky et al., 1983], thus promoting an enhancement in carbohydrate metabolism.

Some suggested effects through which physical activity may contribute to the treatment of obesity are shown in Table III.

TABLE III. Effects of Habitual Physical Activity Upon the Organism

• Beneficial influence upon cardiorespiratory system
• Reduction of body fat mass and development of lean body mass
• Enhancement of carbohydrate and lipid metabolism
• Facilitation of sweating and thermal regulation during exercise
• Reduction of appetite

Obese individuals with a high degree of overweight have difficulties in performing exercise at high work loads due to osteoarticular limitations. Therefore, initial sessions of exercise of light to moderate intensity are recommended. Hiking, swimming, and bicycling are suitable examples. The sessions may start at 60 to 70 percent of the maximal heart rate of the subject increasing up to a gradual achievement of 70 to 80 percent. The duration should be 10 to 15 minutes at first, increasing to 60 minutes at least 3 days a week.

ACKNOWLEDGMENTS

The authors wish to express their gratitude to Prof. Marjorie Moore and Prof. Lourdes Pola for their friendly collaboration in this work.

REFERENCES

Amador M, Bacallao J, Hermelo M, Fernández R, Tolón C (1975): Indice Energia/Proteina: un nuevo aporte para la evaluación del estado de nutrición. I-Valores en niños sanos de edad preescolar. Rev Invest Clin (Mex) 27:247-253.

Amador M, Bacallao J, Flores P (1980): Indice Energia/Proteina: nueva validación de su aplicabilidad en evaluación nutricional. Rev Cubana Med Trop 32: 11-24.

Amador M, González ME, Hermelo M. (1981): Energy/Protein Index: Its usefulness in assessing obesity. Anthrop Közl 25:3-16.

Amador M, Rodriguez C, González ME , Bacallao J, (1982a): Assessing obesity with body weight and height. Act a Paediat Acad Sci Hung 23:381-390.

Amador M, González ME, Córdova L, Pérez N (1982b): Diagnosing and misdiagnosing malnutrition. Acta Paediat Acad Sci Hung 23: 391-401.

Amador M, Bacallao J, Ruiz M (1984): Cambios en los pliegues de grasa durante la reducción de peso en niños obesos. Su relación con la eficiencia del tratamiento. Rev Esp Pediat (in press).

Amador M, (1978): Energy/Protein Index: A new approach for the assessment of the nutritional status. PhD Thesis, Budapest. Hungarian Academy of Sciences Part IV, pp 51-71.

Apfelbaum M, Boudon P, Lacatis D, Nillus P (1970): Effects métaboliques de la diète protéidique chez 41 sujets obeses. Press Med 78:1917-1920.

Apfelbaum M, Bostsarron J, Lacatis D (1971): Effect of caloric restriction and excessive caloric intake on energy expenditure. Am J Clin Nutr 245:1404-1409.

Archibald EH, Harrison JE, Pencharz PB (1983): Effect of a weight-reducing high-protein diet on the body composition of obese adolescents. Am J Dis Child 137:658-662.

Baird IW, Parsons RL, Howard AN (1974): Clinical and metabolic studies of chemically defined diets in the management of obesity. Metabolism 23:645-657.

Beyer PL, Flynn MA (1978): Effects of high and low fiber diets on human feces. J Am Dietet 72:271-277.

Björntorp P (1981): Effects of exercise and training on fat metabolism in normal and obese man. In di Prampero PE, Poortmans JR (ed): "Physiological chemistry of exercise and training." Basel: S. Karger, pp 63-65.

Blackburn L, Bistrian R, Flatt JP (1975): Role of a protein sparing modified fast in a comprehensive weight reduction programme. In Howard AN (ed): "Recent Advances in Obestiy Research: I. Proceedings of the First International Congress on Obesity." London: Newman Publishing Ltd, pp 279-281.

Bogin B, MacVean RB (1981): Nutritional and biological determinants of body fat patterning in urban Guatemalan children. Human Biol 53:259-268.

Boileau RA, Wilmore JH, Lohman TG, Slaughter MH, Riner WF (1981): Estimation of body density from skinfold thicknesses, body circumferences and skeletal widths in boys aged 8 to 11 years: comparison of two samples. Human Biol 53:575-592.

Bray GA (1983): The energetics of obesity. Med Sci Sports Exerc 15:32-40.

Bray GA, Davidson MB, Drenick EJ (1972): Obesity a serious symptom. Ann Intern Med 77:797-805.

Bray GA, Whipp BJ, Koyal SN, Wasserman K (1977): Some respiratory and metabolic effects of exercise in moderately obese men. Metabolism 26:403-412.

Bülow J (1982): Adipose tissue blood flow during exercise. (thesis) Laegeforeningens forlag, University of Copenhague.

Burkitt DP (1979): The protective value of plant fibre against many modern western diseases. Qual Plant—Pl Fds Hum Nutr XXIXl:39-48.

Burkitt D, Morley D, Walder A (1980): Dietary fibre in under- and overnutrition in childhood. Arch Dis Child 55:803-807.

Burmeister W, Fromberg G (1970): Depotfett, bestimunt nach der Kalium 40 methode und seine bezfelnung zur hautfaltendicke bei 4-19 jährigen. Arch Kinderheilkunde 180; 228-236.

Calloway DH, Spector H (1954): Nitrogen balance as related to caloric and protein intake in active young men. Amer J Clin Nutr 2:405-411.

Cheek DB (1979): Body composition studies (letter). Am J Clin Nutr 32:2060-2061.

Cohn SH, Vartsky D, Yasumura S, Vaswani AN, Ellis KJ (1983): Indexes of body cell mass: nitrogen versus potassium. Am J Physiol 244 (Endocrinol Metab 7): E305-E310.

Dedoyard E, Ghesquiere (1980): Evaluation of aerobic power and physical working capacity of female and male Zairians. In Ostyn M, Beunen G, Simons J (eds): "Kinanthropometry II." Baltimore: University Park Press, pp 129-141.

Dempsey JA (1964): Anthropometrical observations on obese and non obese young men undergoing a program of vigorous physical exercise. Res Q 35:275-287.

Dugdale AE, Griffiths M (1979): Estimating fat body mass from anthropometric data. Am J clin Nutr 32:2400-2403.

Durnin JVAG, Rahaman MM (1967): The assessment of the amount of fat in the human body from measurements of skinfold thickness. Br J Nutr 21:681-689.

Durnin JVAG, Womersley J (1974): Body fat assessed from total body density and its estimation from skinfold thickness measurements on 481 men and women aged from 16 to 72 years. Br J Nutr 32:77-97.

Edwards KA (1978): An index for assessing weight change in children: weight/height ratios. J Appl Behav Anal 11: 421-429.

Epstein LH, Koeske R, Zidansek J, Wing RR (1983): Effects of weight loss on fitness in obese children. Am J Dis Child 137:654-657.

Flatt JP, Blackburn GL (1974): Metabolic fuel regulatory system: implication for protein-sparing therapies during caloric deprivation and disease. Amer J Clin Nutr 27:175-187.

Forbes GB, Amirhakimi GH (1970): Skinfold thickness and body fat in children. Human Biol 42: 401-418.

Forbes GB (1981): Body composition in adolescence. In: Tsang RC, Nichols BL, Jr. (eds): "Nutrition and child health: Perspectives for the 1980's." New York, Alan R. Liss, pp 55-72.

Franklin B, Buskirk E, Hodgson J, Gahagan H, Kollias J, Mendez J (1979): Effects of physical conditioning on cardiorespiratory function, body composition, and serum lipids in relatively normal-weight and obese middle-aged women. Int J Obesity 3: 97-105.

Garn SM, (1955): Relative fat patterning: an individual characteristic. Human Biol 27:75-89.

Garn SM, Clark DC, Guire KE (1975): Growth, body composition and development of obese and lean children. In Winick M. (ed): "Childhood Obesity." New York: John Wiley & Sons, pp 23-46.

Garrow JS (1978) "Energy balance and obesity in man." Amsterdam: Elsevier/North Holland Biomedical Press, pp 163-169.

Genuth SM, Castro JG, Vertes V (1974): Weighty reduction in obesity by outpatient starvation JAMA 230: 987-991.

Gisolfi CB (1983): Temperature regulations during exercise: directions—1983. Med Sci Sports Exerc 15:15-20.

Goldman RF (1975) Introduction to bioenergetics. In Bray GA (ed): "Obesity in Perspective, Vol 2." Fogarty International Center Series on Preventive Medicine. DHEW. Publication # 75-708 Washington, D.C. United States Government Printing Office, pp 119-120.

Gurney JM, Jelliffe DB (1973): Arm anthropometry in nutrition assessment: Nomogram for rapid calculation of muscle circumference and cross-sectional muscle and fat area. Am J Clin Nutr 26:912-915.

Harrison GG, Van Itallie TB (1982): Estimation of body composition: a new approach based on electromagnetic principles. Am J Clin Nutr 35:1176-1179.

Heaton KW, (1973): Food as an obstacle to energy intake. Lancet 2:1418-1420.

Heraief E, Burckhardt P, Mauron C, Wurtman JJ, Wrutman RJ (1983): The treatment of obesity by carbohydrate deprivation suppresses plasma tryptophan and its ratio to other large neutral amino acids. J Neural Transmission 57:187-195.

Heymsfield SB, Olafson RP, Kutner MH, Nixon DW (1979): A radiographic method of quantifying protein-calorie undernutrition. Am J Clin Nutr 32: 693-698.

Himes JH, Roche AF, Webb P (1980): Fat areas as estimates of total body fat. Am J Clin Nutr 33: 2093-2100.

Johnson ML, Buke BS, Mayer J (1956): Relative importance of inactivity and overeating in the energy balance of obese high school girls. Am J Clin Nutr 4: 37-44.

Johnston FE (1981): Studies on the relationship between anthropometry and densitometry. Key lecutre presented at 3rd International Symposium on Human Biology. Bozsok, Hungary.

Jourdan M, Margen S, Bradfield RB (1974): Protein-sparing effects in obese women fed low calorie diets. Amer J Clin Nutr 27:3-12.

Kelsay JL (1981): Effect of diet fiber level on bowel function and trace mineral balances of human subjects. Cereal Chem 58: 2-5.

Klein Rf, Troyer WG, Back KW, Hood TC, Bogdonoff MD (1965): Experimental stress and fat mobilization in lean and obese subjects. Metabolism 14: 17-24.

Krotkiewski M, Byhind-Fallenius Ac, Holm J, Björntorp P, Grimby G, Mandroukas K (1983): Relationship between muscle morphology and metabolism in obese women: the effects of long term physical training. Eur J Clin Invest 13: 5-12.

Lee CJ, Lawler GS (1983): Nutrient intakes in relation to body weight of nonobese and obese elderly females. Nutr Res 3: 149-155.

Lesser GT, Deutsch S, Markofsky J (1971): Use of independent measurement of body fat to evaluate overweight and under weight. Metabolism 20: 792-804.

Malina R (1980): A multidisciplinary biocultural approach to physical performance. In Ostyn M, Beunen G, Simons J (eds): "Kinanthropometry II." Baltimore: University Park Press, pp 33-68.

McLaren DS, Read WWC. (1975): Weight/Length classification of nutritional status. Lancet 2: 219-221.

Minuk HL, Hanna AK, Marliss EB, Vranic M, Zinman B (1980): Metabolic response to moderate exercise in obese man during prolonged fasting. Am J Physiol 238: E322-E329.

Mueller W (1982): The use of multivariate biometric methods for the analysis of human growth data. Paper presented at the III International Congress of Auxology. Brussels, Belgium.

Newmark SR (1981): Obesity: Recent developments in concepts of pathogenesis and treatment. J Okla State Med Assn 74: 357-361/

Parizková J (1961): Total body fat and skinfold thickness in children. Metabolism 10: 794-807.

Parizková J (1977): "Body fat and physical fitness." The Hague: Martinus Nijhoff Publ, Martinus Nijhoff Publ, Medical Division, pp 169-196.

Parizková J, Roth Z (1972): The assessment of depot fat in children from skinfold thickness measurements by Holtain (Tanner/Whitehouse) caliper. Human Biol 44: 613-620.

Peña M (1982): Anthropometric aspects and physical fitness in obese children. PhD Dissertation, Budapest.

Peña M, Bacallao J (1983): Changes in body composition and physical fitness in obese children with different treatments. In: "Human Growth and Development." Proceedings of the third International Congress of Auxology. New York: Plenum Press, pp 471-484.

Peña M, Barta L, Regöly-Mérei A, Tichy M (1980): The influence of physical exercise upon the body composition of obese children. Acta Paediat Acad Sci Hung 21: 9-14.

Peña M, Blanco J, Padrón P (1982): Physical fitness in obese, non obese, and specially trained boys. Anthrop Közl 26: 59-67.

Pencharz PB, Motil KJ, Parsons HG, Duffy BJ (1980): The effect of an energy-restricted diet on the protein metabolism of obese adolescents: nitrogen-balance and whole body nitrogen turnover. Clin Sci 59: 13-18.

Pirnay F, Lacroix M, Mosora F, Luycx A, Lefebre P (1977): Effect of glucose ingestion on energy substrate utilization during prolonged muscular exercise. Europ J Appl Physiol 36: 247-254.

Pringle TH, Scobie IN, Murray RG, Kesson CM, Maccuish AC (1983): Prolongation of the QT interval during therapeutic starvation: a substrate for malignant arrhytmias. Int J Obesity 7: 253-261./

Rauh JH, Schumsky DA (1969): Relative accuracy of visual assessment of juvenile obesity. J Am Diet Assoc 55: 459-464.

Roche AF, Siervogel RM, Chumlea WC, Webb P: (1981): Grading body fatness from limited anthropometric data. Am J Clin Nutr 34: 2831-2838.

Rolland Cachera MF, Deheeger M, Bellisle F, Sempé M, Guilloud-Bataille MN, Patois F (1984): Adiposity rebound in children: a simple indicator for predicitng obesity. Am J Clin Nutr 39: 129-135.

Rolland Cachera MF, Sempé M, Guilloud-Bataille M, Patois E, Péquignot-Guggenbuhl F, Fautrad V (1982): Adiposity indices in children. Am J Clin Nutr 36: 178-184.

Scheen AJ, Pirnay F, Luyckx AS, Lefebvre PJ (1983): Metabolic adaptation to prolonged exercise in severely obese subjects. Int J Obesity 7:221-229.

Schweizer TF, Bekhechi AR, Koellreuter B, Reimann S, Pometta D, Bron BA (1983): Metabolic effects of dietary fiber from dehulled soybeans in humans. Am J Clin Nutr 38: 1-11.

Siervogel RM, Roche AF, Himes JH, Chumlea WC, McCammon R (1982): Subcutaneous fat distribution in males and females from 1 to 39 years of ages. Am J Clin Nutr 36: 162-171.

Spencer IOB (1968): Death during therapeutic starvation for obesity. Lancer 1: 1288-1290.

Sprynarová S, Parizková J (1965): Changes in the arerobic capacity and body composition in obese boys after reduction. J Appl Physiol 20: 934-937.

Trowell HC (1976): Dietary fibre: metabolic and vascular disease. In "The present state of knowledge." No. 7, London: Norgine Ltd.

Van Itallie TB (1978): Dietary fibre and obesity. Am J Clin Nutr 31: 543-552.

Van Soest PJ (1978): Dietary fibers: their definition and nutritional properties. Am J Clin Nutr 31: 512-520.

Vroman NB, Buskirk ER, Hodgson JL (1983): Cardiac output and skin blood flow in lean and obese individuals during exercise in the heat. J Appl Physiol: Respirat Environ Exercise Physiol. 55: 69-74.

Vu Tran Z, Weltman E, Glass GV, Mood DP (1983): The effects of exercise on blood lipids and lipoproteins: a meta-analysis of studies. Med Sci Sports Exerc 15: 393-402.

Wadden TA, Stunkard AJ, Brownell KD (1983): Very low caloric diets: Their efficacy, safety, and future. Ann Intern Med 99: 675-684.

Watson PE, WAtson ID, Batt RD (1979): Obesity indices. Am J Clin Nutr 32: 736-737.

Waxman M, Stunkard AJ (1980): Caloric intake and expenditure of obese boys. J Pediatr 96: 187-193.

Wilmore JH (1983): Body composition in sport and exercise: directions for future research. Med Sci Sports Exerc 15: 21-31.

Ylitalo V (1981): Treatment of obese school-children with special reference ot the mode of therapy, cardiorespiratory performance, and the carbohydrate and lipid metabolism. Act Paediatr Scand (Suppl) 290: 1-108.

Yuhasz MS, Eynon RB, MacDonald SB (1980): The body composition, fat pattern, and somatotype of young female gymnasts and swimmers. Anthorp Közl 24: 283-289.

Nutritional Anthropology, pages 277-294

Intervention Advocacy for Action

John W. Townsend, PhD

The Population Council, Apartado 105-152, 11560 Mexico D.F., Mexico

INTRODUCTION

This volume has examined in a critical fashion the interacting themes of anthropology, nutrition, and ecology. In the face of unprecedented population growth, inadequate world food production and inequitable food distribution, the World Food Congress reviewed these same issues in a distinct forum nearly 10 years ago. Upon concluding their deliberation, the international community resolved that by 1984, no child would have to go to bed hungry, no family would have to fear the loss of their daily sustenance, and no one would see their future capacity compromised by malnutrition [Grant, 1984].

Although massive efforts during the past decade in developing countries have augmented annual food production by 2.8% and the prevalence of contraceptive practice has dramatically increased, reducing annual population growth to 2.2%, children in 1984 still go to bed hungry [World Bank, 1984]. As a manifestation of the poverty cycles, malnutrition remains a cruel specter in the lives of poor families in both developing and developed worlds. In 1980, the World Bank estimated that nearly 800 million persons in the Third World were living in conditions of poverty, insufficient to meet the basic necessities of life. This implies that nearly 40% of the world's southern hemisphere faces daily food shortages, overcrowding, inadequate housing, and increased risk of death from illnesses for which low cost, simple remedies are available in the northern hemisphere [Brandt, 1980]. And within the developed world, poverty and malnutrition also affect many families due to the inequitable income distribution, chronic unemployment, and illness.

On the positive side, the past two decades have witnessed a proliferation of research on the interaction of nutrition and human development and, in general, an increasing awareness of the scope of nutritional problems. The relationships between nutrition, infection, physical and cognitive development, mortality, and fertility are now surprisingly well documented, due to intensified research and evaluation. Unfortunately, the harnessing of this wealth of information to reduce the incidence of malnutrition has been less successful. Although a wide variety of development strategies have been applied to the problem of chronic malnutrition, the results have generally fallen far short of expectations, despite large financial investments in their implementation [Mahler, 1980]. The major constraints in the search for effective interventions have included the low political priority placed on nutrition; the lack of appropriate technology and necessary infrastructure to make nutrition programs effective; relatively high costs compared to available budgets; and, finally, the low coverage of existing services.

The complexity of these operational issues has led some to argue for more research. Although appropriate research is still required, more recently emphasis has shifted towards examining the successful components of simpler interventions. The belief is that interventions now exist with predictable positive impacts on child health and development that merit wide application in large populations. The current political and economic costs of these measures are sufficiently low to demand immediate action [Grant, 1984]. Moreover, development of new management tools has vastly simplified the control of once unwieldy program interventions.

The purpose of this chapter is to explore the basis for intervention, provide some broad guidelines for intervention planning, and management, and address some of the political and ethical issues in which interventions in conditions of poverty become embroiled.

ISSUES IN INTERVENTION

Despite increase awareness of the magnitude of the world hunger problem, the questions remains, "What should be done first?" Some argue that an improved world economy and a healthy private sector will produce the bounties and appropriate distribution of wealth needed to reduce the incidence of malnutrition. Others argue that it is the responsibility of the state to ensure that a "safety net" of food and basic services is available to those in greatest need, regardless of the state of the economy.

This call to action is often cast in terms of the need to intervene. Strictly speaking, an intervention is any action that may affect the interest and welfare of others. In the case of malnutrition, interventions seek to modify existing social and economic conditions that may constrain individuals or communities from obtaining and maintaining an adequate nutritional status. Interventions are often discussed in terms of experiments in which the intervention is the treatment. In the context of projects, the intervention is most commonly conceived as the goods or services delivered. However, because of the range of factors which may affect nutritional status, interventions can range from policy development to direct infant feeding.

A conceptual model for affecting nutritional status is presented in Figure 1. As can be observed, the network of contributing causes is quite complex, including factors which affect the quantity and quality of nutrient intake (e.g. food availability) as well as those affecting their biological utilization (e.g., the frequency and duration of illness).

Historically, intervention efforts were first focused on nutritional rehabilitation or on emergency responses to widespread famine as, for instance, in

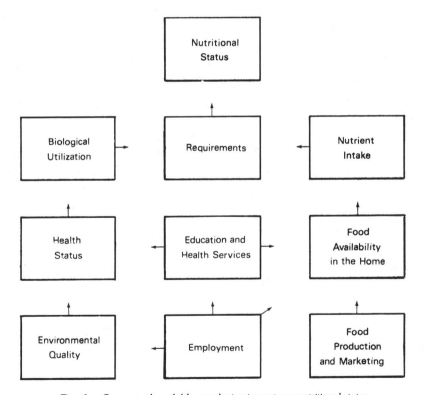

Fig. 1. Conceptual model for producing impacts on nutritional status.

Biafra in the 1970s and more recently in Ethiopia and Chad. The prevention of malnutrition is a relatively more recent notion. The most common preventive interventions carried out in the developing world in recent years have included food and nutrition planning; supplementary feeding programs for children and pregnant women; fortification of staples such as sugar, salt, and flour; nutrition-targeted agricultural programs and marketing strategies; food and nutrition education; and integrated health, sanitation and nutrition programs [Underwood, 1983]. Among integrated programs, family planning, oral rehydration, and the treatment of parasitic infections are frequently employed as indirect interventions because of their capacity to increase the biological utilization of food. Family planning, too, is cited as an indirect intervention because it promotes the health of the mother by increasing birth intervals and by reducing the fertility rate, allowing restricted food supplies to be shared among a smaller number of family members.

How can the most appropriate interventions be selected in developing countries in which poverty is not limited merely to family income but extends to information, skilled manpower and public institutions [Caiden and Wildavsky, 1973]? Because of this poverty, uncertainty often characterizes the design of interventions in low-income countries, both in terms of the unavailability of accurate information and of qualified persons for its analysis. Given the obvious limits on resources, infrastructure, and unpredictable political systems, the task of selecting appropriate interventions should be directed toward reducing this uncertainty. This effort should take into account several issues.

Importance of the Problem

The first issue to be addressed is the prevalence and severity of malnutrition: Does the problem exist to a degree and extent that warrants the mobilization of the resources required for its treatment? What are the personal and social costs of existing levels of malnutrition? What are the costs and consequences of waiting a few months before providing food relief? These costs include increased rates of morbidity and mortality, prevalence of retarded physical and mental development of children, lower productivity of the labor force, and increased potential for social unrest. Using these criteria, for example, in most developing countries interventions such as the iodizing of salt to reduce the prevalence of endemic goiter would be less significant than an agricultural program designed to reduce the prevalence of energy-protein malnutrition by increasing food availability to individuals at greatest risk. Of course, differences of opinion exist between policy makers, advocates identified with distinct disciplines, and potential beneficiaries in their assessment of the severity of the problem, the priority it should be given, and the resources required to remedy the damage. The effort to reach a consensus and to make explicit the views of distinct groups often contributes to a better conceptualization of the problem and provides a broader base for the examination of need and proposed intervention strategies [Townsend, 1984].

Effectiveness of the Solution

Nutrition interventions have been subject to severe criticism due to their often limited impact on the nutritional status of large populations, their potential disincentive effects on local agriculture, and their support of the political status quo [Lappé and Collins, 1977]. For example, Beaton and Ghassemi [1982] report that in many supplementary feeding programs minimal impact on the physical growth of the target population is detected in response to the food distributed, largely due to their inability to attract children at highest risk.

However, recent reviews of major nutritional experiments provide a more promising picture of the effectiveness of nutrition interventions. Kielman et al [1982] conclude that outside of disaster situations, nutritional supplements to preschool children reduce the rates of death and promote growth; in effect, lowering the prevalence but not the incidence of malnutrition. Gwatkin and collaborators [1980] estimate that one third to one half of deaths in children 0 to 5 years of age can be prevented by health and nutrition interventions costing approximately 2% of per capita income. The most powerful components cited are maternal supplementation, maternal immunization against tetanus, nutrition monitoring, and reliance on community health workers. Walsh and Warren [1979] include the promotion of breastfeeding in their proposed selective primary health care priorities, comprising the most cost-effective medical intervention for least-developed countries.

Pollitt [1981] maintains that monofocal interventions produce statistical but not biological impacts on the physical growth and psychosocial development of children, suggesting that interventions should be integrated to include nutrition education, food supplementation to the mother and child, and medical care.

There is not a great deal of data on the nutritional impacts of large-scale development projects. The effects of the nutrition education components are particularly difficult to determine. For example, nutrition education programs are commonly a subcomponent of a larger integrated social development project whose interventions may be more clearly defined (e.g., the use of fertilizers, improved seeds, and soil conservation techniques) and certainly more powerful in producing changes in food availabilty. Under these circumstances it is difficult to estimate what portion of subsequent changes in health or nutritional status can be attributable to the educational component [Klein et al., 1982]. Nevertheless, when combined with nutrition monitoring, education should provide a more powerful vehicle for intervention. Based on these results, UNICEF and WHO have been promoting the mix of a few low-cost, low-technology treatments, whether alone or as part of larger integrated interventions. They are commonly referred to as GOBI, that is, growth monitoring, oral rehydration, breastfeeding, and immunization. When funding and local priorities permit, this mix extends to early childhood stimulation, feeding, and family planning [Grant, 1984].

Demand for Nutrition Services by the Community

Because of the high prevalence of chronic malnutrition in developing countries, subclinical malnutrition often remains undetected by communities. As a result, with the exception of conditions of acute undernutrition or obesity, nutrition is rarely cited as a priority community problem. The literature is also replete with examples of underutilized food programs in areas with endemic malnutrition. In Indonesia, for example, improvements in nutritional status were not a sufficiently strong incentive for small landholders to increase production in home gardens. Although it could be argued that low utilization is largely a result of inappropriate program design and poor management, community demand for services must be a prime consideration in the selection of interventions. This is not to say that malnourished populations are indifferent to their status, merely that other vehicles may provide greater stimulus to community participation and more immediate action.

Consequently, the selection of the appropriate intervention must consider the demand for nutritional services by the community as well as the technical resources of the implementation team to provide them. On the one hand, one might expect, for example, that preventive services such as nutritional surveillance would be of less interest to the community than an income transfer program with potential for more direct payoff. On the other hand, if the implementation team is left without training, supervision, or support, the possibility of producing impacts with innovative nutrition programs is equally low.

Simplicity of the Intervention

One of the key features of successful programs is their simplicity. This virtue is not a product of shallow thinking, but it is rather a consequence of strong theory and clarity required to operationally define the components of the intervention. Moreover, in deciding between interventions with potentially equal impact on nutritional status, the intervention which presents the fewest operational limitations and relies on a minimum of infrastructure should be the treatment of choice. Simplicity should be expressed at virtually all stages of the intervention, e.g., during the formulation, training of personnel, supervision through management information systems, and evaluation. Many intervention planners concerned with the macroanalysis of interventions ignore the difficulty of providing a wide range of services given the kind and length of training personnel need. For example, in one primary health care program in Guatemala, training proved to be extremely difficult as rural promotors were asked to perform over 300 tasks as community volunteers. A simpler set of tasks with clear priorities would have been much more effective.

Logistics

In order for any program to function, it must be able to transport, store, and distribute supplies. Resources either as inputs (e.g., seeds and fertilizers) or products must be handled securely so they are not ruined by moisture, rodents, or are subject to theft. Equally important, the supplies must be delivered to the community at the appropriate intervals. Agricultural interventions are commonly plagued with ill-timed technical assistance or the limited capacity of existing markets to distribute additional production. The stronger the supply system and the greater reliance on local resources, the better. Those interventions which offer multiple vehicles for resupply or clearly identify fallback positions in case of disruptions in logistical support are more likely to endure the rigor of field operation.

Costs

Generally, the lower the cost for a given level of effectiveness, the better the intervention. Costs may be divided into start-up costs and maintenance costs. Large initial investments in nutritional interventions may make sense if the costs of maintaining services can be kept low and benefits projected over a longer period of time.

This effort is really more difficult than it appears. In most developing countries, data on service costs and expenditures for health and nutrition interventions are generally unavailable. Often current costs are grossly underestimated and assumptions about the stability of national budgets are overly optimistic. The selection of specific interventions thus should ensure that self-sufficiency is an ultimate goal and that service programs can continue to operate once external support is withdrawn.

FROM POLICY TO PRACTICE

The systematic preselection of potential interventions based on the forementioned criteria, though necessary, is insufficient in the political and budgetary arena. The task of defining strategic policies and specifying interventions must be made part of the policy process.

That is not to say that social and biomedical scientists should abandon their fields, merely that quality interventions require a closer association between science and politics. Anthropologists should continue to shed light on the cultural context of hunger and the anthropometric consequences of intervention. But applied scientists should also demonstrate a bias for mobilizing knowledge in service of social and political action. Policies imply theories and identify a chain of determinants relating current conditions and inputs to future consequences [Pressman and Wildavsky, 1973]. Programs make theories operational by tying them to objectives, implementation schemes and budgets.

Figure 2 illustrates the transition from the identification of problems and the formulation of policy ideas to the more orderly specification of alternatives and the decision on what policies should be tested in the field. How this is done varies dramatically between prevailing political systems. Once nutritional problems are identified, local program experiences are frequently examined as potential intervention alternatives, exploring constraints to implementation as well as their potential constituencies. The private sector and innovative semi-autonomous institutions in the public sector often provide valuable lessons on practical and field-tested solutions to obvious problems faced by service programs in transportation, supplies, and training. The capacity of policy makers and administrators to influence priorities and budgets provides some guidelines for whether the intervention should be tested in the public or private sector and determines the resources available for demonstrations.

Part of this decision process is making the transition from broad statements of intention, e.g., to increase employment among the rural poor, to concrete actions, e.g., setting up microbusinesses in rural areas. Sometimes small-scale demonstrations must be mounted only to prove to policy makers that certain services can be provided. These opportunities also allow intervention designers to determine the degree to which policy specifications are clear and precise and whether the organizational and personnel resources will allow the policy to be implemented in its bureaucratic and political setting. During field testing, close supervision should be maintained to determine the degree to which field activity corresponds to the guidelines provided and that progress toward a viable intervention is measurable. Thus, in practice, implementation starts with the development of broad program guidelines and moves through a period of testing and resolving the countless technical, administrative, and institutional problems that each new activity presents.

The dynamics of this formative process are complex but essential prior to the approval of a fully operational intervention. The need is not for disciplinary

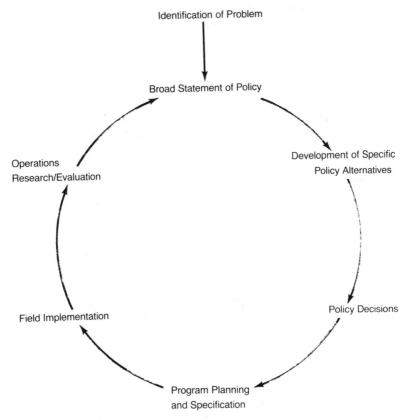

Fig. 2.   Diagram of the policy process.

giants to make new discoveries in dynamic social theory but for sensible persons with knowledge of program areas and experience in the management of organizations to ask if the people in the field can really do what is being proposed [Williams, 1976].

Two relatively new activities accompany the field testing of interventions. While operations research and evaluation have conceptually played a role in the policy process, it has only been recently that program administrators, legislators, and policy makers have acknowledged their utility by allocating funds for their operations. The basic notion is that problems in service delivery can be identified and solutions proposed through the use of social science research techniques. The systematic testing of alternative solutions proposed by operations research is one mechanism for comparing the cost-effectiveness of distinct service strategies. The use of these techniques depends largely on the availability of personnel with research skills and managers with an honest interest in information on the impact of program efforts. Ultimately, the knowledge generated by a closer examination of the effects of intervention contributes to a better understanding of the health and nutritional problems in the target population and also as a test of the robustness of the intervention theory.

Although this process seems reasonable in the abstract, in practice interventions have been plagued by a series of problems both in their design and implementation. The following are a few of the issues encountered in the review of AID financed primary health care programs in developing countries [Parlato and Favin, 1982].

Lack of Solid Criteria for Creating Projects

This problem is largely political in nature and has two manifestations. First, projects are often initiated in response to pressures to "do something," without consideration of their adequacy from a policy perspective. Given the conditions of poor populations, such a response is understandable but often is costly and ineffective in producing the change desired. The second manifestation is the tendency to rapidly expand projects to the national level without evaluative information on the impacts of smaller scale efforts, without considering the administrative and logistic costs of radical changes in scope. Rigid budgets and massive training needs rarely permit high-quality small projects to be adopted rapidly at the national level.

Lack of Participation in Program Planning and Design

When projects are planned solely from above or, perhaps worse, from abroad, implementation problems abound. Frequently key managers and organizations involved in the implementation process are systematically excluded from the planning process. This leads to poor site selection, intervention strategies ill suited to the cultural and political context of the country, and insufficient analysis of the strengths and weaknesses of the implementing agency. Likewise, implementation has been severely hampered when sites are not politically acceptable to national governments or appropriate for local service agencies. Target areas must at least meet the minimal infrastructure requirements for transportation and communications. The probability of success of most interventions may be enhanced if service delivery is coordinated with other development projects in the area selected.

Unrealistic Project Targets and Schedules

For political and bureaucratic reasons, often more services are promised than ever delivered and each step in program implementation takes longer than planned. Projects of short duration are commonly linked to political rather than technical time horizons. Five to ten years is a much more realistic time frame in which to build the infrastructure needed for major nutrition interventions, for increased agricultural production, or the development of effective marketing mechanisms. At least this amount of time is required to see an impact. When international funding prohibits such medium-range plans, a well-integrated series of small projects would be preferable. Funding of additional services to increasingly large populations should be contingent on demonstrated success in the smaller scale institutions.

Lack of Supervision of Project Implementation

Two mechanisms were found in need of strengthening in nearly all projects observed. First, more adequate supervision systems are required to monitor the coverage and quality of services. Interventions in developing countries are commonly designed without explicit supervision components to detect and characterize the problems encountered in service delivery or without funds to maintain this function. The principal consequence of lack of supervision is the irrational development of high-cost services with little concern for quality. The other mechanism is the analysis of information provided by routine supervision so that management decisions can be made to correct problems encountered once service delivery begins. The use of data for decision making is the key to the fine tuning of operations and should receive greater emphasis in the training of program managers.

Basically, the elements which determine the success of the policy process are quite simple: personnel, budgets, and the political context. As in the literature on the utilization of evaluation information [Patton, 1978], nutrition policy leads to interventions when some individual takes direct, personal responsibility for getting information to decision makers, for clarifying the consequences of alternative service strategies, and for pushing budget author-izations through the bureaucracy. The success of this process is not the result of official mandates but of the sweat and tears of concerned advocates.

Secondly, program budgets in poor countries are increasingly prey to the restrictions of finance ministries and the demands of foreign banks. The lower the true cost of reaching a development objective, e.g., reducing deaths due to malnutrition, the greater the contribution of the program to the goals of poorly financed service agencies. Because plans and programs in developing countries frequently are developed without the guarantee of funding for their maintenance, nutrition interventions should be designed either to minimize costs given the impact desired or to produce revenues to support their opera-tion in the vent of adoption. Mechanisms may include, for example, progressive taxes on agriculture production destined for export or the local sale of processed foods made possible by increased production. Unfortunately, pilot projects that do not take into account explicit national priorities and the structural and budgetary limitations of both the public and private sectors are unlikely to be adopted by governments, even if desirable impacts are obtained in the short term.

The third element is the political context. According to Ugalde and Emrey [1979], "the latin american experience has been characterized by an outpouring of hastily conceived policies, plans and programs to satisfy immediate political needs or the will of international leading agencies. However, what was gained at this phase of the policy process was lost during the implementation phase." No one denies that political commitment on the part of national government is essential for the development of nutrition interventions, but it is not sufficient. The political viability of nutrition interventions depends on developing a consensus between the recipients of services and other groups whose interests are also affected, e.g., politicians, taxpayers, and other agencies whose collaboration is essential to the maintenance of services. How this is accomplished is intimately tied to the specific political mechanisms and reality of each country, but without this consensus the work of concerned individuals and limited funds will be ephemeral and ineffective.

RECENT TRENDS IN INTERVENTION DESIGN

One strategy for the design of interventions is to examine recent trends in the delivery of human services so that operations more closely reflect the way in which communities and service organizations confront local needs. Though subtle and not without conflict, these trends can be found in both developing and more developed countries. Although the goals and context of the services are essentially the same, they represent adjustments to past obstacles and the promise of greater future impacts. Their most obvious manifestations are evolving values and program structures, emerging technologies, and changing administrative practices [Demone et al., 1978].

Evolving Values and Program Structure

One increasingly powerful value is that of equity in access to services. Despite inevitable questions of priority in human services, it is now commonly agreed that all groups should have access to high-quality services based upon need and the right to care rather than on social status or financial condition. In terms of nutrition, that means that sufficient food be made available to all and that individuals suffering from malnutrition, whether it is undernutrition or obesity, should have equal access to rehabilitation. Concretely, this value is expressed in the recent development of policies for local food security as well as in the detection, treatment, and referral of persons in traditionally underserved groups such as migrants, refugees, or women as heads of households in marginal urban areas.

A closely related value is the recognition of the client's right to know about the nature of his or her problem and to participate in the formulation and informed choice of treatment. When linked with the notion of community participation, this implies that individuals should participate in the planning, development, and operation of the services designed to address their needs. The promotion of growth monitoring in the child's home is one example of this trend. This involves the mother directly in the primary diagnosis of growth retardation as well as motivates the family to action in addressing at least the immediate causes of growth failure.

At the institutional level, this trend leads to decentralization and the transferral of responsibilities to more effective or less costly agents. There was a time when nearly all treatment for malnourished persons was provided in specialized institutions such as hospitals and nutrition recuperation centers. This regimen was costly both in terms of the construction and maintenance of facilities as well as in terms of personnel and supplies per individual treated. Moreover, the separation of the child or mother from the family contributed little to changing the immediate conditions in the home which led to the episode. Community-based detection and treatment of malnourished persons is now more widely employed, relying on the human resources of the community and locally available foods as the principal treatment medium. Small but longer term investments at the local level are now providing those services that costly national facilities can no longer provide.

Another manifestation of this trend is the emergence of treatment networks and self-help groups. Most nutrition and health facilities cannot provide the range of services required for comprehensive care, both for financial and human resource limitations. As a result, service agencies are forming consortia which agree upon the limits of catchment areas and priority target populations as well as the mix of services which can be provided by each agency. This clarification of roles leads to the local definition of appropriate levels of care and referral systems for specialized needs. Similarly self-help groups are flourishing in some countries on the assumption that persons with similar needs and relatively simple treatment routines can be of greater help to each other than irregular and expensive professional care. These groups are particularly effective in dealing with changes in food habits and lifestyle, when the continuous presence of professional personnel is less important than the motivation and support provided by peers.

These changes have stimulated new efforts toward the purchase of service. Though the private sector has long ignored the social consequences of malnutrition, more recently private for-profit groups are entering the "nutrition business." Their entry has been made possible through three mechanisms. The first is providing nutrition recuperation services on a contract basis at a lower cost than state facilities can. Thus the state becomes a purchaser rather than a direct provider of services. It also reinforces the government's functions in planning, regulating, and monitoring the quality of service. As a corollary action, public agencies are looking at commercial models for the delivery of certain services, such as the subsidized commercial marketing of oral rehydration salts, contraceptives, and simple pharmaceuticals.

The second change is in health maintenance organizations, whereby employers benefit by maintaining employees and their families in good health. Prepaid medical services are increasingly common in more advanced developing countries, e.g., Brazil and Mexico. The third important change is through community level micro businesses which are able to provide employment by producing and distributing simple processed foods with high nutrient value. For example, in Peru one such microenterprise run by a women's cooperative is producing quinua (a local grain) cookies, which are both rich in protein and energy and relatively low in cost. The profit obtained from their sale is a source of capital for other service activities in their urban marginal communities.

Emerging Technologies

With respect to technology, trends can be observed in health/agricultural practice, legal dispositions relating to nutrition, and methods for information dissemination. Health services in general have improved tremendously in the past 20 years due to technological innovations. The trend in non hospital care is toward simpler, less expensive treatment of specific nutritional deficiencies as well as toward pharmaceuticals that enhance the biological utilization of food, e.g., antihelmintic drugs and oral rehydration salts. Another example is the fortification of sugar, salts, and flours with micronutrients which has provided a relatively low-cost vehicle for intervention in large population groups while taking advantage of existing marketing systems.

The use of arm circumference [Vaquera et al, 1983] and low-cost weight/height charts [WHO, 1981] in the detection of children at risk of malnutrition are but two simple methods now being widely used by community health workers in developing countries. In agriculture, the technology developed for preservation of production after harvest (e.g., using appropriate technology for drying and storage) has improved both the conservation and palatability of grains and legumes [IDRC, 1982].

More recently, a new hybrid corn developed by the International Maize and Wheat Improvement Center in Mexico offers promise as a high-yielding yet amino acid balanced staple for corn and bean cultures in Mesoamerica [IN-CAP, 1983]. Progress is slow and the promise of the Green Revolution has yet to be fulfilled, so that there continues to be a need for technological innovations to make interventions more robust and less expensive.

Legal innovations have also begun to appear in developing contries. In Panama, for example, the recently approved constitution specifically guarantees the population the right to a nutritionally adequate diet. In Colombia, legal action is being taken by labor organizations to tie the minimum wage to the cost of housing and feeding an average family. Although prices may fluctuate due to supply and inflation reduces the purchasing capacity of wages, they argue that the state should guarantee the laborer's ability to provide for the basic needs of his/her family.

The technology applied to the dissemination of information on successful interventions continues to change dramatically from nearly exclusive dependence on the printed media to the more recent use of video, theater, and micro media (e.g., games and, puppets) for nonliterate populations. The nonexperimental use of mass communications and personal computers in nutrition service agencies is just beginning to be exploited.

Changing Administrative Practices

Administrative practices have not escaped this trend toward innovation. Due to the increasing limitations in agency budgets and often as a requirement of funding agencies, new administrative practices are being applied which are having substantial impacts on service delivery systems. Although these practices may be common in industry, the health sector has been slow in adopting modern management tools. For example, human service agencies have been reluctant to establish clear goals and objectives which could be used as a basis for evaluation. More recently, perhaps due to the mandate of federally funded contracts and grants, evaluation techniques are being applied with increasing regularity. In order to qualify for additional funding, agencies must now demonstrate the cost-effective nature of their operations. Because the methods being used are more rigorous, agencies have begun to employ specialized personnel in evaluation units to identify problems in service delivery and work with managers in the development of operational solutions. Related progress has been made in the application of management information systems, more explicit program controls and budgets and the use of operations research as a management tool. Although the costs of these innovations remains relatively high, the potential savings in improved program performance appears to be worth the investment. For example, simple management information systems are being established in response to the high cost of maintaining independent nutrition surveillance systems. In this fashion, service providers and supervisors jointly collect, analyze, and interpret the comprehensive information on both inputs and impacts needed for efficient program management.

REMAINING CHALLENGES

What then are the challenges that still must be met? If we can agree upon the model specified earlier, the problem of hunger must be addressed with three priority areas of intervention: 1) improving infant and child feeding practices through the promotion of breastfeeding, appropriate weaning practices, and growth monitoring; 2) primary health care to reduce the incidence and severity of preventable diseases affecting children and women (e.g., diarrhea, tetanus, measles, and respiratory infections), and 3) efforts to insure food security at the local level through increasing food production by the families at risk of malnutrition, reducing post-harvest losses, and improving distribution through more equitable marketing mechanisms.

However, two specters loom as factors that may dramatically influence the success of these efforts. The first is the disastrous condition of the economies of the Third World. The issue of the massive international debt of the developing southern hemisphere, regardless of its causes, must be resolved if local economies are to provide for the basic needs of their populations. In many countries in Latin America, the interest payments alone would be sufficient to cover the marginal costs for the health and nutrition interventions recommended previously. The other major factor is population growth. By the year 2000, nearly 90 million additional persons will inhabit the earth, of which over 80 million will be in developing countries. Population issues must be a fundamental part of development planning, not only because women and children are the principal victims of uncontrolled fertility but because policies, plans, and interventions themselves must reflect the inexorable relationship between population size, available resources, the quality of the environment, and existing levels of development [International Population Conference, 1984].

Certainly research is still needed both to document the cost-effectiveness and benefits of existing policies and to provide a more solid base for the selection, operation, and management of new efforts. By increasing the sensitivity of the public and policy makers to the problem of hunger, research may contribute to the development of a more equitable society. Admittedly this process is long and arduous but progress can be made. Salk [1973] described the megatrends he perceived in the world community as follows:

"we are moving from an epoch preoccupied with notions of anti-death, anti-disease, death control, self-repression and external restraint to a new epoch devoted to distinct values, pro-life, pro-health, birth control, self-expression and self-restraint. We are entering a new epoch in which the individual identifies with the world community, where consensus, collaboration and interdependence are the essence of our dealings with our neighbor." Perhaps this last note is overly optimistic given the prevalence of hunger and social unrest in much of the world. Nevertheless, if concerted efforts are made now to intervene wherever poverty and hunger threaten the lives and well-being of our neighbors, by 1994 we can hope again that because of our efforts, no child will go to bed hungry.

REFERENCES

Beaton GH, Ghassemi H (1982): Supplementary feeding programs for young children in developing countries. Am J Clin Nutr, Supplement 35:864-916.

Brandt W (1980): "North-South: a program for survival." Report of the Independent Commission on International Development Issues. Cambridge, MA: MIT Press, pp 90-104.

Caiden N, Wildavsky AB (1974): "Planning and Budgeting in Poor Countries". New York: Wiley, pp 45-46.

Demone HW, Schulberg HC, Broskowski A (1978): Evaluating the context of developments in human services. In Attkinsson CC, Hargreaves WA, Horowitz MJ, Sorensen JE (eds): "Evaluation of Human Service Programs". New York: Academic Press, pp 27-41.

Grant JP (1984): "Estado Mundial de la Infancia" New York: UNICEF.

Gwatkin DR, Wilcox JR, Wray JD (1980): The policy implications of field experiments in primary health and nutrition care. Soc Sci Med Vol 14C, pp 121-128.

Institute of Nutrition for Central America and Panama (1983): Annual Report, Guatemala City, INCAP.

International Development Research Center (1982): "A Decade of Learning: the first ten years of the Division of Agricultural, Food and Nutrition Sciences." Ottawa: IDRC, pp 25-136.

International Population Conference (1984): "Declaration in The City of Mexico on Population and Development." Mexico D.F.: United Nations, pp 1-7.

Kielman AA, Ajello CA, Kielman NS (1982): Nutrition intervention: an evaluation of six studies. Studies in Family Planning 13:246-257.

Klein RE, Townsend JW, Praun A, Fischer M (1982): The practice of impact evaluation of nutrition education programs. Paper presented to the Workshop on Evaluation of Nutrition Education in Third World Communities, Nestle Foundation, Lausanne, Switzerland, 16-17 September.

Lappé FM, Collins J (1977): "Food First: beyond the myth of scarcity." Boston: Houghton Mifflin.

Mahler H (1980): Forward. In Gwatkin DR, Wilcox JR, Wray JD (eds): "Can Health and Nutrition Interventions Make a Difference." Washington D.C.: Overseas Development Council, pp vi-ix.

Parlato MB, Favin MN (1982): "Primary Health Care: Progress and Problems." Washington DC: American Public Health Association, pp 85-91.

Patton MQ (1978): "Utilization Focused Evaluation." Beverly Hills, CA: Sage, pp 59-76.

Pollitt E (1981): Estudios experimentales y programas pilotos de intervención: un exámen de lo avanzado. In Galofré F (ed): "Pobreza Critica en la Niñez: America Latina y el Caribe." Santiago: CEPAL-UNICEF, pp 348-367.

Pressman JL, Wildavsky A (1973): "Implementation: How Great Expectations in Washington Are Dashed in Oakland, or, Why It's Amazing That Federal Programs Work at All." Berkely, CA: University of California Press, pp xi-xviii.

Salk JL (1973): "The Survival of the Wisest." New York: Harper and Row.

Townsend JW (1984): Social significance of nutrition-related programs. In Brozek J. Schurch B (eds): "Malnutrition and Behavior: Critical Assessment of Key Issues." Lausanne: Nestle Foundation, pp 615-620.

Townsend JW, Farrell WT, Klein RE (1979): Special issues for the measurement of program impact in developing countries. In Klein RE, Read MS, Reicken HW, Brown JA, Pradilla A, Daza CH (eds): "Evaluating the Impact of Nutrition and Health Programs." New York: Plenum Press, pp 99-123.

Ugalde A, Emrey R (1979): Political and organizational issues in assessing health and nutrition interventions. In Klein RE, Read MS, Reicken HW, Brown JA, Pradilla A, Daza CH (eds): "Evaluating the Impact of Nutrition and Health Programs." New York: Plenum Press, pp 309-331.

Underwood BA (1983): "Nutrition Intervention Strategies in National Development." New York: Academic Press.

Vaquera M, Townsend JW, Arroyo JJ, Lechtig A (1983): The relationships between arm circumference at birth and early mortality. J Trop Ped 29 (3):167-174.

Walsh JA, Warren KS (1979): Selective primary health care: an interim strategy for disease control in developing countries. New Engl J Med, 301 (18):967-974.

Williams W (1976): Implementation analysis and assessment. In Williams E, Elmore RF (eds): "Social Program Implementation." New York: Academic Press, pp 267-292.

World Bank (1984): "Report on World Development." Washington DC: World Bank, pp 90-121.

World Health Organization (1981): "Guidelines for Training Community Health Workers in Nutrition." WHO Offset Publication No. 59, Geneva: WHO.

Index

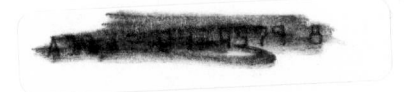